# Global Maternal and Child Health

# Medical, Anthropological, and Public Health Perspectives

**Series Editor**

David A. Schwartz
Medical College of Georgia
Augusta University
Atlanta, GA, USA

*Global Maternal and Child Health: Medical, Anthropological, and Public Health Perspectives* is a series of books that will provide the most comprehensive and current sources of information on a wide range of topics related to global maternal and child health, written by a collection of international experts.

The health of pregnant women and their children are among the most significant public health, medical, and humanitarian problems in the world today. Because in developing countries many people are poor, and young women are the poorest of the poor, persistent poverty exacerbates maternal and child morbidity and mortality and gender-based challenges to such basic human rights as education and access to health care and reproductive choices. Women and their children remain the most vulnerable members of our society and, as a result, are the most impacted individuals by many of the threats that are prevalent, and, in some cases, increasing throughout the world. These include emerging and re-emerging infectious diseases, natural and man-made disasters, armed conflict, religious and political turmoil, relocation as refugees, malnutrition, and, in some cases, starvation. The status of indigenous women and children is especially precarious in many regions because of ethnic, cultural, and language differences, resulting in stigmatization, poor obstetrical and neonatal outcomes, limitations of women's reproductive rights, and lack of access to family planning and education that restrict choices regarding their own futures. Because of the inaccessibility of women to contraception and elective pregnancy termination, unsafe abortion continues to result in maternal deaths, morbidity, and reproductive complications. Unfortunately, maternal deaths remain at unacceptably high levels in the majority of developing countries, as well as in some developed ones. Stillbirths and premature deliveries result in millions of deaths annually. Gender inequality persists globally as evidenced by the occurrence of female genital mutilation, obstetrical violence, human trafficking, and other forms of sexual discrimination directed at women. Many children are routinely exposed to physical, sexual, and psychological violence. Childhood and teen marriages remain at undesirably high levels in many developing countries.

*Global Maternal and Child Health: Medical, Anthropological, and Public Health Perspectives* is unique in combining the opinions and expertise of public health specialists, physicians, anthropologists and social scientists, epidemiologists, nurses, midwives, and representatives of governmental and non governmental agencies to comprehensively explore the increasing challenges and potential solutions to global maternal and child health issues.

More information about this series at http://www.springer.com/series/15852

# Series Editorial Advisory Board

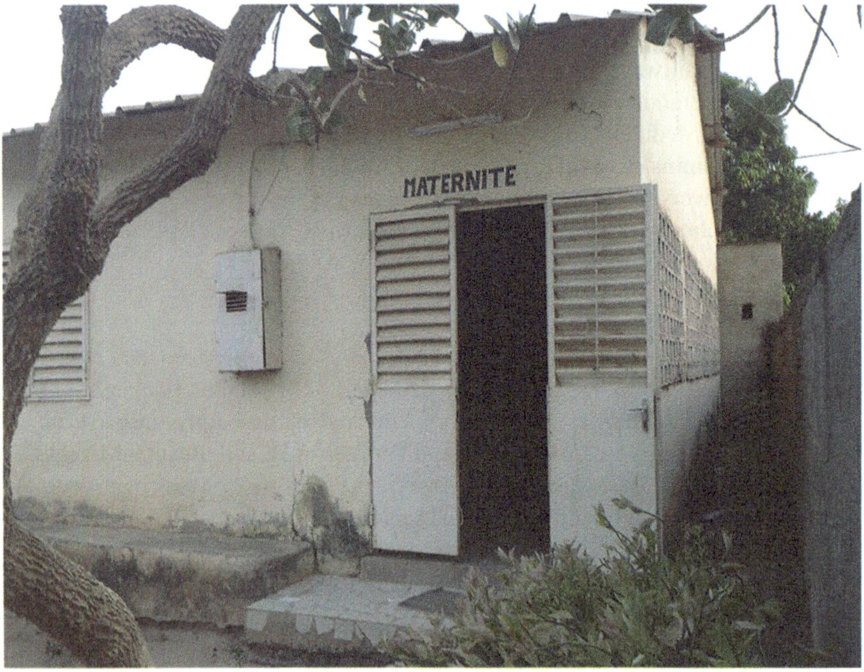


The maternity ward of a Health Post (Poste de Santé) in rural Senegal. (Photo: M. MacDonald)

Lauren J. Wallace
Margaret E. MacDonald • Katerini T. Storeng
Editors

# Anthropologies of Global Maternal and Reproductive Health

## From Policy Spaces to Sites of Practice

Springer

*Editors*
Lauren J. Wallace
Department of Anthropology
McMaster University
Hamilton, ON, Canada

Margaret E. MacDonald
Department of Anthropology
York University
Toronto, ON, Canada

Katerini T. Storeng
Centre for Development & the Environment
University of Oslo
Oslo, Norway

ISSN 2522-8382 ISSN 2522-8390 (electronic)
Global Maternal and Child Health
ISBN 978-3-030-84513-1 ISBN 978-3-030-84514-8 (eBook)
https://doi.org/10.1007/978-3-030-84514-8



This Springer imprint is published by the registered company Springer Nature Switzerland AG
The registered company address is: Gewerbestrasse 11, 6330 Cham, Switzerland

# Foreword

One of the more important lessons I learned as a medical anthropologist came from work on maternal mortality that Oyuna Chuluundorj and I did in Mongolia. Oyuna, who had left her position as an Obstetrician Gynecologist in the Mongolian health system to study medical anthropology, was troubled by increases in maternal morbidity and mortality after Mongolia transitioned from Soviet-style socialism to neoliberal capitalism. As we began to investigate this problem it became increasingly clear that we were not simply dealing with a public health or health system problem, but with a complex set of linked social, economic, and political processes that were increasing the vulnerability of women, particularly those living in rural areas. We learned how fraught the policy-making process is in the domain of maternal and reproductive health given its entanglements with local social norms as well as global ideologies. In short, we learned, as the authors of this volume show clearly across multiple contexts, that a focus on maternal and reproductive health is a powerful and revealing lens through which one can investigate social changes, power, gender relations, political economy, and institutional dynamics within particular contexts. It throws into sharp relief the contested and error-prone terrain of global health policy as it is implemented in different places, and questions the conventional wisdom that maternal and reproductive health are simply the province of health (medical) care systems.

The contributors to this volume underscore the need to engage with "sites of practice," local contexts, and lived experiences. They show how policies are created and implemented, questioning both the evidence base drawn upon in crafting policy and the problems that occur when policies travel globally without critical appraisal of variable relevance or implementation processes. Importantly, this volume moves medical anthropology in a useful new direction, showing how bridging and blending health policy and systems research with ethnography can yield useful insights about what works – or does not – to improve maternal and reproductive health, and why. It adds additional voices and perspectives on the policy process as it looks from "below." Yet while we might hope for a world where local voices and lived experience comprise the primary evidence base for developing policy, in fact policymaking is far more complicated than this and requires both careful analysis and advocacy. This volume offers steps forward for doing this.

Precisely because ethnography has proven to be such a useful approach to understanding the "local" manifestations of health policy, medical anthropology has emerged as what I believe is the leading social science of global health. This volume clearly advances this contribution. In order to understand the impact of health policies on maternal and reproductive health, the key features of a critical global health are identified and examined. These include careful considerations of the social patterning of risk and response; the global circulation of technologies, including pharmaceuticals; the politics of evidentiary processes – what evidence counts, why, and to what effects; exposure of how universal, global policies have uneven, unanticipated, and potentially harmful effects; and the many ethical concerns that emerge with any indiscriminate implementation of policy created in the absence of contextual grounding. The problems of rights, of fairness, and of socially and economically structured inequalities emerge again and again as obstacles to the development of accessible, effective, responsive, and salutogenic health systems.

Of concern, and despite decades of work exhibiting the importance of a biosocial approach, the authors demonstrate that the field of maternal and reproductive health remains prone to the continual and contested pull of technocratic, biomedical solutions. Although there is clear evidence that non-biomedical approaches to birth – for example, midwifery, "humanized" birth, baby-friendly hospitals, doula programs – contribute to better outcomes in terms of maternal and neonatal health, the biomedical imperative of many health systems persists in capturing and regulating reproductive processes. We continue to grapple with global health policies that mandate single-mindedly and uncritically skilled attendance at birth, even though this is only one means for safe and humane delivery, not to mention that what counts as "skill" can be questioned, particularly if there is little attention to other needs – safe, clean, and properly equipped facilities, for example.

Given the subject of inquiry and its centrality to health and, more broadly, the human condition, a focus on maternal and reproductive health is shot through with politics, ideologies, and moral judgments. Controversy emerges here and there: misoprostol, a life-saving drug when used to control postpartum bleeding, for example, may also be deployed as an abortifacient and subject to legal proscriptions; instances of maternal mortality may be used as instruments to discipline providers and government officials, as Oyuna and I found in Mongolia, leading to blame-shifting and underreporting rather than efforts to address causes and identify solutions.

Maternal and reproductive health policy contends with a domain where health outcomes in terms of death and disability reveal astonishing and deeply troubling levels of inequity. It is well known that the risk to a woman in the global "south" of dying in childbirth or suffering a life-changing and stigmatizing disability such as obstetric fistula is many hundreds of times greater than the risk faced by a woman in Europe or North America. These epidemiologic facts reveal a level of social suffering that has no parallel in global health. While there has been some improvement over the past few decades, much more needs to be done. Questioning maternal and reproductive health policy is a critically important area of work. The contributions to this book reveal some of the paths we may take to move toward a healthier world.

Craig R. Janes
Professor and Director
School of Public Health Sciences
University of Waterloo
Waterloo, ON, Canada

# Acknowledgments

The editors and authors thank participants in the "Ethnographic Examinations of Global Maternal and Child Health Policy and Practice" panel at the American Anthropological Association annual meeting in Washington, DC, in 2017, many of whom have contributed in various ways to this book. We extend our thanks to numerous anonymous chapter reviewers, and to Jean-Pierre Olivier de Sardan, D. Ann Herring, Philip B. Adongo, and Bregje de Kok for insightful comments. The editors would like to express their gratitude to their Springer Editor, Janet Kim, who patiently provided editorial expertise, and our energetic and sage Springer Series Editor, David Schwartz, who contributed kind advice without which the book would not have come to fruition. We would also like to thank our families for loving support during the preparation of this book.

We are grateful to York University; the Centre for Development and the Environment at the University of Oslo; the Division of Social and Behavioural Sciences, School of Public Health and Family Medicine, University of Cape Town; the University of Sussex; and the Wellcome Trust [105011/Z/14/Z], in addition to Ljiljana Pantović, Priscilla Magrath, Lauren J. Wallace, and Meredith G. Marten, who generously contributed funds to make this book open access.

# Contents

# Editors and Contributors

## About the Editors

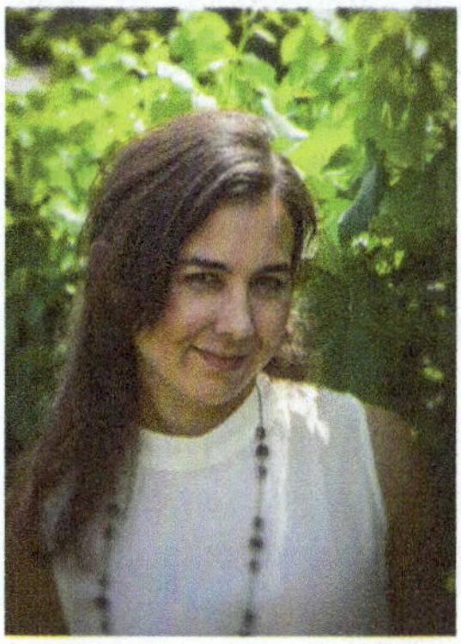

**Lauren J. Wallace, PhD,** is a Senior Researcher at Dodowa Health Research Centre in Accra, Ghana. She is a medical anthropologist whose research critically examines the making and implementation of maternal and reproductive health policies at national and subnational levels. Her PhD (2017, McMaster University, Canada), funded by a Vanier Scholarship from the Canadian Institutes of Health Research, was an ethnographic study of family size and family planning in northern Ghana. She has since "studied up" to examine the dynamics of national priority setting for maternal and reproductive health in Ghana and Uganda ethnographically. Dr. Wallace is currently the Ghana Principal Investigator of the COVID-19 in West and Central Africa (CATALYSE) study, in which she examines policy and systems responses to COVID-19 and their intended and unintended effects in Ghana, in collaboration with national policymakers. She has also worked on other large-scale, interdisciplinary global health studies. Presently, she is also a Researcher at the University of Ghana's School of Public Health, where she examines responsive and effective primary health care programs in urban settlements in Accra, in collaboration with local governments. Dr. Wallace is presently an Adjunct Assistant Professor in the Department of Anthropology at McMaster University, where she has also held an appointment as an instructor in the Midwifery Education Program.

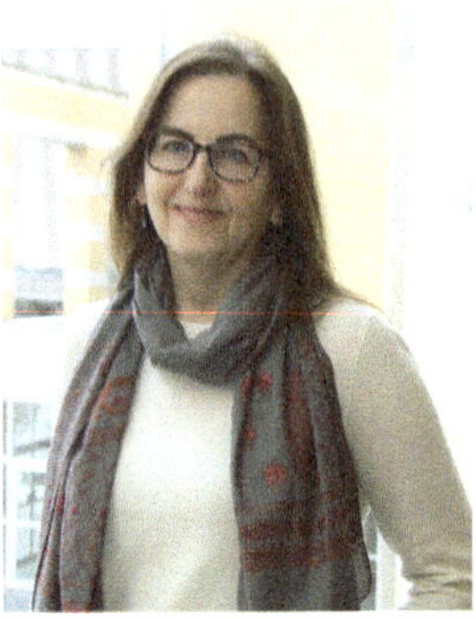

**Margaret E. MacDonald, PhD,** is Associate Professor and Graduate Program Director in the Department of Anthropology at York University in Toronto, Canada. As a medical anthropologist, her interests lie in how cultures of biomedicine, science, and technology shape ideas, practices, and materialities of gender, health, and reproduction. She conducts research in a range of settings across the globe: with midwives and their clients in Canada; within a community of global maternal health advocates and policymakers; and in rural and remote Senegal where non-governmental organizations implement interventions to improve maternal health. Her work in the global health arena has focused on key debates and emerging tools in the campaigns to improve maternal health care and reduce maternal death in low-resource settings: the controversial place of traditional birth attendants in maternal health; the production and uses of photography, film, and infographics as affective, aesthetic information about sexual and reproductive health; and the emergence of new biomedical-technical solutions embedded in feminist politics. She currently leads a collaborative project looking at the work of midwives and the experiences of clients under COVID-19 with particular attention to the impacts of the pandemic on marginalized and racialized groups.

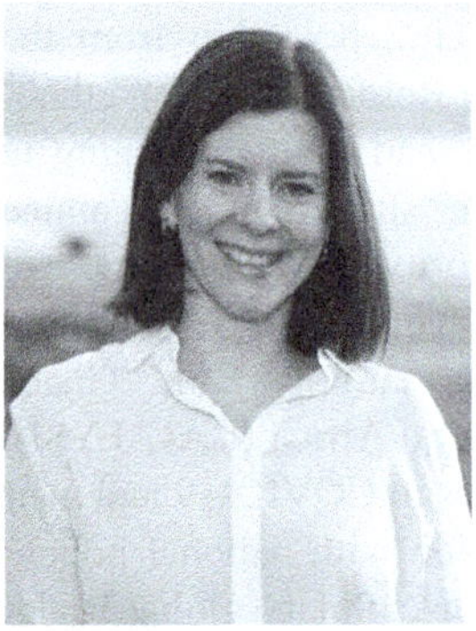

**Katerini T. Storeng, PhD, MSc.,** is Associate Professor at the University of Oslo's Centre for Development and the Environment, and Head of its interdisciplinary Global Health Politics research group. She is a medical anthropologist whose ethnographic research takes a critical perspective on how global norms, values, and power relations influence debates about evidence and health policy processes and practice. Her PhD (2010, University of London, UK) was an ethnographic study of the making of the global Safe Motherhood Initiative. She has since studied the social and political dynamic of global public-private partnerships in global health governance, including Gavi, the Vaccine Alliance, regarding how such partnerships engage civil society. Her current research, funded by the Research Council of Norway, examines new forms of partnerships between public health agencies and pharmaceutical and technology corporations established in response to COVID-19. As former staff and Honorary Associate Professor at the London School of Hygiene & Tropical Medicine, Dr. Storeng has also collaborated on several large-scale, interdisciplinary studies on maternal health, notably longitudinal research into the social consequences of pregnancy-related illness, unsafe abortion, and catastrophic healthcare expenditure in Burkina Faso.

## Contributors

**Christopher J. Colvin, PhD, MPH** Department of Public Health Sciences, University of Virginia, Charlottesville, VA, USA

Division of Social and Behavioural Sciences, School of Public Health and Family Medicine, University of Cape Town, Cape Town, South Africa

**Robbie Davis-Floyd, PhD** Department of Anthropology, Rice University, Houston, TX, USA

**Seydou Drabo, PhD, MPhil** Faculty of Medicine, Institute of Health and Society, University of Oslo, Oslo, Norway

**Alice Emasu, MSW, MBA** TERREWODE, Soroti, Uganda

**Lucy C. Irvine, PhD** Institute for Global Health, University College London, London, UK

**Craig R. Janes, PhD** School of Public Health Sciences, University of Waterloo, Waterloo, ON, Canada

**Margaret E. MacDonald, PhD** Department of Anthropology, York University, Toronto, ON, Canada

**Priscilla Magrath, PhD** Department of Health Promotion Sciences, Mel and Enid Zuckerman College of Public Health, University of Arizona, Tucson, AZ, USA

**Meredith G. Marten, PhD** Department of Anthropology, University of West Florida, Pensacola, FL, USA

**Ljiljana Pantović, PhD** Institute for Philosophy and Social Theory, University of Belgrade, Belgrade, Serbia

**Bonnie Ruder, PhD, MPH, CPM** Terrewode Women's Fund, Eugene, OR, USA

**Katerini T. Storeng, PhD, MSc.** Centre for Development and the Environment, University of Oslo, Oslo, Norway

Faculty of Epidemiology and Population Health, London School of Hygiene and Tropical Medicine, London, UK

**Maya Unnithan, PhD** Department of Anthropology, University of Sussex, Sussex, UK

**Lauren J. Wallace, PhD** Department of Anthropology, McMaster University, Hamilton, ON, Canada

Dodowa Health Research Centre, Research and Development Division, Ghana Health Service, Accra, Ghana

# Chapter 1
# Introduction

**Lauren J. Wallace, Margaret E. MacDonald, and Katerini T. Storeng**

## Introduction

This book treats policy as an ethnographic object. Its ten chapters examine global policies for improving maternal and reproductive health, tracking the processes and politics of their making, the mechanisms of their implementation in diverse contexts, and people's intimate encounters with their consequences and effects. Doing so is timely since there is a growing appreciation that the success of health policies and interventions hinges on issues that are at the core of medical anthropological inquiry: the complexities of program implementation, the impact of socio-political contexts, and issues of local agency, equity and accessibility. Indeed, the burgeoning subfield of health policy and systems research views an interpretive and critical inquiry that draws on multiple disciplines, not least anthropology, as essential to understanding and informing effective policy (Gilson et al., 2011; Ghaffar et al., 2016).

The inspiration for this book was a double panel at the American Anthropological Association annual meeting in Washington, DC, in 2017 convened by Lauren

L. J. Wallace (✉)
Department of Anthropology, McMaster University, Hamilton, Ontario, Canada

Dodowa Health Research Centre, Research and Development Division,
Ghana Health Service, Accra, Ghana
e-mail: wallalj@mcmaster.ca

M. E. MacDonald
Department of Anthropology, York University, Toronto, Ontario, Canada
e-mail: maggie@yorku.ca

K. T. Storeng
Centre for Development and Environment, University of Oslo, Oslo, Norway

Faculty of Epidemiology and Population Health, London School of Hygiene and Tropical
Medicine, London, UK
e-mail: katerini.storeng@sum.uio.no



L. J. Wallace et al. (eds.), *Anthropologies of Global Maternal and Reproductive Health*,
Global Maternal and Child Health, https://doi.org/10.1007/978-3-030-84514-8_1

Wallace, entitled 'Ethnographic Examinations of Global Maternal and Child Health Policy and Practice', for which Maggie MacDonald and Katerini Storeng served as discussants. The panel sought to honour recent ground-breaking studies in which anthropologists had exposed the logic, values and practices of global health. As the book took shape, we sought to bring current medical anthropological research on global maternal and reproductive health into more direct conversation with anthropological studies of policy and with health policy and systems research. Our goal was for these conversations to produce more nuanced, more useful accounts of the making and implementation of global health policy than one field alone.

Reproduction is a unique entry point for anthropological analysis and critique of global health policy because it is a key site of social reproduction in every society. By focusing on reproduction, this book raises vital social and cultural concerns relevant to individuals, families, communities and nations: the meaning of life, personhood and death; moral regimes of gender and sexuality; the complexity of kinship and familial relations; and the intersectionality of gender, class and race. Reproduction is also a site of governance of women's bodies and lives (Jordan, 1978; Ginsburg & Rapp, 1995; Locke & Schepher-Hughes, 1987; Morgan & Roberts, 2012). Policies and interventions designed to improve maternal and reproductive health connect intimately with all levels of health system functioning (Storeng & Béhague, 2017) and are entangled with some of the most fundamental and long-standing tensions in global health including how to balance community versus facility-based health services; targeted interventions versus health systems strengthening; selective versus comprehensive primary care; the distribution of scarce resources across competing actors and needs; and contestation over what constitutes evidence (McCoy et al., 2010). Not unlike other global health interventions, maternal and reproductive health policies are also often framed by perceived wisdom and evidence that has been generated by a narrow set of research methods, often making it difficult to derive solutions relevant to the local context (Béhague & Storeng, 2008; Olivier de Sardan, Diarra & Moha, 2017).

As this book goes to press, the global COVID-19 pandemic is in its second year. The pandemic has disrupted routine reproductive, maternal, newborn, and child health (RMNCH) services, especially in low resource settings, threatening hard-won gains in maternal mortality reduction (Robertson et al., 2020). The pandemic has also exacerbated larger social and economic challenges that underlie weak health systems and poor access to quality of care, laying bare the structural violence that creates vast inequities between nations and within nations along intersectional lines of race, class and gender. At the same time, the pandemic has reinforced the need for critical social science research on the workings of health policy and health systems to be part of the evidentiary mix upon which people-centred and equitable health policy and systems everywhere are built. It is a key moment of reckoning for maternal and reproductive health policy, and for global health more broadly.

## The Anthropology of Global Maternal and Reproductive Health Policy

Policy is a social and political construct. It is a window into larger processes of governance – the mechanisms of power, knowledge, values and vested interests that are used by social actors, including governments, and corporations, to conceptualise, organise and regulate human life and relationships. An anthropological approach to policy contrasts with the instrumental, linear-rational model of the policy process that is often seen in policy analyses rooted in political science. It entails taking on the often complex, ambiguous and messy nature of policy by studying *through* and *across* the multiplicity of actors and interests, locales of power and influence and cycles of policy proposal and revision. The anthropology of policy takes a capacious approach to what counts as policy, including documents and clinical guidelines, laws, position statements, political speeches and declarations. Ethnographic fieldwork is particularly well suited to following policies into their 'implementation contexts' where they are interpreted, adapted, worked around or ignored in the context of practical norms and professional cultures (Shore & Wright, 1997; Wedel & Feldman, 2005, p. 2; Olivier de Sardan, Diarra & Moha, 2017; Fassin, 2013).

Anthropological critique often reveals the *local* consequences of global health, countering the 'master narratives' and working assumptions of the global health enterprise including the dominance of biomedical approaches to understanding health and illness and technocratic approaches to organising care (Nichter, 2008; Whiteford & Manderson, 2000; Castro, 2004). Working in the political economy of health tradition, critical medical anthropologists have also sought to connect the macro-level politics of structural violence and inequality to the micro-level of embodied experience (Singer & Baer, 1995; Farmer, 2004). Such efforts have shifted anthropologists' gaze beyond the local setting and its immediate context, towards an appreciation and analysis of the deeper economic, political and historical underpinnings of health and illness. This shift has involved looking directly at the 'global health enterprise' itself to unpack the complex assemblages of social networks, power relations, ideologies, funding flows, documents, things, knowledge claims and epistemic discourses that constitute it (Pfeiffer & Nichter, 2008, p. 413; Ong & Collier, 2005; Janes & Corbett, 2009). Most recently, the term 'critical global health' has emerged to capture the expansive approach taken by many anthropologists to understanding the 'policy space' of global health (Biehl & Petryna, 2013).

Some of the earliest work in the field of critical global health focused squarely on maternal health. Judith Justice's detailed examination of the planning and implementation of a program to train and disperse Assistant Nurses Midwives throughout the Nepalese countryside (1989) and Brigitte Jordan's classic critique of training courses for traditional birth attendants in Mexico (1978) both clearly illustrate the lack of consideration of local context in national-level policies meant to improve maternal health care. These studies and a small body of ethnographic work that followed explored the interface between the technical logics of global health policy and programs and the material and sociocultural realities that produce poor maternal health. In so doing, they pointed to stark disjunctures between global 'safe motherhood' policy and the lived experiences of women, health workers and their communities (Pigg, 1997; Allen, 2002; Foley, 2007; Berry, 2010; MacDonald, 2017; Olivier de Sardan, Diarra & Moha, 2017). The interest in policy as a site of ethnographic inquiry within medical anthropology and critical global health studies has expanded greatly over the past decade; attention to metrics and the datafication of global health playing no small part (Storeng & Béhague, 2014; Adams, 2016).

The chapters in this edited book contribute to a growing body of knowledge illuminating global maternal and reproductive health policies through close attention to their formation and implementation in particular contexts. This volume offers ethnographic insights into the mechanisms by which global maternal and reproductive health policies are formed and implemented in diverse locales around the world, from India to Burkina Faso, Tanzania and Uganda, Switzerland and Serbia, the United States and Brazil. They will be of interest to scholars working in the overlapping subject areas of critical global health, medical anthropology, and the anthropology of reproduction and health policy and systems research. It is our intention that these chapters also speak to and inform the work of global public health experts and the development of guidelines and interventions. In short, we hope that these chapters can contribute to improved knowledge as well as actual practice.

## Implementation Disconnects and Policy Rhetoric

The disjuncture between policy ideals and their implementation in practice – a longstanding concern of anthropological critiques of global health – is taken up by several authors in this volume. The notion of a 'travelling model' whereby an intervention developed by international experts is introduced in a standardised format in many settings, without consideration for specific, local, implementation contexts, analytically captures this situation. Travelling models have long been taken to be intrinsically effective, and therefore universally applicable; yet in reality, they ignore or underestimate the particularities of social and cultural context, resulting in disconnect on the ground (Olivier de Sardan, Diarra & Moha, 2017; see also MacDonald, 2017).

The trouble with travelling models is illustrated in **Ljiljana Pantović's** chapter on the implementation of the international Baby Friendly Hospital Initiative (BFHI) in a Serbian hospital. Pantovic shows how the social, political and economic conditions in Serbia – namely the devastating effects of the civil war, international sanctions in the 1990s and the deleterious effects of IMF policies on the Serbian healthcare system since the 2000s – have severely hindered the uptake of the BFHI by frontline health workers. The ten steps meant to foster the uptake of breastfeeding by new mothers, she observes, are both thinly learned and thinly applied by healthcare workers struggling to manage high workloads in understaffed hospitals, in combination with unsustainable national funds for implementation.

**Bonnie Ruder and Alice Emasu's** chapter on the global push to bring surgical repair to obstetric fistula similarly reveals the failure of a travelling model to solve a complex problem. Their ethnography examines a donor-funded treatment model in Uganda that focusses on surgical camps but without follow-up or patient tracking. While the majority of women who receive the surgery experience its life-changing benefits, a sizeable minority experience residual incontinence and complications – something that the surgical camp model does not fund or even measure. Poor outcomes are underreported and thus women suffering from residual incontinence fade from view in the story of a global health intervention defined by its success. Consequently, limited attention and resources are dedicated to residual incontinence, leaving many women without alternative treatment options.

New drugs and devices are key features of health policies and projects as they circulate around the world. Getting them to have the effect that policymakers intended, however, is a process often met with roadblocks, gaps and diversions (Russel, Sobo & Thompson, 2000; Suh, 2015). This is starkly relayed in **Seydou Drabo's** ethnographic fieldwork on access to a drug, misoprostol, for medical abortion in Ouagadougou, Burkina Faso, where abortion is illegal in most circumstances. Growing evidence for the safety and effectiveness of misoprostol for use in the prevention and treatment of postpartum haemorrhage and unsafe abortion – two major causes of maternal death worldwide – have persuaded global and national level institutions to recommend its use. As Drabo explains, women seeking abortions in Ouagadougou are able to access misoprostol through unofficial channels, including intermediaries such as health workers and drug sellers, sex workers and friends. However, he describes a landscape of deeply unequal and frequently unsafe access to the drug depending on one's social position. Drabo concludes that even as global policy hails misoprostol as a revolution in terms of its safe and effective biochemical effects on the body and simple and low cost features, the matter of safe access to safe abortion for all women in settings like Burkina Faso has not been addressed.

Like travelling models, the 'key social representations' and 'master narratives' in global health that surround them often frame problems in ways that limit thinking about potential solutions, leading to implementation gaps and distortions, unintended consequences and failed projects (Nichter, 2008; Inhorn, 2006). **Meredith Marten's** chapter examines the impact of the circulation of buzzwords, master narratives and policy rhetoric – in her case the push amongst global donors to implement 'sustainable' maternal health programs and projects in Tanzania. By describing programmes focused on prevention of mother-to-child transmission of HIV, (PMTCT), Basic Emergency Obstetric and Newborn Care (BEmONC) and Respectful Maternity Care (RMC), she reveals how donors' unrealistic yet frequently replicated 'doctrine of sustainability' paradoxically seems to undermine the strength of the health systems that donors claim to support. Marten argues that the sustainability doctrine fails to challenge neoliberal and philanthrocapitalist models of health care, advancing funding and implementation models more accountable to donors than to the public health systems providing care.

## Policy Ambivalence

Global health has been characterised by several enduring debates about how best to deliver health care and improve health outcomes in low resource settings – comprehensive versus selective primary health care, community versus facility-based health, targeted interventions versus health systems strengthening (McCoy et al., 2010). Several authors in this book trace the arc of interventions intended to address major maternal and reproductive health challenges back to the 1970s, showing how they have played out against this backdrop over time. These authors reflect upon and illuminate the retreat, ambivalence, and in some cases, return, of previously contested policy approaches.

The theme of policy ambivalence surrounding community and facility-based approaches to care is taken up in **Maggie MacDonald's** chapter, which follows the story of the traditional birth attendant (TBA) in global maternal health from the launch of the Safe Motherhood Initiative (SMI) in 1987 to the present. MacDonald argues that the original shift away from training TBAs within safe motherhood programs and their subsequent loss of legitimacy in global health was influenced by weak and inconclusive evidence, flawed conceptualizations of TBAs and the lack of consideration for the role of the larger political and economic context in which they worked – all of which was shaped by the re-organisation of the safe motherhood movement at the global level. MacDonald discusses how the recent repositioning of TBAs in maternal health policies and guidelines as potentially useful providers has been informed by a growing evidence base pointing to the effectiveness of TBAs, as well as the advent of high tech, cost effective, point of use technologies, which have led to the decentring of health facilities and professional health providers as the sole locus of clinical care.

Policy ambivalence is also illustrated in **Maya Unnithan's** account of the conflicting approaches to reproductive health that have played out in India since the 1990s. On the surface, India's family planning program seems to have undergone radical shifts from a population control model implemented through 'targets', to the abolition of targets and an integrated reproductive and child health model that upholds the rights of women to contraceptive choice. Yet, looking deeper, policy documents themselves offer clear indications of a return to state-promoted sterilisation, including cash incentives to clients to enhance contraceptive uptake and the introduction of new metrics to evaluate health worker performance. Unnithan shows how on the ground, these metrics are still perceived by Auxiliary Nurse Midwives as 'targets'. Pressure on these community-level health workers from state directives to fulfil targets, and their experiences and perceptions of the lack of safety of reversible forms of contraception, combine to create a contraceptive bias towards sterilisation, even as Indian family planning takes on a new rights-based discourse.

## Contesting Authoritative Knowledge and Practice

An enduring theme in critical anthropological studies of global health policy and implementation has been how the dominance of biomedicine tends to discredit local health knowledge and practitioners (Davis-Floyd & Sargent, 1997). In maternal and reproductive healthcare, this trend has been characterised by the consolidation of power away from traditional birth attendants and other lay healers and towards biomedical health facilities as the only safe place to give birth. Contestations around the professionalisation of maternity care are contests about authoritative knowledge and practice; that is, whose knowledge and authority counts and what counts as care. Global health interventions into maternal and reproductive health care are typically accompanied by the medicalisation and technocratic management of birth, with myriad and complex consequences for quality of care in underfunded, under-resourced healthcare systems.

Extending the discussion of the role of community-level birth attendants, **Priscilla Magrath** analyses Indonesia's national policy to improve maternal health by promoting an official partnership between 'skilled birth attendants' (SBAs) and 'traditional birth attendants'. In West Java, where she conducted ethnographic fieldwork, the local district health office engaged in 'policy entrepreneurship' to resolve enduring contests over the professionalisation of maternity care and promoted the partnership regulation throughout the region. Taking the local district as her starting point, Magrath maps the dense networks of national and global policies and pressures that exert themselves in local health governance and clinical practice: global policies promoting SBAs and sidelining TBAs; pressure on individual nations to reach the Millennium Development Goal on reducing maternal mortality; and the limited financial power and decision space afforded to districts under decentralisation in Indonesia. She concludes that by spotlighting the relationship between SBAs and TBAs as a key strategy to improve maternal health, attention was diverted from other health system challenges including under-resourced medical facilities and a weak referral system.

## The Rise of Evidence and Its Uses

An empirical focus on reproductive and maternal health also provides a lens through which to see transformations in the global governance of health through the rise of metrics and the epistemic communities who uphold evidence-based policymaking as evidence of success and impact. Anthropologists have highlighted how the 'fetishization' of indicators such as the maternal mortality ratio (MMR) within global efforts to improve maternal health, while conveying accountability, may actually serve to regulate reproductive health behaviour in limiting ways, casting aside certain types of reproductive bodies as unworthy of protection, damaging health systems and deflecting attention away from the realities of mothers and health workers (Storeng & Béhague, 2017; Adams, 2016; Brunson & Suh, 2020; de Kok, 2019).

**Christopher Colvin's** chapter provides insights into why it is important to challenge narrowly defined standards of what constitutes evidence and describes the partial moves underway to incorporate social scientific evidence in a research tradition traditionally dominated by positivist methodologies. He provides an autoethnographic account of an effort to integrate qualitative evidence synthesis (QES) into the World Health Organization's global OptimizeMNH guidelines for task shifting in maternal and newborn health (MNH). Colvin describes the delicate balance between adopting quantitatively inspired methods for evidence synthesis and innovating new methods that would both suit the project needs and be seen as legitimate by qualitative researchers, such as recognition of the critical role of local context in explaining the findings from individual studies. Colvin concludes that the rise of QES indicates growing room for the inclusion of potentially transgressive forms of knowledge within the often conservative world of health policy.

**Robbie Davis Floyd's** chapter offers another insider perspective on the uses of evidence in advocacy coalitions in global health. An applied anthropologist, Davis-Floyd recounts how, as a member of an activist organisation with a critical stance towards the mainstream biomedicalisation of pregnancy and birth, she came together with the International Federation of Gynecology and Obstetrics (FIGO) to develop a set of global guidelines for improving the quality of maternity care. This process brought to the fore many of the core debates in the history of global maternal health, notably what to do about traditional birth attendants and what counts as quality of care. She argues that the coalition found agreement on these issues through a commitment to the key values of the women's health and midwifery movements: a process which seems to have brought ethnographic knowledge, activist commitments and mainstream biomedical authority into productive conversation with each other.

Finally, **Lucy Irvine's** research from Brazil explores how natural birth activists are trying to get women-centred evidence to successfully inform policies at the national level. She provides a local-level analysis of 'evidence-based advocacy' by the movement for humanised care in childbirth in São Paulo. Scientific evidence is used strategically in developing specific policy programmes to optimise the use of medical interventions in childbirth and to lend authority in clinical encounters alongside rights-based language such as 'obstetric violence'. However, when faced with resistance from pro-C-section doctors, movement members make use of other strategies to improve access to quality care, such as stimulating demand for humanised birth in the private health sector, which can serve to reinforce existing inequalities in access to high-quality maternity care.

## Conclusion

The ten chapters in this book explore the making and doing of global health policy in a range of geographical settings, cutting across global, national and local levels, and in doing so, they make evident four key ways in which anthropological knowledge contributes meaningfully to the analysis of global health policy. First, ethnography is unique amongst qualitative methods in terms of its long duration and depth of engagement; triangulation and data saturation are inherent features of the method and are highly effective at yielding detailed insights into people's actions, interactions, moral dilemmas, and beliefs, as well as the sights and sounds of the locations they inhabit. Second, these authors show that knowledge generated at the level of the particular – while not necessarily replicable – can nonetheless provide insights that can contribute to national and global level health policy and practice beyond a given location.

Third, the authors tend to analyse policy development and its unfolding within a holistic 'health systems' framework that considers health policies in terms of their impacts on the entire health system. This involves the capture and critical interrogation of multiple scales and their interconnections at once (Feierman et al., 2010; see also Lee, Buse & Fustukian, 2002). Such an approach endeavours to include the global flows of financial and political arrangements, rationalities, technologies and regimes of actors and agendas that configure health practices and inequalities rather than imagine phenomena as confined by spatial and geographic boundaries.

Fourth, the authors advance a much-needed critical perspective to the study of global health policy. They turn their gaze beyond the cultural beliefs of lay communities to examine how health, illness and healing systems are socially, culturally, historically and politically situated. In unpacking the complex 'how' of policy, including the workings of policy communities, governance processes and the social lives of policies, authors in this volume take note of both the weaknesses of policy processes and their accomplishments. A critical approach is also about the kinds of questions that are posed and the analytical work undertaken to make sense of the data. Critical investigations of global health policy are carried out from the premise that there are important things happening in the spaces rendered invisible by medical and public health frameworks or off to the side of the main social arenas created by global health activities (Pigg, 2013, p. 128, 133). Ultimately, a critical perspective can serve as a powerful corrective to the tendency within global health scholarship to displace policy debates from the political realm and recast them as technical debates about healthcare delivery (Mishra & Storeng, 2014; see also Li, 2007).

## *An Agenda for Future Research on Global Maternal and Reproductive Health Policy*

Medical anthropologists' research on global health has much to contribute to the emerging interdisciplinary field of health policy and systems research (HPSR), defined by Sheikh and colleagues (2011) in terms of its attention to wider influences and micro-processes that shape the multiple levels of policy decisions and practices (see also Gilson et al., 2011). A key insight that anthropological research brings to this field is that techno-scientific solutions alone will not improve health and health care and that critical attention to the making and practice of policy should inform the policymaking process itself. Indeed, HPSR views an interpretive and critical inquiry that draws on multiple disciplines, not least anthropology, as essential to understanding and informing effective policy.

In order to refine useful conceptual and empirical insights about policymaking in global health, anthropologists must be prepared to work more judiciously at the juncture between medical anthropology and anthropology of policy, and in closer partnership with local policymakers and experts. Even as anthropologists tend to see themselves as already allied with local players and therefore critical of the global health enterprise writ large, entrenched power asymmetries in global health whereby funded researchers in higher resource settings partner with those in lower resource settings, often set the research agenda. As Jean-Pierre Olivier de Sardan has observed (2021), weak understandings of specific and varied implementation settings lead to the 'revenges of the context', an idea not confined to local sociocultural context but to the politics of knowledge production in global health more seriously. Relative to anthropology, more has been done within the field of HPSR to go beyond critique and imagine how to build the capacities and collaborative possibilities of researchers and policymakers in lower resource contexts for generating, and using, relevant evidence (Bennett, Frenk & Mills, 2018; Agyepong et al., 2021).

We hope that this book sheds new light on old problems in global health policy through ethnographic attention to both policy spaces and sites of practice. The success of health policies and interventions meant to improve reproductive health and reduce maternal suffering and death, we believe, will be aided by greater and more direct engagement between the often separate worlds of policymaking and the practices of interpretive and critical inquiry. Critical, collaborative, multi-disciplinary engagement is the future of global health policy.

## References

Adams, V. (2016). *Metrics: What counts in global health*. Duke University Press.

Agyepong, I. A., Godt, S., Sombie, I., Binka, C., Okine, V., & Ingabire, M.-G. (2021). Strengthening capacities and resource allocation for co-production of health research in low and middle income countries. *British Medical Journal*, 372. https://doi.org/10.1136/bmj.n166

Allen, D. R. (2002). *Managing motherhood, managing risk: Fertility and danger in West Central Tanzania*. University of Michigan Press.
Béhague, D. P., & Storeng, K. T. (2008). Collapsing the vertical–horizontal divide: An ethnographic study of evidence-based policymaking in maternal health. *American Journal of Public Health, 98*(4), 644–649. https://doi.org/10.2105/AJPH.2007.123117
Bennett, S., Frenk, J., & Mills, A. (2018). The evolution of the field of health policy and systems research and outstanding challenges. *Health Research Policy and Systems, 16*, 43. https://doi.org/10.1186/s12961-018-0317-x
Berry, N. (2010). *Unsafe motherhood: Mayan maternal mortality and subjectivity in post-war Guatemala*. Berghan Books.
Biehl, J., & Petryna, A. (2013). *When people come first: Critical studies in global health*. Princeton University Press.
Brunson, J., & Suh, S. (2020). Behind the measures of maternal and reproductive health: Ethnographic accounts of inventory and intervention. *Social Science and Medicine, 254*. https://doi.org/10.1016/j.socscimed.2019.112730
Castro, A. (2004). Contracepting at childbirth: The integration of reproductive health and population policies in Mexico. In A. Castro & M. Singer (Eds.), *Unhealthy health policy: A critical anthropological examination* (pp. 133–134). Altamira Press.
Davis-Floyd, R. E., & Sargent, C. (Eds.). (1997). *Childbirth and authoritative knowledge: Cross-cultural perspectives*. University of California Press.
de Kok, B. C. (2019). Between orchestrated and organic: Accountability for loss and the moral landscape of childbearing in Malawi. *Social Science and Medicine, 220*, 441–449. https://doi.org/10.1016/j.socscimed.2018.09.036
Farmer, P. (2004). An anthropology of structural violence. *Current Anthropology, 45*(3), 305–325. https://doi.org/10.1086/382250
Fassin, D. (2013). A case for critical ethnography: Rethinking the early years of the AIDS epidemic in South Africa. *Social Science & Medicine, 99*, 119–126. https://doi.org/10.1016/j.socscimed.2013.04.034
Feierman, S., Kleinman, A., Stewart, K., Farmer, D., & Das, V. (2010). Anthropology, knowledge- flows and global health. *Global Public Health, 5*(2), 122–128. https://doi.org/10.1080/17441690903401338
Foley, E. (2007). Overlaps and disconnects in reproductive health care: Global policies, national programs, and the micropolitics of reproduction in northern Senegal. *Medical Anthropology, 26*(4), 323–354. https://doi.org/10.1080/01459740701619830
Ghaffar, A., Gilson, L., Tomson, G., Viergever, R., & Rottingen, J.-A. (2016). Where is the policy in health policy and systems research agenda? *Bulletin of the World Health Organisation, 94*(4), 306–308. http://dx.doi.org/10.2471/BLT.15.156281
Gilson, L., Hanson, K., Sheikh, K., Agyepong, I. A., Ssengooba, F., & Bennett, S. (2011). Building the field of health policy and systems research: Social science matters. *PLoS Medicine,* 8(8), e100179. https://doi.org/10.1371/journal.pmed.10001079
Ginsburg, F., & Rapp, R. (Eds.). (1995). *Conceiving the new world order: The global politics of reproduction*. University of California Press.
Inhorn, M. C. (2006). Defining women's health: A dozen messages from more than 150 ethnographies. *Medical Anthropology Quarterly,* 20(3), 345–378.
Janes, C. R., & Corbett, K. K. (2009). Anthropology and global health. *Annual Review of Anthropology, 38*, 167–183. https://doi.org/10.1146/annurev-anthro-091908-164314
Jordan, B. (1978). Revised and updated by Robbie Davis-Floyd in 1993 for the 4th edition. *Birth in four cultures: A cross-cultural investigation of childbirth in Mexico, Holland, Sweden, and the U.S.* Waveland Press.
Justice, J. (1989). *Policies, plans and people: Culture and health development in Nepal*. University of California Press.
Lee, K., Buse, K., & Fustukian, S. (Eds.). (2002). *Health policy in a globalising world*. Cambridge University Press.

Li, T. (2007). *The will to improve. Governmentality, development and the practice of politics*. Duke University Press.

Locke, M. M., & Schepher-Hughes, N. (1987). The Mindful Body: A prolegomenon to future work in medical anthropology. *Medical Anthropology Quarterly, 1*(1), 6–41.

MacDonald, M. (2017). Why ethnography matters in global health. *Journal of Global Health, 7*(2), 020302. https://doi.org/10.7189/jogh.07.020302

McCoy, D., et al. (2010). Maternal, neonatal and child health interventions and services: Moving from knowledge of what works to systems that deliver. *International Health, 2*(2), 87–98. https://doi.org/10.1016/j.inhe.2010.03.005

Mishra, A., & Storeng, K. (2014). Politics and practices of global health: Critical ethnographies of health systems. *Global Public Health, 9*(8), 858–864. https://doi.org/10.1080/17441692.2014.941901

Morgan, L. M., & Roberts, E. F. S. (2012). Reproductive governance in Latin America. *Anthropolology & Medicine, 19*(2), 241–254. https://doi.org/10.1080/13648470.2012.675046

Nichter, M. (2008). *Global health: Why cultural perceptions, social representations, and biopolitics matter*. University of Arizona Press.

Olivier de Sardan, J.-P. (2021). *La revanche des contextes: Des mésaventures de l'ingénierie sociale, en Afrique et au-delà*. Katharla.

Olivier de Sardan, J. P., Diarra, A., & Moha, M. (2017). Travelling models and the challenge of pragmatic contexts and practical norms: The case of maternal health. *Health Research Policy and Systems, 15*(Suppl 1), 60. https://doi.org/10.1186/s12961-017-0213-9

Ong, A., & Collier, S. J. (Eds.). (2005). *Global assemblages: Technology, politics, and ethics as anthropological problems*. Blackwell.

Pfeiffer, J., & Nichter, N. (2008). What can critical medical anthropology contribute to global health? A health systems perspective. *Medical Anthropology Quarterly, 22*, 410–415. https://doi.org/10.1111/j.1548-1387.2008.00041.x

Pigg, S. L. (1997). Authority in translation: Finding, knowing, naming and training "traditional birth attendants" in Nepal. In R. Davis-Floyd & C. Sargent (Eds.), *Childbirth and authoritative knowledge: Cross-cultural perspectives* (pp. 233–263). University of California Press.

Pigg, S. L. (2013). On sitting and doing: Ethnography as action in global health. *Social Science & Medicine, 99*, 127–134. https://doi.org/10.1016/j.socscimed.2013.07.018

Robertson, T., et al. (2020). Early estimates of the indirect effects of the COVID-19 pandemic on maternal and child mortality in low-income and middle-income countries: A modelling study. *Lancet Global Health*. https://doi.org/10.1016/S2214-109X(20)30229-1

Russel, A., Sobo, E. J., & Thompson, M. S. (2000). *Contraception across cultures: Technologies, Choices, Constraints*. Routledge.

Sheikh, K., Gilson, L., Agyepong, I. A., Hanson, K., Ssengooba, F., & Bennett, S. (2011). Building the field of health policy and systems research: Framing the questions. *PLoS Medicine, 8*(8), e100179. https://doi.org/10.1371/journal.pmed.10001079

Shore, C., & Wright, S. (1997). Policy: A new field of anthropology. In *Anthropology of policy: Critical perspectives on governance and power* (pp. 3–39). Routledge.

Singer, M., & Baer, H. (1995). *Critical medical anthropology*. Baywood Publishing.

Storeng, K. T., & Béhague, D. P. (2017). "Guilty until proven innocent": The contested use of maternal mortality indicators in global health. *Critical Public Health, 27*(2), 163–176. https://doi.org/10.1080/09581596.2016.1259459

Storeng, K. T., & Béhague, D. P. (2014). 'Playing the numbers game': Evidence-based advocacy and the technocratic narrowing of the safe motherhood initiative. *Medical Anthropology Quarterly, 28*, 260–279. https://doi.org/10.1111/maq.12072

Suh, S. (2015). 'Right tool,' wrong 'job': Manual vacuum aspiration, post-abortion care and transnational population politics in Senegal. *Social Science and Medicine, 135*, 55e66. https://doi.org/10.1016/j.socscimed.2015.04.030

Wedel, J. R., & Feldman, G. (2005). Why an anthropology of public policy? *Anthropology Today, 21*(1), 1–2.

Whiteford, L. M., & Manderson, L. (Eds.). (2000). *Global health policy, local realities: The fallacy of the level playing field*. Lynne Rienner.

# Part I
# Implementation Disconnects and Policy Rhetoric

# Chapter 2
# Baby (Not So) Friendly: Implementation of the Baby-Friendly Hospital Initiative in Serbia

**Ljiljana Pantović**

## Introduction

> *Diši! Diši!Ajmo sad, gurajte glavica samo što nije!*
> *Breath! Breath! Let's push now the head is almost here!*

During my fieldwork in one of the largest maternity hospitals in the Balkans, with over 6000 births per year and 20–25 births per day, these were the most frequently uttered sentences in the delivery ward. When the baby is born, it is 'not like in Hollywood movies, where you hear crying instantly', said Sandra, a new mother describing her birthing experience. She went on to tell me that: 'the seconds you wait before the baby takes its first breath feel like hours'.

'Don't worry, baby needs a moment to get their bearings'. Mara,[1] the nurse-midwife, comforts Sandra as she suctions the baby's nose and swiftly and with such dexterity cuts and ties the umbilical cord. The baby is not on Sandra's chest while Mara is completing these procedures but on the edge of the gynaecological bed. Sandra's husband is not there; he is home waiting for Sandra to be allowed to turn

[1] All names and other personal identifiers in the chapter have been changed to protect privacy and confidentiality.

This research was supported by the Klinzing Grant for Dissertation Research, European Studies Centre, University of Pittsburgh, Social Sciences Doctoral Dissertation Fellowship, University of Pittsburgh. This article was realised with the support of the Ministry of Education, Science and Technological Development of the Republic of Serbia, according to the Agreement on the Realisation and Financing of Scientific Research.

L. Pantović (✉)
Institute for Philosophy and Social Theory, University of Belgrade, Belgrade, Serbia
e-mail: ljiljana.pantovic@instifdt.bg.ac.rs



L. J. Wallace et al. (eds.), *Anthropologies of Global Maternal and Reproductive Health*, Global Maternal and Child Health, https://doi.org/10.1007/978-3-030-84514-8_2

her phone back on so she can call him with the good news. The baby starts to cry and Mara hands the baby over to Sandra.

Sandra was right, those seconds feel like hours, while the time the baby spends on the mother's chest, between 1 and 3 min, passes in a heartbeat. 'Congratulations! Here is your baby. Look here, ten fingers and ten toes. What is the baby's name?' said Mara. 'Can you please repeat to me the number on your wristband?' she asks Sandra. This is a scripted conversation for Mara that she has done too many times to count.

It was a routine that I witnessed more than a hundred times during the births that I attended during my fieldwork in the hospital. Mara asks these questions to make sure there are no mistakes in the moments when the baby and mother are separated. It is not a question of if they will be separated, but when. Sandra repeats the number on her wristband to Mara while simultaneously trying to take her first look at the child she has been carrying in her body all these months. There is no discussion of breastfeeding, it was not a part of Mara's script. 'Is that the same number as the number we just gave baby? Can you tell us that number?', asks Mara again.

I started a timer on my watch when the baby was given to Sandra and observed the same routine pattern. In less than 3 min, the baby is taken from the mother's arms, weighed and measured, and put under the heater on the table on the far wall of the delivery cubicle. The mother is encouraged to stay on the delivery bed and rest. She is given her cell phone back so she can call her partner and family to tell them the birth went well. Partners and other family members are not allowed in the hospital and will only see both mother and child in 2–4 days' time when they are discharged from the hospital.

Most of the time, the newborns cry while under the lights until they tire themselves out. Mother and baby stay like this, in the same space but too far apart to see each other for another 1–2 h. The mother is waiting for the placenta to be delivered, to be inspected by the doctor and to have her episiotomy sewn up, and having her blood pressure measured every 30 min. After those 2 h pass and both mother and child are in good health, the baby is put back into the mothers' arms. In a wheel bed, the pair are taken downstairs to the *'bejbifrendli'* ward on the first floor of the hospital. There they will be rooming in with at least one but as many as three more babies and mothers for the remainder of their time in the hospital.

This is what a typical birth and hospital stay look like for most mothers in maternity hospitals in Serbia that once were certified by the WHO/UNICEF Baby-Friendly Hospital Initiative (BFHI). When I asked Mara why this hospital was not following all the steps prescribed by the initiative, she stated: 'Oh, we are following them. We must adapt them a little. International standards get a bit fuzzy here'. At the centre of this chapter is the following question: What does being a Baby-Friendly Hospital look like in practice?

I show the important insight ethnography provides in understanding the implementation and evaluation of the global Baby-Friendly Hospital Initiative (BFHI) in the context of the European semi-periphery. In Serbia today, less than 13% of children are exclusively breastfed for the first 6 months of life (Ministry of Health, 2018). And yet, Serbia has officially been a part of the BFHI for over 26 years. We know little about why Serbia's implementation of the BFHI has been so challenging. There is little, current published literature on the implementation of the BFHI in Serbia or breastfeeding more generally. During the almost 30-year period since the BFHI was adopted in Serbia, there was one external evaluation (Becker & Zisovska, 2009) of the country's BFHI implementation process; however, it was conducted over 10 years ago and failed to take into account the local socio-political context under which this initiative had been implemented. Without understanding these contexts, one cannot fully appreciate why the initiative had only moderate success in the country or propose effective solutions.

I combine analysis of global BFHI policy with a historical overview of the socio-political context in which it was implemented and ethnographic observations to show that in Serbia the global BFHI has been 'thinly' implemented. It has not had substantive buy-in from healthcare workers in maternity hospitals, nor has it resulted in significant changes in the routines on the hospital floor that would positively promote and support breastfeeding. Despite a renewed national-level commitment to breastfeeding promotion, the policies are still thinly learned and implemented.

The global Baby-Friendly Hospital Initiative implemented in Serbia in the early 1990s and the national-level policies which renewed it in 2018 have been constrained by social, political and economic conditions that hindered the uptake of the program by frontline health workers – namely the devastating effects of the civil war and international sanctions in the 1990s, and the deleterious effects of IMF policies on the Serbian healthcare system since the 2000s. I suggest that the pressure of time due to high workloads, and understaffed hospitals, in combination with unsustainable national funds for implementation may contribute to the reality of the thin implementation of BFHI.

After describing my research methods, I briefly present the key tenets of the global BFHI. I then address some of the key policy literature on the initiative and breastfeeding more generally. I describe three key socio-political periods from 1994 through to the present that have impacted the BFHI and health care more broadly in Serbia. I then juxtapose this review of the published literature and policy documents with my observations of the lack of internalisation of the ten steps of the BFHI visible in the everyday routines of one maternity ward.

## Methods

My analysis of the BFHI is based on a year of ethnographic fieldwork conducted during 2016–2017 in a large city in Serbia as part of a larger research project on maternal health care (Pantovic, 2016, 2018, 2019). I spent 4 months of participant observation in one of the largest maternity hospitals in Serbia, observing over 150 births, and 8 months in birthing classes taught by nurse-midwives. Inside the hospital, I shadowed various doctors, mostly residents, three to four times a week to learn what their typical workday was like. I was there to give a supportive smile to the women during delivery, and to help out the nurses when they made gauze and other materials. I took the first pictures of newborns so their mothers could share them with their families and partners. I made and drank coffee with the medical staff, and in general, I spent time observing the daily routines in the ward. I conducted semi-structured interviews with 14 gynaecologists and with 80 women who had given birth during that year, and unstructured interviews with four nurse-midwives and three owners and non-medical staff of privately-owned institutions, centred on maternal care. I also analysed relevant documents, including policies and reports on maternity care in Serbia. The transcribed interviews and field notes were entered into qualitative research NVivo software for managing, analysing and interpreting the data. The data were analysed using a mixture of deductive and inductive codes. Since this chapter is based on a larger study on privatization and consumerism of maternal health care, initially the data were analysed based on deductive codes focusing on patient provider relationships, continuity of care and birthing experiences. What emerged out of my field notes and interviews were inductive codes around breastfeeding, skin-to-skin contact in the delivery ward and working conditions in the maternity hospital. These inductive themes form the centre of the data presented in this chapter.

## The Global Baby-Friendly Hospital Initiative

In 1991, due to a decline in breastfed children across the world, the WHO and UNICEF launched the Baby-Friendly Hospital Initiative. The momentum behind the initiative was a long-standing grassroots movement that became prominent in the 1970s; the movement was fuelled, in particular, by a call by North American mothers to boycott baby formula sold by big corporations such as Nestle, who had been producing infant foods since the start of the twentieth century (Van Esterik, 2006). Their lobbying was successful and lead to the creation of the 1981 *International Code of Marketing of Breast Milk Substitutes* (WHO, 1981) which discouraged the advertising and privileging of formula over breast milk. WHO and UNICEF published the Ten Steps to Successful Breastfeeding in 1989, as part of a set of policies and procedures for maternity facilities to implement in order to support and improve breastfeeding. In 1990, the *Innocenti Declaration On The Protection, Promotion and Support of Breastfeeding* called for all governments to implement the ten steps within their maternity and newborn programs. The Baby-Friendly Hospital Initiative, launched by WHO and UNICEF in 1990, is a set of guidelines intended to motivate facilities worldwide to implement the Ten Steps to Successful Breastfeeding and comply with the International Code of Marketing of Breast-milk Substitutes (WHO, 2017).

1a. Comply fully with the International Code of Marketing of Breast-milk Substitutes and relevant World Health Assembly resolutions.
1b. Have a written infant feeding policy that is routinely communicated to staff and parents.
1c. Establish ongoing monitoring and data-management systems.

2. Ensure that staff have sufficient knowledge, competence and skills to support breastfeeding.
3. Discuss the importance and management of breastfeeding with pregnant women and their families.
4. Facilitate immediate and uninterrupted skin-to-skin contact and support mothers to initiate breastfeeding as soon as possible after birth.
5. Support mothers to initiate and maintain breastfeeding and manage common difficulties.
6. Do not provide breastfed newborns any food or fluids other than breast milk, unless medically indicated.
7. Enable mothers and their infants to remain together and to practice rooming-in 24 hours a day.
8. Support mothers to recognize and respond to their infants' cues for feeding.
9. Counsel mothers on the use and risks of feeding bottles, teats and pacifiers.
10. Coordinate discharge so that parents and their infants have timely access to ongoing support and care.

The Baby-Friendly Hospital Initiative was meant to not only promote breastfeeding but also to empower women to feel confident in this process. The BFHI focuses on reforming maternity care institutions and educating medical providers, and the wider community to support breastfeeding. For a hospital to receive the status of 'baby-friendly', the staff must be educated on the benefits of breastfeeding and the risks associated with supplementary bottle feeding. Promoting or advertising formula is banned in baby-friendly hospitals. The hospital has to provide rooming-in for mother and infant and enable breastfeeding on demand starting with the newborn latching on within the first hour after birth (WHO/UNICEF, 2009). Women have to be educated about breastfeeding as well and have access to lactation specialists to support them in using breastfeeding techniques (WHO, 2017).

Several studies have shown that hospitals that are BFHI-accredited have higher breastfeeding rates than hospitals that do not or have not been renewed (Bartington et al., 2006; Abolyan, 2006; Bagci Bosi et al., 2016; Pérez-Escamilla, Martinez & Segura-Pérez, 2016; Braun et al., 2003). However, policy analyses report 'baby-friendly fatigue' in various countries – a term used to describe the waning interest in the initiative at the national level (2017). WHO (2017) estimates that only about 10% of babies in the world are born in a facility currently designated as baby friendly.

Public health and anthropological studies that examine the implementation of global breastfeeding texts such as the BFHI identify a number of challenges. Anthropological studies in particular demonstrate the social and cultural distance between the producers of global guidelines and their recipients, outlining how global texts misalign with local realities, including the contexts and needs of mothers and frontline workers (Dykes, 2006; Desclaux & Alfieri, 2015; Blystad et al., 2010; Gottschang, 2000). Ethnographic accounts of the implementation of breastfeeding policies focus on how the process of breastfeeding has been undermined by capitalist regimes. This includes the negative impacts of the influences of industrialisation and medicalisation on post-natal wards, which shape the use of time and space, and decisions surrounding infant feeding (Dykes, 2006) and the reinforcement of inequities in the division of labour, gender roles and power relations through breastfeeding discourses communicated by the public and in health promotion literature (Maher, 1992; Faircloth, 2013; Tomori, 2014; Stearns, 2009; Haraway, 2013). Numerous studies have traced the disconnect between specific WHO infant feeding guidelines and the way breastfeeding is actually experienced as a culturally and socially embedded practice (Desclaux & Alfieri, 2015; Blystad et al., 2010; Gottschang, 2000). Desclaux and Alfieri (2015), for instance, argue that HIV-positive women in West Africa did not apply medical recommendations regarding infant feeding since none of the infant feeding practices recommended were common in the lay culture of feeding. Similarly, Gottschang (2000) examines the conflict between global BFHI guidelines and local realities for Chinese mothers whose economic realities make breastfeeding difficult.

Numerous public health studies also identify challenges that negatively impact the implementation of the BFHI. At the national level, funding constraints are a major barrier (Saadeh, 2012; UNICEF & WHO, 2017). The 2nd Global Nutrition Policy Review, implemented by WHO in 2016–2017, a multi country evaluation of the implementation of the BFHI, notes that with the exception of a few countries, sustainable national funding for BFHI implementation is rare. In many settings, the initiative was funded from government or other sources when it was initiated; however, due to various issues, including changes in national leadership, shifting national priorities or tight budgets, funding is no longer available (UNICEF & WHO, 2017). The BFHI works best when it is endorsed and funded by national authorities; however, there is often low awareness or acceptance of the need for the initiative among government departments and, as a result, government ownership of the initiative can be lacking (Wieczorek et al., 2015; Saadeh, 2012; UNICEF & WHO, 2017). In countries where the BFHI has been less successful, government ownership is often less compared to the ownership demonstrated by external bodies such as donors and NGOs (UNICEF & WHO, 2017).

National funding constraints often trickle down to the facility level, where there is a lack of resources for the assessment and designation process, or for training staff (UNICEF & WHO, 2017). Even where funding and national political coordination exists, the individual experiences and attitudes of health workers and hospital management are also important issues influencing the implementation of the BFHI (Wieczorek et al., 2015; Nickel et al., 2013; Abolyan, 2006; UNICEF & WHO, 2017; Walsh et al., 2011). The attitudes of administrators influence the commitment of health workers to implement the steps (Nickel et al., 2013; Schmied et al., 2011; Wieczorek et al., 2015). For instance, some studies describe the action of an individual change agent, who facilitates implementation of the steps by promoting the initiative among managers of professional groups and units, requiring staff to participate in hands-on breastfeeding trainings, and including breastfeeding support in staff members' annual performance reviews (Nickel et al., 2013; Wieczorek et al., 2015).

Misunderstanding of the BFHI on the part of health workers can also pose a challenge to BFHI implementation (Abolyan, 2006; Nickel et al., 2013; UNICEF & WHO, 2017; Walsh et al., 2011; Wieczorek et al., 2015). For instance, in North Carolina, night shift nurses thought that supplemental artificial feeds had few if any negative consequences, and felt that providing the mother an opportunity to rest (by removing the baby) was more beneficial than supporting breastfeeding (Nickel et al., 2013). Rather than using the BFHI as a strategy to improve health professionals' practices, nurses in Australia tended to 'focus on the ten steps as a set of tasks to be accomplished' (Schmied et al., 2011, p. 9). They interpreted the BFHI as a tool to convey the message that breastfeeding was the only way to properly feed a baby and then used it to influence infant feeding decisions, giving women little choice in their feeding method (Schmied et al., 2011).

Systemic issues, including a high workload for health facility staff and their lack of time, have also been identified as causes of the thin implementation of the BFHI (Reddin, Pincombe & Darbyshire, 2007; Taylor et al., 2011; Schmied et al., 2011; Semenic et al., 2012; Thomson et al., 2012; Nickel et al., 2013; Abolyan, 2006). In some contexts, health workers often perceive the BFHI in a positive way and are committed to BFHI implementation, but the pressure of time leads them to take shortcuts or seek a 'quick fix'. In Serbia, the BFHI has been constrained by social, political and economic conditions that hindered the commitment to the program at the national level as well as its uptake by facilities and frontline health workers.

## The History of the Baby-Friendly Hospital Initiative in Serbia

I describe three key socio-political periods that impacted the BFHI and health care more broadly in Serbia: the 1990s, early 2000s and the current political regime from 2012 onwards. Larger social, economic and political contexts shape the implementation of global maternal health policies; my descriptions of these three periods provide crucial historical context, shedding important light on the low prioritization of the BFHI at the national level, and its thin implementation in health facilities.

### *The 1990s*

During the 1990s, Serbia was under international isolation. The wars and international sanctions left the previously 'generous' healthcare sector of Yugoslavia in severe crisis (Perišić, 2014). The Milošević regime tried to maintain the illusion of the status quo, but in reality, the country's infrastructure was deteriorating (Perišić, 2016). All of the hospitals in Serbia lacked basic supplies, and medical staff experienced significant delays in receiving their salaries (Stambolovic, 2003). The last decade of the twentieth century was a harsh one for Serbian citizens. The old millennium ended with the 1999 NATO bombing campaign that devastated the country. One of the gynaecologists I spoke to remembers working in a large maternity hospital during the sanctions and the bombing:

> During the sanctions, it became increasingly difficult to work. There were no medications, no resources. During the bombing, it was the worst. We would frequently lose electricity. Imagine doing a C-section under candlelight! No one did this except us! We worked, without water or power but we worked.

Milošević's regime led the country into sanctions and 'had taken Serbia from the largest republic in the internationally respected and cosmopolitan Socialist Federal Republic of Yugoslavia to a pariah country plagued by nationalism, haunted by war crimes, and devastated by economic insecurity' (Greenberg, 2014, p. 5). It was during this period of upheaval that the country formally adopted the WHO Baby-Friendly Hospital Initiative with the aim of ameliorating the low rates of breastfeeding and high mortality rate of infants and young children (Chalmers, 1997). When Becker and Ziskova's (2009) evaluation came out, Dr. Durda Kisin from the Public Health Institute in Serbia stated that 'this initiative was implemented in a time when most hospitals did not have running hot water. The idea was to encourage mothers to breastfeed, but the times were tough' (RTS. Problemi u srpskim porodilištima 2010, translated by the author).

## *The Early 2000s*

The new century brought about a feeling of hope and change in Serbia that could have led to a better implementation of the policy than the previous period. People stormed the nation's capital of Belgrade on 5 October 2000 and ousted Milošević. The new democratically-elected Serbian government had high hopes for overall change. The new post-Milošević government slowly managed to lift the international sanctions and started negotiations of their own with the International Monetary Fund (IMF). The goal of the post-Milošević government was to 'create a real market economy' (Perišić, 2016, p. 649), emphasizing market and economic stability. When it came to reforms in health care, this government tried to maintain at least the perception of universal healthcare coverage. The government sought help from various international aid organisations to re-build essential healthcare infrastructure. Most notably, the World Health Organization (WHO) and the World Bank provided humanitarian aid to Serbian hospitals, with special attention to the maternity wards. At this time, the UNICEF country office was still providing support for the implementation of the BFHI Initiative (Becker & Zisovska, 2009, p. 41). As of 2005, the largest number of public maternity wards and hospitals, 84%, were certified as baby-friendly (Ministry of Health, 2018). At this time, 91% of women were breastfeeding exclusively upon discharge in Baby-Friendly designated facilities and 78% of births were taking place in facilities certified as meeting and maintaining Baby-Friendly criteria (Becker & Zisovska, 2009).

Even though hopes were high right after the revolution in Serbia, they quickly grew into disappointment. Along with the rest of the world, Serbia felt the impact of the 2007/2008 global economic crisis that shattered the already fragile and still recovering economy. In this period, the WHO and UNICEF officially stopped funding the BFHI and national public health officials noted a drop in children exclusively breastfed in the first 6 months of life, from 15.1% to the current 12.8% (Ministry of Health, 2018). It is unclear if the national government provided any funding for the BFHI afterwards. Still recovering from the wars and sanctions, at this time the International Monetary Fund imposed reforms that have had a severe impact on healthcare provisioning (Perišić, 2014, 2016; Stambolieva, 2016). Every one of these reforms hurt healthcare provisioning for most of the population of Serbia. These reforms included further containing public healthcare spending and imposing a cap on the duration of sick leave benefits, increasing the level of co-payments, and downsizing the number of medical and nonmedical staff in public health care, as well as speeding up reforms of public enterprises and the privatization process. Reforms also included severe cuts in public healthcare funding and imposition of a ban on new hires within the public sector by the right-wing government, at the time led by then Prime Minister (now President) Aleksandar Vučić. While there are no official reports as to how many public healthcare providers have immigrated to Western European countries, the public and media narrative describes the current state of the Serbian healthcare system as on the brink of collapse (Arsenijevic, Pavlova & Groot, 2013; Hyde, 2016; Vasiljevic-Prodanovic, 2015).

As Becker and Zisovska note, BFHI designations have an expiration date, and only half of the initially awarded hospitals were re-appraised in the period between 2002 and 2010 (Ministry of Health, 2018). By 2009 most of the hospitals no longer met the standard (Becker & Zisovska, 2009). On behalf of UNICEF and WHO, in 2009, Becker and Zisovska carried out an evaluation of the BFHI from 1995 to 2008. Drawing on interviews with managers, health workers and mothers, observations, and desk review, the aim of the evaluation was to assess the status of the initiative and provide guidance and recommendations to the newly formed government working group for BFHI (Becker & Zisovska, 2009). Becker and Zisovksa (2009, p. 25) concluded that the initiative was supported by the national government but that the program itself was only 'moderately effective until about 2003 when support was reduced and activity curtailed, though low-level activity continued in some areas due to the commitment of individuals'. They reported that the current practices in the observed hospitals were well below the standards expected by WHO/UNICEF global criteria, and noted that there 'are misperceptions of what the BFHI is by many mothers, staff, and managers as well as the wider community' (Becker & Zisovska, 2009, p. 2). Hospital staff, as well as mothers, had limited knowledge on the benefits of the BFHI practices, only that it should be done, and women and providers equated the entire initiative with step seven: the rooming-in recommendation. Women were left to care for their babies on their own without any education or support on breastfeeding. Both managers and staff often misunderstood whether their facility was actually accredited (Becker & Zisovska, 2009). The low activity and low profile of the BFHI was attributed both to lack of funds for national coordination and local implementation (Becker & Zisovska, 2009). In accordance with the recommendation given in the Becker report in 2009, a National Committee on Breastfeeding was formed (Ministry of Health, 2018).

## *2012 to the Present*

From 2012 onwards, the Serbian government has made several attempts to revive the BFHI, but these attempts have been unsystematic, hard to document and follow up on and have resulted in little to no actual change. In 2012 and 2013, the public Institute for the Care of Mothers and Children conducted training with 600 medical providers, educating them on infant nutrition (Ministry of Health, 2018). But adherence to standards that encourage breastfeeding was not mandatory in the new accreditation process of public hospitals. As it stands, not one of the previously certified Baby-Friendly hospitals has gotten its status re-confirmed (Ministry of Health, 2018). The program did not continue, nor was there follow up from either the government or UNICEF (Ministry of Health, 2018).

In June 2017, Ana Brnabić became the first woman and the first openly gay prime minister. After her appointment, Brnabić's government set up the National Program to Support Breastfeeding (2018). This program is very self-critical of the current disconnect between the practice and policy, stating in its opening paragraph that: 'the Republic of Serbia has a legal and policy framework around breastfeeding but it is not implemented to the fullest extent' (Ministry of Health, 2018, p. 4).

The national program makes a clear link with the global BFHI and notes the importance of this initiative for maternal care in Serbia (Ministry of Health, 2018, p. 5). The program explicitly states the importance of implementing the Ten Steps in every maternity ward and hospital in Serbia (Ministry of Health, 2018, p. 27). The policy actively supports the idea that mothers and newborns should not be separated during their stay in the hospital along with a list of other 'shoulds' – for maternity hospitals and wards (Ministry of Health, 2018). For example, the hospitals should provide individualised care, should be family-oriented, partners should be present at birth, the first feeding should happen in the first hour of birth, there should be skin-to-skin contact. The program sums up this list of shoulds by stating that it is the state's job to 'support mothers so that they find breastfeeding as a pleasant and useful experience and not a chore and a norm they have to fulfill' (Ministry of Health, 2018, p. 6). As a precursor to the new national program, the Serbian government in 2017/2018, with the support of UNICEF, conducted another round of BFHI training for medical providers (Ministry of Health, 2018), although there is no indication of how many providers were trained and where these providers work. A major insight that ethnography offers for health policymakers is that it can offer an in-depth understanding of what happens in health facilities, and what gets lost when moving from policy to practice. I now turn to my own ethnographic research in one previously accredited Baby-Friendly Hospital in Serbia.

## The Not-So-Baby-Friendly Maternity Hospital

Mothers who gave birth vaginally are now rooming in with their newborns, in accordance with the seventh step for the promotion of breastfeeding. This rooming-in *is* the hospitals' baby-friendly approach. This '*bejbifrendli*' ward consists of around 20 rooms. The rooms have either four or two beds. Each room has a toilet and a shower but sadly not all the rooms' lavatories are functional, so women tend to share and walk to the rooms that do have a working shower and toilet.

Along with sharing the room with at least one another woman, mothers in the *bejbifrendli* ward also room in with their newborns in small cribs that are placed right next to their beds. In the entire hospital, there are no railings. After giving birth, which usually also includes having an episiotomy, women tend to use the crib itself as support to get up in order to get out of bed to pick up their babies or walk to the closest bathroom. Visitors are not allowed in the *bejbifrendli* ward, or in any area of the hospital. This means that the women are completely isolated during their stay from their partners, their family or any kind of support system. The lack of internalization of the Ten Steps is visible in the everyday routines in this ward.

When both women and medical providers use the English term '*bejbifrendli*' what they are referring to is a ward in the maternity hospital where mothers who had given birth vaginally are placed right after delivery. Women who had C-sections are not in this '*bejbifrendli*' ward, they spend the first night in the intensive care ward and the next 3–4 days in the semi-intensive care ward. The C-section newborns are not with their mothers during their stay in the hospital. The C-section ward mothers see their newborns on a fixed feeding schedule of every 3 h. This was the standard in the entire hospital after the BFHI accreditation.

The nurses would bring the newborns to the mothers on a 3-h cycle for around 30 min. Before giving the babies to their mothers the nurses would weigh them. Mothers were told to feed their babies for 5 min on each breast, burp the baby and hand them back to the paediatric nurse. After feeding the baby would be weighed again and if the nurse deemed that the baby was not fed enough, they would give them baby formula.

In the *bejbifrendli* ward of the hospital, women were meant to take care of their infants on their own, including feeding them. But this did not mean they could do whatever they wanted, including breastfeed on demand. Ana was a third-time mother who took the time to inform herself about UNICEF's breastfeeding policies because of her previous birth experiences in the hospital. After her discharge from the hospital, she told me about the nurses' lack of support for her wish to breastfeed on demand.

Having breastfed before, Ana, unlike other women who had just given birth for the first time, had enough hands-on experience when it came to breastfeeding and she felt confident in her ability to care for her baby on her own during her stay in the baby-friendly ward. She wanted to breastfeed her baby more frequently than what women are typically instructed to do during the maternity classes they can attend prior to giving birth. In the classes, women are told that they should feed babies, not on demand but on a 3-h schedule and no more than 5 min per breast. Her breastfeeding more than those prescribed 10 min created problems within the baby-friendly ward.

> I had a bad experience with breastfeeding in the hospital. I was in the baby-friendly ward, the baby was with me. One nurse noticed I wasn't breastfeeding my child during the hospital prescribed time frame but whenever I wanted. She kept telling me that I should not feed the baby whenever I wanted to, that the baby needs time to digest the milk. She told me that I should feed the baby for no more than 5 minutes. I did not want to argue with her, so I said, fine. She saw that I wasn't really going to listen to her really. She sent another nurse in with a stopwatch and she timed me! After five minutes past, she took the baby and placed him on my other breast. After another five minutes, she took him and put him in the crib. I had to secretly breastfeed my child. I was so nervous. I requested a breast pump because I had so much milk and the nurse told me it was my own fault for not listening to their rules. They are supposed to support breastfeeding but not like this.

Ana was one of the few mothers who had attended birthing classes in order to prepare for labour psychologically and physically. These classes are completely free and are covered through the state health insurance. It is during these classes that breastfeeding is discussed the most with pregnant women. These courses are the key sites where women are encouraged to breastfeed, and yet, according to the main coordinator of the classes, less than 30% of the women in the city actually attend these courses because they live too far or have to work during class times.

During the classes that I observed, the quality of information about breastfeeding provided to women varied and depended solely on the attitude and knowledge of the teaching-midwife. Nurse-midwives would always list the medical benefits of breastfeeding from these studies, such as lower rates of middle ear infections, lower cancer rates and other benefits. However, in addition to being told that babies should not be fed on demand, instructors would frequently add claims about the benefits of breastfeeding that were harder to support. For example, during one such lecture, a nurse-midwife told her class that: 'you won't gain weight if you breastfeed and your child won't become a drug addict (*narkoman*)'. A key aspect of the BFHI is teaching medical providers about the medical benefits of breastfeeding for both mother and infant. Yet, when I conducted fieldwork during 2017 there was no mention of or discussion on these trainings in staff meetings.

Feeling safe and supported is a key prerequisite for women to feel empowered to successfully breastfeed (Stankovic, 2017). This support should also entail providing women with ample and adequate information about their birth, breastfeeding, and other concerns, as well as respecting their privacy and wish to rest after giving birth. When asked about breastfeeding support, women replied that their experiences with the staff varied drastically. 'When I just got to the room the nurse was great. She explained things to me and even helped me place the baby properly. The nurse that came in the afternoon shift, she did not even bother' said one woman while trying to soothe her crying newborn. On many occasions I observed that instead of a nurse coming in to help with the first feeding, women were played an old VHS tape about breastfeeding. This appeared to be a WHO breastfeeding video from the 1990s. It was in English with Serbian subtitles. What usually would happen is that the nurse would turn the video on and leave the room. The moment the nurse left, the mothers would show no interest in watching this old video. Some even told me that they looked up how-to tutorials on YouTube rather than watching the VHS, or that they asked for help from their roommate if they were lucky enough to have a roommate who had given birth before.

It would be unjust and a simplification to state that nurses refuse to provide mothers with lactation assistance. That their refusal to teach and encourage women to breastfeed was a matter of active resistance towards the policy and that they do not see the benefits of breastfeeding. We cannot disregard the global and local political and economic constraints that affect their agency as healthcare workers. As described in the background section, there have been radical cuts in Serbia's healthcare sector resulting in shortages of staff, especially gynaecological and paediatric nurses, who are tasked with helping women in the recovery process after giving birth.

The nurse-midwives, along with the residents, were the health workers I spent the most time with in the hospital. Most of the midwives were middle-aged women, and all of them can best be described as women who will not tolerate nonsense. The midwives have their break room within the delivery ward. They would usually make coffee for each other and share a breakfast of *burek,* a type of meat or cheese pie, or some other pastry from the bakery or canned sardines. The conversations in the room were often very lively and jovial, however, the women also frequently used break time to vent about the difficult working conditions they faced in the hospital, especially being overworked and underpaid. While making herself a cup of coffee, one nurse-midwife, Milana, a serious woman with short blond hair, started talking about her feelings about her work.

> It is a hard job, but I love it. The only thing I can complain about is the fact that they cut down our off days. We work 12-hour shifts, plus night shifts twice a month (24h shift) and we used to have three days off; now we have two. That is barely enough for you to get some sleep, not nearly enough time if you have a family as well.

The nurse-midwives I spoke to were all very unhappy with their economic status. I asked Nena, another senior midwife, to compare, in her view, their situation during socialism and now; she said: 'Sure the technology is better now, but our paycheck is not. It is challenging to make ends meet let alone think about things like holidays. Those are luxuries for us'. Milena smirked at that comment and added: 'I am surprised we do not make more mistakes along the way! It is because we are tired! Tired, overworked and severely underpaid'.

During my fieldwork, I observed how the shortage of nursing staff affected women's experiences during their stay in this hospital. Women do not even know the names of the medical staff working in the maternity hospital, the staff do not introduce themselves to the women, nor do they wear name tags. The absence of a friendly, human relationship with the staff, coupled with the poor infrastructure of the hospital left women disappointed with their birthing experience (Arsenijevic, Pavlova & Groot, 2014; Baji et al., 2017; Sekulic, 2016; Pantović, 2016). Frequently they would tell me that they felt as if they were left to fend for themselves.

> When it comes to breastfeeding, they did not explain anything. This is my first baby and I asked the nurse when I should feed the baby for the first time. She told me I could feed her now if I want to. We did try but she (the baby) was not interested. The nurse told me that the baby will be fine even without breast milk in the first 24 hours, that the baby is not hungry that she will let me know when she is hungry. When I asked her to come and help me, she told me that she is too busy to come that I must figure it out on my own.

All the women I spoke to wanted to breastfeed and tried extremely hard to do so in the hospital. Some, like Ana, persisted and breastfed on demand despite the nurses, while others complied with the unwritten rules of the hospital that told them their child needed to supplement their feeding with formula. When leaving the hospital, the struggle continues. 'People think that I am crazy for still breastfeeding my one-year-old!' one mother told me during our follow-up interview. Although there are no studies on public perceptions of breastfeeding in Serbia, my conversations with mothers and media reports suggest that there are public misconceptions that also contribute to an environment unsupportive of breastfeeding. For instance, according to a BBC news report (Dojenje na javnom mestu u Srbiji: Beba bira gde i kada će da jede, poručuju mame, 2019) women are often met with negative comments and disdain from the general population when they choose to breastfeed in public.

In the hallways of the baby-friendly ward, there are multiple framed posters outlining the ten steps to successful breastfeeding, posters outlining the importance of breastfeeding in the first 6 months of life. Visually the Baby-Friendly Hospital Initiative was very present in the walls and TV screens of the hospital, but most women did not feel they were informed or encouraged to breastfeed. There was a sharp disconnect between what was written on the walls and in policy documents and what occurred in practice.

## Discussion and Conclusion

Through a review of the history of Serbia's BFHI policy implementation, alongside ethnographic observations of the daily routines in one such designated 'baby-friendly' maternity hospital, this chapter provides insight as to why the implementation of the BFHI in Serbia over the past 30 years has been met with little success. I have described three key socio-political periods that impacted the BFHI and health care more broadly in Serbia (contexts that previous external evaluations of BFHI in Serbia have not fully considered): the 1990s, early 2000s, and the current political regime from 2012 onward. I show that the Baby-Friendly Hospital Initiative implemented in Serbia in the early 1990s and the national-level policies which renewed it in 2018 have been constrained by social, political and economic conditions that hindered the uptake of the programs by frontline health workers – including the devastating effects of the civil war and international sanctions in the 1990s, and the deleterious effects of IMF policies on the Serbian healthcare system since the 2000s.

Dobre (2008) uses the term 'thin learning' to describe how EU policies were adopted in Romania to superficially comply with EU accession without actual implementation and governmental reform. In the case of the BFHI the policy also appears to have become thinly implemented instead of actually promoting breastfeeding in a meaningful way. Within health facilities, I observed a non–evidence-based approach when providing information about breastfeeding, a lack of rooming in and initiation of breastfeeding within a half hour of birth, and lack of breastfeeding on demand. My findings are similar to those reported by Becker and Zisovska (2009) in their evaluation, which took place over 10 years ago, suggesting that, despite a renewed national-level commitment to breastfeeding promotion, breastfeeding policies are still poorly implemented, with the lack of internalization of the ten steps of the BFHI visible in the everyday routines of the maternity ward.

Women like Ana were left on their own to care for their babies with little breastfeeding education or assistance. Even though the ward was called '*bejbifriendli*' and baby formula is not given out routinely, the practice of breastfeeding every 3 h for 10 min describes a more staff-schedule friendly than baby-friendly practice. The rationale for separating mothers with C-section from their infants and feeding infants formula during this period is not clear, but it may have been for the ease of staff in caring for mothers. Allowing for feeding on demand would require restructuring hospital and health worker schedules to fit the needs of each individual breastfeeding woman. Instead, women are disciplined to breastfeed on the demand of the hospital. Based on my observations and interviews with health workers, it seems, as in other contexts, that the pressure of time due to high workloads, and understaffed hospitals (Abolyan, 2006; Schmied et al., 2011; Semenic et al., 2012; Taylor et al., 2011; Thomson, Bilson & Dykes, 2012) in combination with unsustainable national funds for implementation (Saadeh, 2012; UNICEF & WHO, 2017) may contribute to the reality of the thin implementation of BFHI in Serbia.

Taking a closer look at the social, political and economic context in which the initiative was first implemented in Serbia, it is not difficult to understand why it has had so many shortcomings. The initiative was first signed during sanctions and civil wars with the infrastructure in shambles – conditions under which it would have been impossible to succeed. The larger social and political backdrop of the timing of the initiative is linked with Serbia's political and economic trajectory towards the European Union; by initially signing on to the BFHI, Serbia may have also been trying to signal its alignment with European norms and standards such as empowering women to breastfeed. Yet, political support for the BFHI appears to have waxed and waned. As in other country contexts (Saadeh, 2012; UNICEF & WHO, 2017) a consistent source of funding for the initiative has also been a challenge. The period of its initial successes was closely tied with the provision of UNICEF funds, but beyond inconsistent funding from external partners such as UNICEF, the initiative has since never had a consistent source of public funding. Funds have been made available for recent trainings of health providers, however, it is unclear if a consistent source of funds is available for training, and for other activities which are important for the implementation of the BFHI, including for the assessment and designation of facilities (Ministry of Health, 2018; UNICEF & WHO, 2017).

In the past few years, the state of the public maternity hospitals has become a hot-button issue in the country, due partially to intense media scrutiny. Although problems in the maternity hospitals were widely known (Arsenijevic, Pavlova & Groot, 2014), there exists an unwritten rule that women should not speak about them in public. To counter this silence, a grass roots NGO Majka Hrabrost (Mother Courage) collected online surveys from mothers who delivered infants in one of the maternity hospitals in Serbia between 2000 and 2008. It identified three main problems in Serbian maternity care: poor communication, corruption, and outdated medical protocols that are still in use, such as mandatory enemas upon admission (Arsenijevic et al., 2014). These findings confirm the observations I made during my fieldwork, and have also been noted in a more recent survey conducted by another NGO Centar za Mame (Centre for Moms) (Sloboda Rađanju – rezultati o iskustvima žena na porođaju u Srbiji, 2015). In addition to the lack of support for breastfeeding, women are often simply told to endure the lack of support and lack of agency they experience overall during their birthing experience and stay in the maternity hospitals.

Sadly, Mother Courage is no longer working in Serbia and Centre for Moms seems to be the only viable NGO left working on issues around maternity in the country. New problems seem to be emerging while previous issues remain unresolved. Even though the national program for the support of breastfeeding is now over 2 years into implementation, there is no civil sector oversight or analysis of its effects. Furthermore, the Serbian government passed new legislation that effectively slashed maternity leave and pay for most women in Serbia (Apelujemo da se izmene Zakona o finansijskoj podršci porodici sa decom uključe u novi budžet, 2019; Više od 13.000 mama oštećeno Zakonom o finansijskoj podršci porodici sa decom, 2019). With a lack of civil sector oversight, coupled with the poor working conditions in the hospitals and the overall low public interest in promoting breastfeeding, it is difficult to see how the BFHI in Serbia will move beyond thin implementation focused only on written policy documents and lip service by politicians to actual changes in practice.

## References

Abolyan, L. V. (2006). The breastfeeding support and promotion in Baby-Friendly Maternity Hospitals and not-as-yet Baby-Friendly hospitals in Russia. *Breastfeeding Medicine, 1*(2), 71–78. https://doi.org/10.1089/bfm.2006.1.71

Centar za Mame. (2019). Apelujemo da se izmene Zakona o finansijskoj podršci porodici sa decom uključe u novi budžet. http://centarzamame.rs/blog/2019/11/06/da-li-su-najavljene-izmene-zakona-o-finansijskoj-podrsci-porodici-sa-decom-obecanje-ludom-radovanje/. Accessed 7 Aug 2020.

Arsenijevic, J., Pavlova, M., & Groot, W. (2013). Measuring the catastrophic and impoverishing effect of household health care spending in Serbia. *Social Science & Medicine, 78*(1), 17–25. https://doi.org/10.1016/j.socscimed.2012.11.014

Arsenijevic, J., Pavlova, M., & Groot, W. (2014). Shortcomings in maternity care in Serbia. *Birth-Issues in Perinatal Care, 41*(1), 14–25. https://doi.org/10.1111/birt.12096

Bagci Bosi, A. T., Eriksen, K. G., Sobko, T., Wijnhoven, T. M. A., & Breda, J. (2016). Breastfeeding practices and policies in WHO European region member states. *Public Health Nutrition, 19*(4), 753–764. https://doi.org/10.1017/S1368980015001767

Baji, P., Rubashkin, N., Szebik, I., Stoll, K., & Vedam, S. (2017). Informal cash payments for birth in Hungary: Are women paying to secure a known provider, respect, or quality of care? *Social Science & Medicine, 189*, 86–95. https://doi.org/10.1016/j.socscimed.2017.07.015

Bartington, S., Griffiths, L. J., Tate, A. R., & Dezateux, C. (2006). Are breastfeeding rates higher among mothers delivering in Baby Friendly accredited maternity units in the UK? *International Journal of Epidemiology, 35*(5), 1178–1186. doi: 10.1093/ije/dyl155

Becker, G., & Zisovska, E. (2009). *Evaluation of the Baby-Friendly Hospital Initative in Serbia for the period of 1995–2008*. WHO/UNICEF.

Blystad, A., van Esterik, P., de Paoli, M. M., Sellen, D. W., Leshabari, S. C., et al. (2010). Reflections on global policy documents and the WHO's infant feeding guidelines: Lessons learnt. *International Breastfeeding Journal, 5*(18).

Braun, M. L. G., Giugliani, E. R., Soares, M. E. M., Giugliani, C., de Oliveira, A. P., & Danelon, C. M. M. (2003). Evaluation of the impact of the Baby-Friendly Hospital Initiative on rates of breastfeeding. *American Journal of Public Health, 93*(8), 1277–1279.

Chalmers, B. (1997). Changing childbirth in Eastern Europe: Which systems of authoritative knowledge should prevail? In R.E. Davis-Floyd & C.F. Sargent (Eds.), *Childbirth and Authoritative Knowledge: Cross-cultural Perspectives* (pp. 263-83). University of California Press.

Desclaux, A., & Alfieri, C. (2015). Between proscription and control of breastfeeding in West Africa: Women's strategies regarding prevention of HIV transmission. In T. Cassidy & A. El Tom (Eds.), *Ethnographies of breastfeeding: Cultural contexts and confrontations* (pp. 125–144). Bloomsbury.

Dobre, A. M. (2008). Designing and justifying regional reforms: Lessons from Romania. *Policy & Politics, 36*(4), 587–600. https://doi.org/10.1332/147084408X349783

Marinković, L. (2019, July 21). Dojenje na javnom mestu u Srbiji: Beba bira gde i kada će da jede, poručuju mame. *BBC News*. https://www.bbc.com/serbian/lat/srbija-48585987

Dykes, F. (2006). *Breastfeeding in hospital: Mothers, midwives and the production line*. Routledge.

Faircloth, C. (2013). *Militant lactivism? Attachment parenting and intensive Motherhood in the UK and France*. Berghahn Books.

Gottschang, S. Z. (2000). Reforming routines: A Baby-Friendly Hospital in Urban China. In L. M. Whiteford & L. Manderson (Eds.), *Global health policies, local realities: The fallacy of the level playing field* (pp. 265–288). Lynne Rienner Publishers.

Greenberg, J. (2014). *After the revolution: Youth, democracy, and the politics of disappointment in Serbia*. Stanford University Press.

Haraway, D. (2013). *Simians, cyborgs, and women: The reinvention of nature*. Routledge.

Hyde, R. (2016). Mixed diagnosis for Serbian health system. *The Lancet, 388*(10061), 2729–2730. https://doi.org/10.1016/s0140-6736(16)32460-6

Maher, V. (1992). *The anthropology of breast-feeding: Natural law or social construct*. Routledge.

Ministry of Health, Republic of Serbia. (2018). *Uredba o nacionalnom programu podrške dojenju, porodičnoj i razvojnoj nezi novorođenčeta*. Službeni Glasnik RS. https://www.pravno-informacioni-sistem.rs/SlGlasnikPortal/eli/rep/sgrs/vlada/uredba/2018/53/1/%20reg. Accessed 5 Oct 2021.

Nickel, N. C., Taylor, E. C., Labbok, M. H., Weiner, B. J., & Williamson, N. E. (2013). Applying organisation theory to understand barriers and facilitators to the implementation of baby-friendly: A multisite qualitative study. *Midwifery, 29*(8), 956–964. doi: 10.1016/j.midw.2012.12.001

Pantović, Lj. (2016). Buying a connection. Private practice in public health care – The case of a Serbian maternity hospital. *Anthropology of Eastern Europe Review, 34*(1), 25–38.

Pantović, Lj. (2018). Not-so-informal relationships. Selective unbundling of maternal care and the reconfigurations of patient–provider relations in Serbia. *Südosteuropa. Journal of Politics and Society, 66*(3), 371–391. doi: 10.1515/soeu-2018-0029

Pantović, Lj. (2019). Private within the Public: Negotiating Birth in Serbia. [Doctoral Dissertation, University of Pittsburgh] Pitt Campus Repository. http://d-scholarship.pitt.edu/35994/
Pérez-Escamilla, R., Martinez, J. L., & Segura-Pérez, S. (2016). Impact of the Baby-friendly Hospital Initiative on breastfeeding and child health outcomes: A systematic review. *Maternal & Child Nutrition, 12*(3), 402–417. https://doi.org/10.1111/mcn.12294
Perišić, N. (2014). Health care system between the state and the market – The case of Serbia. *Serbian Political Thought, 2*, 193–209.
Perišić, N. (2016). The Serbian welfare state: A transition loser. In K. Schubert, P. de Villota, & J. Kuhlmann (Eds.), *Challenges to European welfare systems* (pp. 647-669). Springer.
Reddin, E., Pincombe, J., & Darbyshire, P. (2007). Passive resistance: Early experiences of midwifery students/graduates and the Baby Friendly Health Initiative 10 steps to successful breastfeeding. *Women and Birth, 20*(2), 71–76. DOI:https://doi.org/10.1016/j.wombi.2007.04.003
RTS. (2010). Problemi u srpskim porodilištima. https://www.rts.rs/page/stories/sr/story/125/drustvo/470991/problemi-u-srpskim-porodilistima.html. Accessed 7 Aug 2020.
Saadeh, R. J. (2012). The Baby-Friendly Hospital Initiative 20 years on: facts, progress, and the way forward. *Journal of Human Lactation, 28*(3), 272–275.
Schmied, V., Gribble, K., Sheehan, A., Taylor, C., & Dykes, F. C. (2011). Ten steps or climbing a mountain: A study of Australian health professionals' perceptions of implementing the baby friendly health initiative to protect, promote and support breastfeeding. *BMC Health Services Research, 11*(1), 208.
Sekulic, N. (2016). O kulturi rađanja – istrazivanje o problemu nasilja nad zenama tokom porođaja 2 -/Culture of giving birth: Research on the issue of violence against women during delivery. *Sociologija, 58*, 260. https://doi.org/10.2298/SOC16S1259S
Semenic, S., Childerhose, J. E., Lauzière, J., & Groleau, D. (2012). Barriers, facilitators, and recommendations related to implementing the Baby-Friendly Initiative (BFI): An integrative review. *Journal of Human Lactation, 28*(3), 317–334. doi: 10.1177/0890334412445195
Centar za Mame. (2015). Sloboda Rađanju – rezultati o iskustvima žena na porođaju u Srbiji. http://centarzamame.rs/blog/2015/03/01/sloboda-radanju-rezultati-o-iskustvima-zena-na-porodaju-u-srbiji/. Accessed 7 Aug 2020.
Stambolieva, M. (2016). *Welfare state transformation in the Yugoslav successor states: From social to unequal*. Routledge.
Stambolovic, V. (2003). Epidemic of health care reforms. *European Journal of Public Health, 13*(1), 77–79. https://doi.org/10.1093/eurpub/13.1.77
Stankovic, B. (2017). Women's experiences of childbirth in Serbian public healthcare institutions: A qualitative study. *International Journal of Behavioral Medicine, 24*(6), 803–814. https://doi.org/10.1007/s12529-017-9672-1
Stearns, C. A. (2009). The work of breastfeeding. *Women's Studies Quarterly, 37*(3/4), 63–80.
Taylor, C., Gribble, K., Sheehan, A., Schmied, V., & Dykes, F. (2011). Staff perceptions and experiences of implementing the Baby Friendly Initiative in neonatal intensive care units in Australia. *Journal of Obstetric, Gynecologic, & Neonatal Nursing, 40*(1), 25–34. doi: 10.1111/j.1552-6909.2010.01204.x
Thomson, G., Bilson, A., & Dykes, F. (2012). Implementing the WHO/UNICEF Baby Friendly Initiative in the community: A 'hearts and minds' approach. *Midwifery, 28*(2), 258–264.
Tomori, C. (2014). *Nighttime breastfeeding: An American cultural dilemma*. Berghahn Books.
UNICEF & WHO. (2017). *Country experiences with the Baby-Friendly Hospital Initiative: Compendium of case studies around the world*. https://www.healthynewbornnetwork.org/hnn-content/uploads/BFHI_Case_Studies_FINAL_.pdf. Accessed 5 Oct 2021.
Van Esterik, P. (2006). *Celebrating the Innocenti declaration on the protection, promotion and support of breastfeeding: Past achievements, present challenges and priority actions for infant and young child feeding 2nd*. UNICEF Innocenti Research Centre Report.
Vasiljevic-Prodanovic, D. (2015). Corruption in health care: Victims of white coat crime in Serbia. *Temida, 18*(1), 97–110. https://doi.org/10.2298/tem1501097v

Dnevni list Danas. (2019, July 16). Više od 13.000 mama oštećeno Zakonom o finansijskoj podršci porodici sa decom. https://www.danas.rs/ekonomija/vise-od-13-000-mama-osteceno-zakonom-o-finansijskoj-podrsci-porodici-sa-decom/

Walsh, A. D., Walsh, A. D., Pincombe, J., Pincombe, J., Henderson, A., & Henderson, A. (2011). An examination of maternity staff attitudes towards implementing Baby Friendly Health Initiative (BFHI) accreditation in Australia. *Maternal and Child Health Journal, 15*(5), 597–609. https://doi.org/10.1007/s10995-010-0628-1

WHO. (2017). *National implementation of the Baby-friendly Hospital Initiative.*

WHO/UNICEF. (2009). *Baby-friendly hospital initiative: revised, updated and expanded for integrated care.* https://apps.who.int/iris/handle/10665/43593. Accessed 5 Oct 2021.

Wieczorek, C. C., Schmied, H., Dorner, T. E., & Dür, W. (2015). The bumpy road to implementing the Baby-Friendly Hospital Initiative in Austria: A qualitative study. *International Breastfeeding Journal, 10*(1), 3. https://doi.org/10.1186/s13006-015-0030-0

# Chapter 3
# The Promise and Neglect of Follow-up Care in Obstetric Fistula Treatment in Uganda

**Bonnie Ruder and Alice Emasu**

## Introduction

In the calm before the afternoon storm, the regional referral hospital in central Uganda was uncharacteristically quiet. The parking lot and hospital grounds were almost completely empty. In the maternity ward, only a few postpartum mothers and family members occupied the otherwise vacant space. Missing were the long lines of women waiting for care—the norm in maternity wards throughout Uganda—along with the chaotic bustle of the hospital grounds that I had grown accustomed to. It was four days into a national doctors' strike, in which doctors were protesting appallingly low wages and a chronically underfunded healthcare system. The news of the strike had spread throughout Uganda, persuading everyone except those with dire emergencies to stay home.

For our study team, the strike meant that the surgeon scheduled to conduct fistula screenings was called away to handle the latest emergency. Several hours passed while I waited with a fistula counselor and translator who works for a local NGO, a nurse, and 12 potential study participants who were waiting to be screened. The study was designed to investigate the etiology, severity, and quality of life for women experiencing persistent residual incontinence after surgical closure of an obstetric fistula. All of these women had undergone surgery for obstetric fistula, yet they were still leaking urine. The women sat next to each other on a long wooden bench and quickly bonded over their shared affliction—their incontinence and the suffering it brought.

B. Ruder (✉)
Terrewode Women's Fund, Soroti, Uganda
e-mail: bruder@terrewodewomensfund.org

A. Emasu
TERREWODE, Soroti, Uganda
e-mail: alice@terrewode.com



L. J. Wallace et al. (eds.), *Anthropologies of Global Maternal and Reproductive Health*, Global Maternal and Child Health, https://doi.org/10.1007/978-3-030-84514-8_3

Many hours later, the doctor appeared ready to screen the women. Fistula screening involves a relatively simple test in which a catheter is inserted into the urethra and the bladder is backfilled with a blue dye that is used to diagnose vesico-vaginal fistulas and stress incontinence. Ten of the 12 women passed the screening; this meant their fistula was closed yet they were still leaking urine, thus they qualified for participation in the study. The two women who did not qualify were informed that their fistulas were still open and that they may need another surgery to close their fistula. The counselor and surgeon met with each woman individually to explain their findings and discuss treatment options. Of the ten women who qualified for the study, several were initially dry upon discharge from their fistula surgery yet started to leak urine again days or months later. Other women started leaking immediately following surgery; however, this screening was the first time a healthcare worker had explained that they were experiencing residual incontinence rather than a failed closure. In both circumstances, the women had either not received follow-up care or returned for follow-up but were still confused about their prospects for treatment. All of the women were clear, however, that they desperately wanted to be cured from the continuous leaking.

– *Fieldnotes, first author, October 2017*

This chapter presents findings from a community-led project with a Ugandan nongovernmental organization (NGO) that was designed to investigate both the clinical profile and qualitative experiences of women with post-repair incontinence. The chapter draws on ethnographic fieldwork and narratives collected through open-ended interviews with fistula surgeons and women suffering from residual incontinence. Based on the emergent themes, we conducted a desk review of international and Ugandan fistula policies and guidelines, tracing fistula policy in Uganda to understand the current approach to follow-up care after fistula treatment. We discovered vague fistula policies, absent guidelines, and unfunded mandates, especially in relation to follow-up care. Ultimately, we argue that an inadequate treatment model that neglects follow-up care exists. We argue that this neglect can be traced to a donor-funded delivery model that fails to prioritize, or fund, follow-up care as an essential component of fistula treatment. As a result, poor outcomes are underreported and women who experience poor outcomes are largely erased from the fistula narrative. This erasure shapes treatment possibilities and research priorities, leaving out women still in need of additional treatment.

## Obstetric Fistula in Uganda

International discussions about maternal health in low-income countries tend to focus on maternal deaths. However, these deaths are only the tip of the iceberg in terms of the health effects of the poor availability and quality of maternity services (Paxton & Wardlaw, 2011; Storeng et al., 2012). Closely entwined with maternal mortality and propelled by the same health system deficiencies are maternal morbidities, injuries women suffer during pregnancy, childbirth, or postpartum. Assumed to be directly or indirectly related to difficult obstetric events, these morbidities/disabilities include conditions such as uterine prolapse, stress incontinence, hypertension, hemorrhoids, perineal tears, urinary tract infections, severe anemia, depression, fistula, and ectopic pregnancy (Koblinsky et al., 2012). The World Health Organization (WHO) estimates that for every maternal death, 30–50% of women who survive suffer humiliating or disabling injuries (WHO, 2015).

Beyond the acute impact of obstetric complications and the potential for future morbidities and disabilities, maternal morbidities have secondary consequences for women and their families. These consequences extend the meaning of loss beyond quantitative indicators such as the maternal mortality ratio or Disability-Adjusted Life Years (DALYs). For instance, studies from Burkina Faso tell of consequences that can span over several years and include catastrophic health expenditure, severe and persistent illness—including increased risk of all cause and pregnancy related death in the ensuing 4 years and mental health problems—stigmatization, violence, isolation and divorce, and loss of family stability and community status (Filippi et al., 2007; Storeng et al., 2010).

The most severe of maternal morbidities is an obstetric fistula. Obstetric fistula is a traumatic childbirth injury caused most often by prolonged, obstructed labor, due to either fetal malpresentation or more commonly, cephalo-pelvic disproportion—where the fetus's head is unable to fit through a woman's pelvis during labor. During the prolonged labor, the continuous pressure of the fetal head on the bladder or rectal tissues causes diminished blood flow. Eventually the tissue becomes necrotic and sloughs off, leaving a small hole, or fistula, between the woman's vaginal walls and the bladder and/or rectum. The result is uncontrollable leakage of urine and/or feces. In most cases of obstetric fistula, the fetus dies. The pressure exerted by the fetus during prolonged labor can also damage nearby organs and nerves. The multisystem injuries, described as the "obstructed labor injury complex," include renal failure, secondary infertility, foot drop from nerve injury, vaginal stenosis, and chronic skin maceration[1] (Arrowsmith et al., 1996).

The social and emotional consequences of living with fistula are also extreme, as the odor from continuous incontinence often leads to discrimination and social shaming from friends, family, and community members. Women with fistula commonly report feeling embarrassment, loneliness, worry, sadness, disappointment, and anger (Mselle et al., 2011; Pope et al., 2011; Weston et al., 2011). Women with fistula also report serious mental health issues, including severe depression and suicidal tendencies (Browning et al., 2007; Khisa et al., 2017). Divorce, separation, and marital discord are common (Ahmed & Holtz, 2007; Barageine et al., 2015;

[1] Foot drop is caused from peroneal-nerve compression during labor and results in weakness or paralysis of the forefoot. Women with foot drop experience difficulty lifting their foot and thus have limited mobility. Chronic skin maceration is the breakdown of skin on the labia and inner thighs which occurs due to the prolonged exposure to moisture. Vaginal stenosis is the narrowing and loss of flexibility in the vagina, resulting in painful intercourse.

Mwini-Nyaledzigbor et al., 2013), though not universal, experiences for women with fistula.

Today, obstetric fistulas are extremely rare in high-income countries. However, in low-resource countries with underfunded and poorly provisioned healthcare systems and limited access to quality emergency obstetric care, especially caesarean delivery, fistula remains a public health problem. The WHO (2018) estimates that in sub-Saharan Africa and Asia more than two million women live with untreated fistula, yet reliable prevalence data on obstetric fistula is unavailable. Prevalence of obstetric fistula is difficult to determine in part because women are often reluctant to reveal their symptoms, and due to the fact that true prevalence can only be confirmed with clinical examination, rendering large community-based prevalence studies cost prohibitive.

The primary intervention for women with obstetric fistula is surgical treatment, with reported success rates between 80% and 97% (Barone et al., 2012; Delamou et al., 2016; Ouedraogo et al., 2018). Following treatment, women typically report improvements in their social life and relationships, income-earning opportunities, and overall quality of life (Drew et al., 2016; El Ayadi et al., 2019; Pope et al., 2011).

However, access to fistula treatment in Uganda, similar to other low-resource countries with high fistula burdens, is severely limited. In Uganda, an estimated 114,000 women currently suffer from fistula with an additional 1,900 new cases annually (UBOS, 2018), yet due to the chronically underfunded and underprovisioned healthcare system, treatment capacity is only estimated at 1,670 cases per year (UBOS, 2018). Health facilities are plagued by a lack of infrastructure and equipment, essential drugs, and even basic supplies. Uganda also struggles with severe health worker shortages and an inadequate distribution of health workers, with the majority of health workers located in urban areas despite a predominantly rural population. Compounding this are the low wages—the major complaint during the national doctors' strike—poor morale, inadequate training, and low-staff competence, all of which result in poor quality of care, which recent studies have shown is even more pronounced in rural health facilities (Kruk et al., 2016).

In response to these healthcare deficiencies, Uganda turned to fistula surgical camps, which were initially promoted by international development agencies, including UNFPA, the African Medical and Research Foundation (AMREF), and the WHO, in Uganda and throughout sub-Saharan Africa as a short-term solution to deal with the huge backlog of patients while simultaneously building surgical capacity in countries most affected by obstetric fistula (Ramsey et al., 2007; Hancock & Collie, 2004). The two-week surgical camps are usually hosted at public hospitals and are offered several times a year at different locations throughout the country with either a foreign surgeon and/or one or more Ugandan surgeons. Promoted via radio announcements, it is common for 50 or more women to receive treatment during this two-week period, though sometimes many more women turn up, resulting in overcrowding, long surgical days that stress support staff at the hospital, and women being turned away when time or funding runs out (Ruder et al., 2018). Routine treatment at referral hospitals has been introduced in Uganda, yet is still not available in most areas of the country.

While the majority of women who have undergone a successful surgical repair will remain continent, as many as 16–55% may experience residual incontinence post-fistula closure in the form of stress incontinence, urge incontinence, and increased urinary urgency and frequency (Murray et al., 2002; Wall et al., 2004). Clinical studies have reported risk factors for developing residual incontinence, which include urethral involvement, reduction in the size of the bladder, the size and location of the fistula, and the extent and severity of vaginal scarring (Browning, 2006; Goh et al., 2008). Studies that describe women's experiences with residual incontinence reveal that they experience a lower quality of life, continued mental health concerns, stigma, and lower levels of social support than women who are successfully repaired (Browning, 2012; Donnelly et al., 2015; El Ayadi et al., 2019; Pope et al., 2011; Wilson et al., 2016).

Despite calls for more research, residual incontinence remains an underexplored and poorly tracked outcome of fistula treatment. In a recent review of current challenges in the field of obstetric fistula, Rane et al. (2020) cite residual incontinence as one of the most pressing problems—one that is not well understood and for which there are no clear treatment solutions. This is due in part to the fact that fistula outcomes and surgical success rates are based on a clinical assessment conventionally conducted at discharge, typically 14 days after the surgery. However, repair breakdowns and residual incontinence may occur up to six months or more after discharge, invalidating these results. Furthermore, for years, treatment success has been narrowly defined solely by the closure of the fistula defect. Thus, "success" rates may fail to provide an accurate account of whether the woman is actually dry following the surgery (versus closed fistula with residual incontinence), and they fail to capture long-term continence of the patient. Despite a call more than a decade ago for data on surgical outcomes based on both closure and continence, the literature on fistula surgery remains plagued by the absence of clear definitions of "success" and "failure" following surgical treatment (Harrison et al., 2015; Wall & Arrowsmith, 2007).

Quality follow-up care for patients could provide a more accurate assessment of long-term continence results, yet the majority of fistula treatment programs lack a systematic follow-up protocol (Morren et al., 2016). Additionally, few studies document follow-up care post-surgery, which many argue is too expensive and impractical to be implemented given the local context—in which women often travel long distances from remote areas to receive treatment (Murray et al., 2002; Lewis & De Bernis, 2006). While the number of studies reporting on long-term follow-up is growing, the vast majority report fistula outcomes upon hospital discharge. To our knowledge, this study is the first to report both women's and surgeons' experiences with follow-up care, and to trace follow-up guidelines in fistula policy.

When speaking of policy, we draw on Gilson (2012) who notes that health policy refers to the formal written documents, rules and guidelines created to promote and improve health. Policy making is often described as a multistep process, two essential features of which are central here: (1) evaluation to assess effectiveness and any unforeseen outcomes; and (2) revision to make necessary adjustments to better achieve desired outcomes (Buse et al., 2005). This study reveals how these essential steps are unattended to in fistula policy—to the detriment of women with residual incontinence.

## Methods

This chapter draws on qualitative results from a community-led project with a Ugandan NGO that provides fistula treatment and reintegration services, including psychosocial counseling, safe motherhood and sexual health and reproductive rights education, and income generating skills training. This study was part of the first author's larger dissertation study that utilized a mixed-method study design to investigate the experiences of women suffering from residual incontinence post-fistula closure (n = 36). We triangulated the findings with semi-structured, open-ended interviews with fistula surgeons—both Ugandan and international surgeons—who work or have worked in Uganda (n = 12).[2]

Participants were recruited using purposive sampling (Bernard, 2006). Data collection took place between October 2017 and September 2018 in eastern and central Uganda, regions chosen due to the high volume of fistula treatment and the established community presence of the Ugandan NGO we collaborated with. Semi-structured interviews lasted an average of one hour and were conducted at the NGO's office or at a local conference room reserved for privacy. The first author, a medical anthropologist and midwife, conducted the interviews with the assistance of local female translators who are also trained fistula counselors, familiar with the sensitive nature of fistula. Interviews were conducted in the participant's native language, *Ateso*, *Kumam*, or *Lugandan*, and audio recorded with their permission, translated into English, and transcribed verbatim. Interviews with fistula surgeons lasted an average of one hour and were conducted in English at a location convenient to the surgeon or via Skype if the surgeon was out of the country.

In order to situate the emergent themes of the findings, we conducted a desk review focused on the broader field of obstetric fistula policy. We searched unpublished ("grey") literature (Google, organizational websites, Ugandan Ministry of Health (MoH) website). We were also able to locate hard copies of Ugandan MoH policy documents that are not available online, looking specifically for policy guidelines for follow-up care post-fistula treatment.

Collectively, we also drew on participant observation from extensive fieldwork on fistula research projects in Uganda, participation in Ugandan MoH and Fistula Technical Working Group (FTWG) meetings, and attendance at international global health and obstetric fistula conferences in order to situate fistula policy.

Transcripts were coded and sorted into emerging themes using Nvivo 12.2. Analysis was conducted using modified grounded theory, an iterative method that requires a close interaction with the data in order to allow emic themes to emerge,

[2] In order to respect confidentially, no identifying details on the surgeons are provided.

followed by theoretical construction based on the emergent themes (Charmaz, 2006). Informed consent was obtained from all participants who enrolled in the study, with signature or thumbprint. The study protocol was approved by the Institutional Review Board at Oregon Health Sciences University, Oregon State University, Makerere University College of Health Sciences, and the Uganda National Council for Science and Technology.

## Obstetric Fistula Emerges as an International Priority

Once virtually unknown, obstetric fistula emerged as an international priority in the early 2000s, following two decades of focus on maternal mortality and safe motherhood. The United Nations Population Fund (UNFPA) was the first to champion the cause on the international stage with their "Campaign to End Fistula" in 2003. They drew in dozens of partners to the campaign, including large funders such as the Gates Foundation, corporate sponsors such as Virgin Atlantic, and celebrity spokespersons such as British-American singer-songwriter Natalie Imbruglia (UNFPA, 2008).

In the early years, the campaign worked with countries to produce baseline needs assessments, and then offered financial and technical assistance to ministries of health to create new national guidelines and strategies to tackle fistula, and to establish national technical working groups (UNFPA & EngenderHealth, 2003; UNFPA, 2008). UNFPA continues to promote and raise funds for the campaign, including serving as the secretariat of the International Fistula Working Group, which coordinates global efforts to eliminate fistula (UNFPA, 2008). The Campaign to End Fistula has led to numerous UN resolutions on supporting efforts to end obstetric fistula (2007, 2010, and 2012) and resolutions on the intensification of efforts to end obstetric fistula (2014, 2016, 2018 & 2020) including the development of a global road map within a decade (UN, 2018). Their goal is to end fistula by 2030 (Anastasi et al., 2017).

## Fistula Policy in Uganda

Obstetric fistula policy has been determined in large part over the years by international development agencies and funding organizations, such as international nongovernmental organizations (INGOs). These agencies and organizations have provided millions of dollars in resources and focused international attention on the issue of obstetric fistula. In many cases, they have provided the only funding for fistula treatment in low-resource countries. These organizations have thus played a critical role in assisting national ministries of health in formulating individual country-level policies regarding fistula treatment.

This is certainly the case in Uganda, where for years international development agencies have worked alongside the Ugandan MoH to formulate a national fistula policy. While fistula treatment started in Uganda in the 1990s with a few dedicated international surgeons providing fistula surgery and training Ugandan surgeons, it was not until the 2000s that Uganda began to formulate fistula guidelines. Uganda was included in UNFPA's initial nine country fistula assessment, conducted in 2002, the year prior to the UNFPA kick-off of their Campaign to End Fistula (UNFPA & EngenderHealth, 2003). Also in 2002, with funding and assistance from the UNFPA, the Ugandan MoH founded the Fistula Technical Working Group (FTWG). The FTWG is made up of a diverse group of stakeholders including MoH representatives, Ugandan fistula surgeons, international development partners such as UNFPA, the African Medical and Research Foundation (AMREF), EngenderHealth, and the WHO, and Ugandan civil society and NGOs (Creanga et al., 2008). The purpose of the FTWG is to coordinate fistula stakeholder activities and integrate fistula services into the maternal healthcare system. Before the group was established, there was no national oversight or coordination for fistula prevention and treatment in Uganda. The group has been instrumental in creating Uganda's fistula policies, such as the *Minimum Package for Conducting Fistula Camps* (Ministry of Health, 2014) and the *National Obstetric Fistula Strategy* (Ministry of Health, 2011).

Aside from establishing standards, guidelines, and protocols to guide the provision of fistula services and "integrating fistula services into the Ugandan health system" the group reports its achievements as "building an information base for obstetric fistula, to better plan for and manage prevention, treatment, and reintegration services," which includes increasing the number of fistula questions on the Ugandan Demographic and Health Survey (a nationally representative household survey conducted every 5 years) from one to three, and beginning the process of integrating key fistula indicators into routine administrative data so that health facilities can regularly report on fistula cases (Fistula Care, 2013, p. 2). However, the group is plagued by a lack of resources and insufficient implementation support from the MoH, and despite their achievements, fistula strategies in Uganda remain poorly implemented and disjointed with specific deficits in "data systems, capacity building, clinical standards, and support by partners" (Ministry of Health, 2011, p. 7).

## In Search of Follow-up Protocols

Surprisingly, an exhaustive search for follow-up care protocols revealed that follow-up care is rarely mentioned in international or Ugandan guidelines. In fact, according to the WHO, "once healed, [women] return to far-off villages in remote regions making follow-up impossible" (Lewis & De Bernis, 2006, p. 71). When follow-up care is included, instructions are often vague, such as in "*The prevention and management of obstetric fistula: A curriculum for nurses and midwives*," which states that follow-up appointments should occur within 3 months and that nurses and midwives are to "*ensure* that the client has the necessary means and transportation to come back for the visit" (emphasis added) (ECSA-HC, 2012, p. 220). Exactly how nurses and midwives are to "ensure" this unfunded mandate is not discussed.

In Uganda's national guidelines, follow-up care often falls under reintegration rather than clinical protocols and is relegated to NGOs and community organizations. For example, *Uganda's Minimum Package for Conducting Fistula Camps* (2014) states "NGOs can follow-up the patients at home at one, three and six months and one year after her return to her village" (p. 13). In *Uganda's National Training Guidelines* (2012b) the responsibility for follow-up care is shifted to village health teams, counselors, and community representatives. No mention of reporting or referral mechanisms for follow-up care is made. As further evidence of the absence, the MoH *Fistula Reporting Data Forms* (2012), developed with development partners EngenderHealth, UNFPA, and AMREF, fail to include follow-up care or outcomes among the reportable data fields.

Even a relatively recent report from Fistula Care and EngenderHealth (2013, p. 5), which celebrated Ugandan achievements and expected progress, and stated: "Health care providers must follow consistent approaches for prevention and treatment that are grounded in current medical knowledge and evidence," failed to include follow-up care in their guidelines and protocols, despite outlining service standards and the importance of quality of care.

The lack of specificity around follow-up care in international and national guidelines comes despite the fact that the International Federation of Gynecologists and Obstetricians (FIGO) *Global Competency-Based Fistula Surgery Training Manual* from 2011 included specific competencies on follow-up care (FIGO, 2011). Likewise, the UN began calling for "careful" follow-up by December 2012, and has continued to do so in every subsequent declaration on obstetric fistula, including the 2016 resolution which stated: "governments of countries affected by fistula should designate obstetric fistula as a nationally notifiable condition, triggering immediate reporting, tracking and follow-up" (UN, 2016, p. 11).

We have observed that the lack of attention to follow-up care in policy documents is also reflected in conference proceedings and meetings. For instance, the biannual International Conference of Obstetric Fistula Surgeons, which began in 2007, has yet to highlight the issue. One notable exception was during the 2014 conference in Kampala, Uganda when a well-respected surgeon took the floor to express his concerns about the lack of follow-up care and demanded to know "Who is paying for follow-up?" (October 2014, fieldnotes, first author). Similarly, at national meetings in Uganda, such as FTWG meetings, follow-up is seldom prioritized, even when guidelines and quality of care strategies are discussed. In the following sections, we share the results from semi-structured, open-ended interviews with women suffering from residual incontinence post-fistula closure and fistula surgeons.

## Women's Experiences with Fistula Follow-up Care

This study offers a unique understanding of barriers to follow-up care because the women in our study were still leaking after their surgery and thus, were especially motivated to attend follow-up appointments. Women often returned multiple times for follow-up care and the majority, 83%, eventually received additional surgery. This corresponds with other studies on residual incontinence. For example, Browning and Menber (2008) found that women with residual incontinence symptoms were twice as likely to return for follow-up than women free of symptoms. At first glance, the high rate of follow-up in this study appears to be a success; however, the in-depth interviews present a more troubling picture of women's experience with follow-up care, which is closely tied with their experience of receiving an unclear diagnosis.

### *Unclear Diagnosis*

The majority of the women who participated in this study were unaware that their fistula was actually closed and still spoke of themselves as having a fistula, as seen in the opening vignette. Here a 45-year-old woman who had eight prior surgeries explains, "When I was discharged on my last treatment, the doctors did not tell me that all my fistulas had been closed. Instead, I only knew it yesterday, when I was screened at the hospital."

Another woman who has had a total of five surgeries shared,

> The last surgery, the doctors did not tell me anything about why I was still leaking. In fact, I was so disappointed. Because after leaving [the regional hospital] and going to Mulago [the national referral hospital], I was thinking that I would come back when I was dry. I got so traumatised. Then after that, they even didn't tell me what I should do.

This finding corroborates our previous research findings, which show that women receive minimal information from medical personnel about their initial diagnosis of fistula (Ruder et al., 2018). The lack of clarity regarding their diagnosis was also a source of distress for the women in this study, and most reported that they were not given medical advice specific to residual incontinence. Very few women understood their fistula was closed and that the cause of the leaking was residual incontinence. Instead of clear medical advice and a diagnosis, the majority were told that maybe something could be done for them in the future; they should go home and wait for an announcement for another camp. This poor understanding of their medical condition led women to repeatedly seek out both follow-up care and additional treatment.

Surgeons who participated in this study did take the time to explain the cause of the incontinence, using hand gestures and easy-to-understand descriptions such as "the fistula is closed, but the 'brakes' which hold in your urine have been damaged and are not working correctly." Women quickly understood this diagnosis was different from a failed fistula repair. This simple explanation seemed to alleviate much of the suffering that resulted from the uncertainty they reported after repeated surgeries without improvement, as this woman shared after her screening: "I'm glad the doctor told me I don't have a hole, it's now the brakes, the muscles that are weak."

## *Barriers to Follow-up*

Both women participants and surgeons identified multiple barriers women experience in receiving follow-up care. According to women, foremost amongst these were transportation costs. As this woman describes clearly: "I did not go back for review because I did not have any money for transport to the hospital." While women are often reimbursed for transportation costs when they travel for a fistula camp, transportation costs for follow-up appointments are not typically reimbursed by donors. For woman with residual incontinence, they have already raised funds needed for the surgery.[3] Now, suffering from what they think of as a "failed surgery," they must again raise funds to return for additional medical care. Additionally, to attend both the fistula camp and follow-up appointments, women often travel long distances on crowded public buses where it is difficult to conceal their incontinence, thus returning six weeks later is a significant burden.

Tenacity and perseverance were common themes in this study however, as women overcame hardship and repeatedly sought additional care. Unfortunately, their stories also highlight the dysfunction with follow-up care in Uganda. A woman who suffered with residual incontinence for six years shared:

> So, the last time I was in hospital for surgery, the doctors advised me to do [Kegel] exercise for one month. He told me in the morning I should do it ten times, the holding of the muscles, then in the evening ten times. He told me to call them after one month, but when I called the sister [nurse], the contact number they had given me, she never picked up her phone.

Kegel exercises are a standard treatment for some forms of residual incontinence, yet in many cases of severe residual incontinence post-fistula closure, prove insufficient as treatment.

Many women were simply told to return home and wait for a call to return for additional treatment, which despite their extreme patience—sometimes after waiting years—never came. Others described poor continuity of care; these women returned to the hospital where they were treated during a fistula camp, only to find that the doctors who conducted their surgery were no longer there. Instead they found junior doctors or clinical officers who were unable to explain to the women why they were still leaking or what course of action they should take. These women were frustrated and often lost hope because of this experience.

[3] Even when surgical costs are covered by a donor, women typically need money for food and upkeep at the hospital, and for the family member who has accompanied them.

## Surgeon's Perspectives on Follow-up

According to surgeons who participated in this study, the standard of practice in Uganda is to recommend a follow-up appointment six weeks post-surgery, though as stated above, unlike fistula treatment, follow-up is not a donor-funded activity. Surgeons report that they routinely ask women treated for fistula to return for follow-up appointments; however, most do not return. They pointed to several structural barriers that impede follow-up visits, including transportation costs, long distances to the hospital, and difficulty missing work or leaving children to attend the appointment. As one surgeon explained,

> They don't have money for transport and that is the limiting factor. If there is a way they can be supported with funds to return for [follow-up], they will come back. But the limiting factor, even to come for care, the biggest limiting factor is transport.

Another surgeon said succinctly, "The biggest challenge is poverty. Poverty. They don't have the means and they don't have the support from their family. They have been sick, they have not been earning any income."

In addition to these barriers, Ugandan doctors also blamed a lack of perceived value around follow-up care in "Ugandan culture," especially for women who are dry after treatment. As one surgeon explained, "And then there's the culture of follow-up in my society. The culture is—'I feel I'm okay, why should I go [for follow-up]?' For as long as somebody feels okay, they don't see the need to come to the hospital." Despite these challenges, the surgeons in this study agreed that follow-up care is important because it has the potential to capture critical health indicators, such as residual incontinence, fertility, sexual function, mental health, and quality of life after fistula repair. According to one senior surgeon,

> We need to follow-up women after fistula repair. It could be three months or six months. The reason is, some of the ladies are discharged when they are dry and they go home. In some cases, you never hear from them again. So surely you cannot know if they are still dry after three, four, or six months. Some of them get pregnant again and we don't even know how they delivered. Did they go hospital, did the fistula recur? So, follow-up is a key component after repair.

## Tracking Residual Incontinence

A greater understanding of the scope of residual incontinence can only be achieved with accurate and thorough evaluation and documentation of surgical outcomes, including long-term outcomes. Yet, despite efforts from the MoH and partners to improve reporting, apparent in the Uganda MoH *Fistula Reporting Data Forms* (2012a), this information is not available. According to the Ugandan *National Obstetric Fistula Strategy* (Ministry of Health, 2011),

> Currently, there is no standard reliable data system for obstetric fistula whether from facilities or Population based. The lack of accurate data on the prevalence, incidence and

> outcomes of repair regarding obstetric fistula is a challenge to informed decisions on support interventions for policy, planning and programming (p. 18).

Ugandan surgeons, when questioned about the prevalence of residual incontinence, agreed that nuanced tracking of patient outcomes is not standard practice in Uganda despite its obvious benefits. As one surgeon stated, "Well, I couldn't give you figures on that, because we haven't consistently followed that up. We don't have that data, and we wouldn't be routinely documenting that. That information is missing."

Clinical data is collected during fistula treatment camps and at hospitals, then reported to funding agencies, yet these metrics often focus on the numbers of women who received surgery, failing to capture the full range of surgical outcomes. According to one surgeon,

> Donors ask, 'How many fistulas did you do last year? How many women did you reach out to? How many operations did you do?' That's what they're interested in. 'Oh, you did 300 last year, okay. We can fund that.'

Another surgeon was even more critical of fistula metrics,

> The metrics are fudgeable, they're easily manipulated. I think most of the time the metrics are reported as the number of surgical operations carried out at a particular camp, or over the course of year. People want to see large numbers, with high success rates. So, the success rates are also fudgeable, if you will. Traditionally people simply talked about fistula closure rates that were successful. So, if the fistula was closed, that was a success, even if the urethra was broken and the patient was as wet after surgery as she was before. So, there's not a lot of transparency. There's not a lot of rigor in any of this data. It's really quite soft.

The role of follow-up care in helping to identify and track long-term continence also emerged in interviews with women who left the hospital dry, yet later started leaking, as this woman's story illustrates:

> I was expecting to get healed from fistula. And true, the day I was discharged, I was really completely dry. I went home dry. But when I reached home, it was after six months that I started seeing leakage of urine. Every day it became worse, until now it is just like before treatment.

Another woman who had two previous surgeries shared a similar experience:

> At my follow-up appointment, they confirmed I still had a fistula. So, I was admitted and they operated on me again. After two weeks I was discharged and I was dry. I went home dry and for the first two days I remained dry. On the third day, I started leaking again.

Despite their current incontinent status, the fact that these women left the hospital dry undoubtedly means that their cases were counted as a "success." Without follow-up care and corresponding tracking mechanisms, their poor outcomes were never reported.

Several doctors offered suggestions to rectify the inconsistencies with, or neglect of, follow-up care, such as additional funds specifically earmarked for follow-up or community-based follow-up care. However, other surgeons were more critical in their assessment, claiming that the lack of follow-up care actually serves donors by maintaining higher success rates for fistula surgery than would be reported with improved adherence to follow-up care. According to one surgeon, the paucity of resources and emphasis devoted to follow-up care is directly linked to the fact that "follow-up doesn't appeal to donors." He argued that a careful counting of women with residual incontinence would force donors to acknowledge "partially failed surgeries."

## Failure of Policy or Priority? Making Sense of the Neglect of Follow-up

Women's stories of residual incontinence are stories no one wants to hear as they complicate and make messy the dominant narrative humanitarian organizations and international donor agencies have popularized. Their stories expose the barriers and challenges women face in seeking quality diagnoses and care when they suffer from complications following obstetric fistula surgery. Likewise, surgeons shared their stories and insights into the challenges with tracking residual incontinence and the dynamics that allow poor follow-up to occur. We did not include donor agencies as participants in this study, and as such, we know little about their perspectives on follow-up care nor their funding motivations. Nonetheless, it is clear that a strong commitment to follow-up care is lacking.

What is assumed to matter to international funders are the number of women "successfully" treated. These numbers bolster donors' goals and serve as a cause for celebration on multiple websites where organizations proudly tally the number of women saved from a life of misery (see Heller, 2018). These achievements are then used to raise funds for more surgeries. Fistula funding depends on this narrative of fistula as highly curable (Del Vecchio Good et al., 1990), thus the message of hope is central to building and maintaining funding streams to finance fistula programming. These are complex ethics—international funding for obstetric fistula programs is critical as programs are not financed by national governments nor are they sustainable without continued input from foreign donors. As such, it is easy to empathize with the need to create a compelling story.

Yet, an unintended consequence of this compelling narrative of success is its power to obscure and silence the experience of women who are not cured; women with residual incontinence are systematically omitted from this narrative. Fistula policies do little to counter this narrative. Findings reveal follow-up policies that are vague, absent, and/or unfunded, and thus, not adhered to. Evaluation and revision, essential steps in policy making, and translation of policy into action, all appear to be missing (Buse et al., 2005; Janes & Corbett, 2009). Results of our study also illuminate the toll failures in clinical assessment of fistula outcomes, data collection, and follow-up care exact on women who are on the receiving end of policies that "exact a type of violence of erasure" (Adams, 2016, p. 226). This violence shapes not only their treatment experience, but also determines what problems go unheard, and which potential solutions are left unexplored. This is evident in the dearth of attention, resources, research, and alternative treatment options dedicated to residual incontinence. Women in this study were offered either additional surgery, which has a diminishing likelihood of success with each attempt due to the build-up of scar tissue, or taught to do Kegel exercises, which, given the extreme incontinence many of the women experienced, seemed wildly insufficient. Doctors were also frustrated and discontented with the options available to treat these women.

Ultimately, the solution involves challenging overly simplistic fistula narratives and the reductive representations of obstetric fistula outcomes they promote. Well-funded fistula policies that seek to provide an accurate and comprehensive account of treatment that also include poor outcomes are needed. Rajkotia (2018) provides insight here, arguing that within the global health community there is intense pressure to report favorable data—so favorable in fact, it may be too good to be true. Surgeons in this study corroborated Rajkotia's argument as they shared their experiences dealing with donors who are predominantly concerned with the number of women treated rather than long-term follow-up or wellbeing. Follow-up care remains an unfunded policy precisely because it has the potential to complicate the narrative of success. Rajkotia also warns that succumbing to the "success cartel" can stifle innovation and progress in global health (2018, p. 1).

Innovation is precisely what is needed to address the pain and suffering associated with residual incontinence. Specifically, there is a need for innovative and context-specific treatment methods that attend to the unique characteristics of residual incontinence post-fistula closure. Both conservative and surgical options need to be explored. Long-term follow-up and accurate assessment of outcomes are critical to these efforts. It is encouraging that several studies have addressed the problem of lack of follow-up, employing not-so-novel strategies such as transportation reimbursement, follow-up via mobile phone, and provision of incentives (Browning & Menber, 2008; Delamou et al., 2015; Donnelly et al., 2015; Drew et al., 2016; El Ayadi et al., 2019; Maulet et al., 2013; Nielsen et al., 2009; Ouedraogo et al., 2018). For example, Barone and colleagues achieved a follow-up adherence of 96% at 3 months by offering transportation reimbursement and small appreciation gifts. These studies show that follow-up is both feasible and critical to furthering our understanding of long-term continence, comorbidities, mental health, and social reintegration after fistula treatment. By amplifying women's voices and relaying their experiences to a wider community, our findings provide evidence upon which to build innovative protocols that will improve care for women suffering from fistula and encourage policies at the donor and national level that take into account a long-term, holistic view of health and continence (Barone et al., 2012; Delamou et al., 2016; UN, 2020).

## References


Adams, V. (2016). *Metrics: What counts in global health*. Duke University Press. https://doi.org/10.1215/9780822374480

Ahmed, S., & Holtz, S. A. (2007). Social and economic consequences of obstetric fistula: Life changed forever?. *International Journal of Gynecology & Obstetrics, 99*, S10–S15. https://doi.org/10.1016/j.ijgo.2007.06.011

Anastasi, E., Romanzi, L., Ahmed, S., Knuttson, A. T., Ojengbede, O., & Grant, K. (2017). Ending fistula within a generation: Making the dream a reality. *The Lancet Global Health, 5*(8), e747–e748. http://dx.doi.org/10.1016/S2214-109X(17)30226-7

Arrowsmith, S., Hamlin, E. C., & Wall, L. L. (1996). Obstructed labor injury complex: Obstetric fistula formation and the multifaceted morbidity of maternal birth trauma in the developing world. *Obstetric and gynecological survey, 51*(9), 568–574.

Barageine, J. K., Beyeza-Kashesya, J., Byamugisha, J. K., Tumwesigye, N. M., Almroth, L., & Faxelid, E. (2015). "I am alone and isolated": A qualitative study of experiences of women living with genital fistula in Uganda. *BMC Women's Health, 15*(1), 73. https://doi.org/10.1186/s12905-015-0232-z

Barone, M. A., et al. (2012). Determinants of postoperative outcomes of female genital fistula repair surgery. *Obstetrics and Gynecology, 120*(3), 524. https://doi.org/10.1097/aog.0b013e31826579e8

Bernard, R. H. (2006). *Research methods in anthropology*. Altamira Press.

Browning, A. (2006). Risk factors for developing residual urinary incontinence after obstetric fistula repair. *BJOG: An International Journal of Obstetrics & Gynaecology, 113*(4), 482–485. https://doi.org/10.1111/j.1471-0528.2006.00875.x

Browning, A. (2012). *The problem of continuing urinary incontinence after obstetric vesicovaginal surgery. Obstetric fistula in developing countries*. RCOG International News.

Browning, A., & Menber, B. (2008). Women with obstetric fistula in Ethiopia: A 6-month follow up after surgical treatment. *BJOG: An International Journal of Obstetrics & Gynaecology, 115*(12), 1564–1569. https://doi.org/10.1111/j.1471-0528.2008.01900.x

Browning, A., Fentahun, W., & Goh, J. T. (2007). The impact of surgical treatment on the mental health of women with obstetric fistula. *BJOG: An International Journal of Obstetrics & Gynaecology, 114*(11), 1439–1441. https://doi.org/10.1111/j.1471-0528.2007.01419.x

Buse, K., Mays, N., & Walt, G. (2005). *Making health policy (understanding public health)*. Bell & Brain Ltd.

Charmaz, K. (2006). *Constructing grounded theory: A practical guide through qualitative analysis*. Sage Publications Limited.

Creanga, A. A., Iliyasu, Z., & Arinaitwe, L. K. (2008). *An evaluation of the United Nations Population Fund/Uganda's Obstetric fistula program*. UNFPA Publication. http://web2.unfpa.org. Accessed 22 July 2018.

Del Vecchio Good, M.-J., Good, B. J., Schaffer, C., & Lind, S. E. (1990). American oncology and the discourse on hope. *Culture, Medicine and Psychiatry, 14*(1), 59–79. https://doi.org/10.1007/BF00046704

Delamou, A., Delvaux, T., Utz, B., Camara, B. S., Beavogui, A. H., Cole, B., et al. (2015). Factors associated with loss to follow-up in women undergoing repair for obstetric fistula in Guinea. *Tropical Medicine & International Health, 20*(11), 1454–1461. https://doi.org/10.1111/tmi.12584

Delamou, A., Delvaux, T., Beavogui, A. H., et al. (2016). Factors associated with the failure of obstetric fistula repair in Guinea: Implications for practice. *Reproductive Health, 13*, 135. https://doi.org/10.1186/s12978-016-0248-3

Donnelly, K., Oliveras, E., Tilahun, Y., Belachew, M., & Asnake, M. (2015). Quality of life of Ethiopian women after fistula repair: Implications on rehabilitation and social reintegration policy and programming. *Culture Health & Sexuality, 17*(2), 150–164. https://doi.org/10.1080/13691058.2014.964320

Drew, L. B., Wilkinson, J. P., Nundwe, W., Moyo, M., Mataya, R., Mwale, M., et al. (2016). Long-term outcomes for women after obstetric fistula repair in Lilongwe, Malawi: A qualitative study. *BMC Pregnancy Childbirth, 16*, 2–2. https://doi.org/10.1186/s12884-015-0755-1

ECSA-HC, F. C. E. (2012). *The prevention and management of obstetric fistula: A curriculum for nurses and midwives*. C. East, and Southern African Health Community/EngenderHealth/Fistula Care. www.engenderhealth.org/files/pubs/fistula-care-digitalarchive/3/3.1/Prevention-Management-Nursing-Curriculum-English. Accessed 23 March 2018.

El Ayadi, A. M., Barageine, J., Korn, A., Kakaire, O., Turan, J., Obore, S., et al. (2019). Trajectories of women's physical and psychosocial health following obstetric fistula repair in Uganda: A longitudinal study. *Tropical Medicine & International Health, 24*(1), 53–64. https://doi.org/10.1111/tmi.13178

FIGO. (2011). *Global competency-based fistula surgery training manual*. International Federation of Gynecology and Obstetrics. www.figo.org. Accessed 1 March 2018.

Filippi, V., Ganaba, R., Baggaley, R. F., Marshall, T., Storeng, K. T., Sombié, I., et al. (2007). Health of women after severe obstetric complications in Burkina Faso: A longitudinal study. *The Lancet, 370*(9595), 1329–1337. https://doi.org/10.1016/s0140-6736(07)61574-8

Fistula Care. (2013). *Creating an enabling environment for Fistula prevention and treatment in Uganda*. EngenderHealth_USAID. www.fistulacare.org. Accessed 1 Sept 2018.

Gilson, L., & World Health Organization. (2012). *Health policy and systems research: A methodology reader*. World Health Organization. https://www.who.int/alliance-hpsr/resources/reader/en/ Accessed 3 Oct 2018.

Goh, J. T., Browning, A., Berhan, B., & Chang, A. (2008). Predicting the risk of failure of closure of obstetric fistula and residual urinary incontinence using a classification system. *International Urogynecology Journal, 19*(12), 1659–1662. https://doi.org/10.1007/s00192-008-0693-9

Hancock, B., & Collie, M. (2004). Vesico-vaginal Fistula surgery in Uganda. *East and Central African Journal of Surgery, 9*(2), 32–37.

Harrison, M. S., Mabeya, H., Goldenberg, R. L., & McClure, E. M. (2015). Urogenital fistula reviewed: A marker of severe maternal morbidity and an indicator of the quality of maternal healthcare delivery. *Maternal Health, Neonatology and Perinatology, 1*(1), 20. https://doi.org/10.1186/s40748-015-0020-7

Heller, A. (2018). *Fistula politics: Birthing injuries and the quest for continence in Niger*. Rutgers University Press. https://doi.org/10.2307/j.ctt2111gvj

Janes, C. R., & Corbett, K. K. (2009). Anthropology and global health. *Annual Review of Anthropology, 38*, 167–183. https://doi.org/10.1002/9781444395303.ch7

Khisa, W., Wakasiaka, S., McGowan, L., Campbell, M., & Lavender, T. (2017). Understanding the lived experience of women before and after fistula repair: A qualitative study in Kenya. *BJOG: An International Journal of Obstetrics & Gynaecology, 124*(3), 503–510. https://doi.org/10.1111/1471-0528.13902

Koblinsky, M., Chowdhury, M. E., Moran, A., & Ronsmans, C. (2012). Maternal morbidity and disability and their consequences: Neglected agenda in maternal health. *Journal of Health, Population, and Nutrition, 30*(2), 124. https://doi.org/10.3329/jhpn.v30i2.11294

Kruk, M. E., Leslie, H. H., Verguet, S., Mbaruku, G. M., Adanu, R. M., & Langer, A. (2016). Quality of basic maternal care functions in health facilities of five African countries: An analysis of national health system surveys. *The Lancet Global Health, 4*(11), e845–e855. http://dx.doi.org/10.1016/S2214-109X(16)30180-2

Lewis, G., & De Bernis, L. (2006). *Obstetric fistula: Guiding principles for clinical management and programme development*. Geneva: World Health Organization. https://www.who.int/reproductivehealth/publications/maternal_perinatal_health/9241593679/en. Accessed 3 September 2018.

Maulet, N., Keita, M., & Macq, J. (2013). Medico-social pathways of obstetric fistula patients in Mali and Niger: An 18-month cohort follow-up. *Tropical Medicine & International Health, 18*(5), 524–533. https://doi.org/10.1111/tmi.12086

Ministry of Health. (2011). *National Obstetric Fistula Strategy 2011/2012–2015/2016*. Government of Uganda. https://fistulacare.org/archive/files/5/5.4/Uganda_National_Obstetric_Fistula_Strategy.pdf. Accessed 3 Oct 2018..

Ministry of Health. (2012a). *Fistula reporting data forms*. Government of Uganda, Department of Clinical Services.

Ministry of Health. (2012b). *National training guidelines and standards for treatment of female Genital Fistula*. Government of Uganda. https://fistulacare.org/archive/files/8/8.1/8.1.9/Fistula-training-guidelines.pdf. Accessed 3 Oct 2018.

Ministry of Health. (2014). *Minimum Package for conducting Fistula Camps*. Government of Uganda.

Morren, G., van den Boogaard, W., & Dominguez, E. (2016). *Management of Obstertic Fistula in Burundi: The experience from a multidisciplinary approach over five years*. M.-O. M. Department MSF Project in Gitega Province. Medecins Sans Frontieres. http://www.endfistula.org/sites/default/files/pub-pdf/MSF_Fistula%20in%20Burundi_EN-WEB.pdf. Accessed 1 Oct 2018.

Mselle, L. T., Moland, K. M., Evjen-Olsen, B., Mvungi, A., & Kohi, T. W. (2011). "I am nothing": Experiences of loss among women suffering from severe birth injuries in Tanzania. *BMC Womens Health, 11*(1), 49. https://doi.org/10.1186/1472-6874-11-49

Murray, C., Goh, J. T., Fynes, M., & Carey, M. P. (2002). Urinary and faecal incontinence following delayed primary repair of obstetric genital fistula. *BJOG: An International Journal of Obstetrics & Gynaecology, 109*(7), 828–832. https://doi.org/10.1111/j.1471-0528.2002.00124.x

Mwini-Nyaledzigbor, P. P., Agana, A. A., & Pilkington, F. B. (2013). Lived experiences of Ghanaian women with obstetric fistula. *Health Care Women International, 34*(6), 440–460. https://doi.org/10.1080/07399332.2012.755981

Nielsen, H. S., Lindberg, L., Nygaard, U., Aytenfisu, H., Johnston, O. L., Sorensen, B., et al. (2009). A community-based long-term follow up of women undergoing obstetric fistula repair in rural Ethiopia. *BJOG: An International Journal of Obstetrics & Gynaecology, 116*(9), 1258–1264. https://doi.org/10.1111/j.1471-0528.2009.02200.x

Ouedraogo, I., Payne, C., Nardos, R., Adelman, A. J., & Wall, L. L. (2018). Obstetric fistula in Niger: 6-month postoperative follow-up of 384 patients from the Danja Fistula Center. *International Urogynecology Journal, 29*(3), 345–351. https://doi.org/10.1007/s00192-017-3375-7

Paxton, A., & Wardlaw, T. (2011). Are we making progress in maternal mortality? *New England Journal of Medicine, 364*, 1990–1993. https://doi.org/10.1056/NEJMp1012860. PMID:21612467.

Pope, R., Bangser, M., & Requejo, J. H. (2011). Restoring dignity: Social reintegration after obstetric fistula repair in Ukerewe, Tanzania. *Global Public Health, 6*(8), 859–873. https://doi.org/10.1080/17441692.2010.551519

Rajkotia, Y. (2018). Beware of the success cartel: A plea for rational progress in global health. *BMJ Global Health, 3*(6), e001197. https://doi.org/10.1136/bmjgh-2018-001197

Ramsey, K., Iliyasu, Z., & Idoko, L. (2007). Fistula Fortnight: Innovative partnership brings mass treatment and public awareness towards ending obstetric fistula. *International Journal of Gynecology and Obstetrics, 99*, 130–136. https://doi.org/10.1016/j.ijgo.2007.06.034

Rane, A., Browning, A., Majinge, P., & Pope, R. (2020). Challenges in the field of obstetric fistula. *International Journal of Gynecology & Obstetrics, 148*, 6–8. https://doi.org/10.1002/ijgo.13032

Ruder, B., Cheyney, M., & Emasu, A. A. (2018). Too long to wait: Obstetric Fistula and the sociopolitical dynamics of the fourth delay in Soroti, Uganda. *Qualitative Health Research, 28*(5), 721–732. https://doi.org/10.1177/10497323177540

Storeng, K. T., Murray, S. F., Akoum, M. S., Ouattara, F., & Filippi, V. (2010). Beyond body counts: A qualitative study of lives and loss in Burkina Faso after 'near-miss' obstetric complications. *Social Science & Medicine, 71*(10), 1749–1756. https://doi.org/10.1016/j.socscimed.2010.03.056

Storeng, K., Drabo, S., Ganaba, R., Sundby, J., Calvert, C., & Filippi, V. (2012). Mortality after near-miss obstetric complications in Burkina Faso: Medical, social and health-care factors. *Bulletin of the World Health Organization*, 418–425. https://doi.org/10.2471/BLT.11.094011

UBOS. (2018). *Uganda Demographic and Health Survey 2016*. Uganda Bureau of Statistics and ICF. https://dhsprogram.com/publications/publication-fr333-dhs-final-reports.cfm. Accessed 10 Oct 2018.

UN. (2016). *Intensifying efforts to end obstetric fistula*. United Nations. https://www.unfpa.org/resources/intensifying-efforts-endobstetric-fistula. Accessed 10 Oct 2018.

UN. (2018). *Intensification of efforts to end obstetric fistula*. United Nations. https://digitallibrary.un.org/record/1660278?ln=en. Accessed 4 Jan 2019.

UN. (2020). *Intensification of efforts to end obstetric fistula*. United Nations. https://digitallibrary.un.org/record/3896019?ln=en. Accessed 11 Nov 2020.

UNFPA. (2008). *Campaign to end fistula: The year in review*. UNFPA. https://www.unfpa.org/publications/campaign-end-fistulayear-review. Accessed 7 March 2016.

UNFPA & EngenderHealth. (2003). *Obstetric fistula needs assessment report: Findings from nine African countries*. UNFPA.

Wall, L. L., & Arrowsmith, S. D. (2007). The "continence gap": A critical concept in obstetric fistula repair. *International Urogynecology Journal, 18*(8), 843–844. https://doi.org/10.1007/s00192-007-0367-z

Wall, L. L., Karshima, J. A., Kirschner, C., & Arrowsmith, S. D. (2004). The obstetric vesicovaginal fistula: Characteristics of 899 patients from Jos, Nigeria. *American Journal of Obstetrics and Gynecology, 190*(4), 1011–1016. https://doi.org/10.1016/j.ajog.2004.02.007

Weston, K., Mutiso, S., Mwangi, J. W., Qureshi, Z., Beard, J., & Venkat, P. (2011). Depression among women with obstetric fistula in Kenya. *International Journal Gynaecology Obstetrics, 115*(1), 31–33. https://doi.org/10.1016/j.ijgo.2011.04.015

WHO. (2015). *Trends in maternal mortality: 1990–2015: Estimates from WHO, UNICEF, UNFPA, World Bank Group and the United Nations Population Division: Executive summary*. https://www.unfpa.org/publications/trends-maternal-mortality-1990-2015. Accessed 3 Sept 2018.

WHO. (2018). *Obstetric Fistula*. https://www.who.int/news-room/facts-in-pictures/detail/10-facts-on-obstetric-fistula. Accessed 3 Sept 2018.

Wilson, S. M., Sikkema, K. J., Watt, M. H., Masenga, G. G., & Mosha, M. V. (2016). Psychological symptoms and social functioning following repair of obstetric fistula in a low-income setting. *Maternal and Child Health Journal, 20*(5), 941–945. https://doi.org/10.1007/s10995-016-1950-z

# Chapter 4
# The Domestication of Misoprostol for Abortion in Burkina Faso: Interactions Between Caregivers, Drug Vendors and Women

**Seydou Drabo**

## Introduction

Misoprostol has been hailed as a revolution for maternal health globally because of its potential to reduce mortality and morbidity from post-partum haemorrhage and unsafe abortion (Potts, 2006), providing relatively safe and discreet termination of pregnancy (Winikoff & Sheldon, 2012). Since 2005, the World Health Organization (WHO) has recognized misoprostol as a lifesaving drug and recommended that it be included on the list of essential medicines, although only 'where permitted under national law and culturally acceptable' (World Health Organization, 2006). Advocates of safe abortion services, however, fought for its inclusion in the treatment of post-partum haemorrhage in countries with restrictive abortion laws, with the expectation that once it is in the health system, women will be able to access it and thereby avoid harmful abortion procedures (Fernandez et al., 2009; Hofmeyr, 2012).

A recent report examining the safety of abortion globally suggests that clandestine abortion in legally restrictive settings is becoming relatively safer as misoprostol replaces harmful methods (Singh et al., 2018). However, we know little about how women actually use misoprostol to induce abortion. This chapter addresses this knowledge gap by examining how misoprostol is acquired and used by women, drug vendors and healthcare workers to manage unwanted pregnancy in Ouagadougou, the capital of Burkina Faso in West Africa. Previous studies have shown that privileged individuals are able to circumvent Burkina Faso's restrictive abortion law by resorting to private clinics that offer clandestine abortions (Storeng & Ouattara, 2014). Misoprostol is marketed in pharmacies and drug stores, enabling women to avoid clinics altogether and access the drug in secrecy (Moland et al.,

S. Drabo (✉)
Faculty of Medicine, Institute of Health and Society, University of Oslo, Oslo, Norway
e-mail: seydou.drabo@medisin.uio.no



L. J. Wallace et al. (eds.), *Anthropologies of Global Maternal and Reproductive Health*, Global Maternal and Child Health, https://doi.org/10.1007/978-3-030-84514-8_4

2018). This chapter shows how the uses of misoprostol to induce abortion depend less on the formal policies designed to regulate its use than on women's 'informal' use of the drug.

I analyse how misoprostol circulates outside Ouagadougou's formal healthcare system as a form of 'pharmaceutical diversion'. Ann Lovell defines pharmaceutical diversion as a process that connects formal healthcare providers and pharmacists with networks of individuals who 'diffuse the product and knowledge about it' beyond the clinic (Lovell, 2006, p.156). Thus, the chapter focuses on the micro-level of the everyday practices of individuals who seek to acquire, circulate and use diverted pharmaceuticals outside their formal regulated circuits, uses and applications. Similarly, women's uses of misoprostol can be conceptualized as what Childerhose and MacDonald (2013) call 'domestication' – how consumers create new uses for biomedical goods, including drugs and devices that were never intended by manufacturers or regulators and are not overseen by professionals. The notion of domestication has particular relevance for how consumers bring biomedical goods into their homes for reasons of privacy and personal agency, in the sense of the ability to influence one's life by acting independently (Mortimer & Shanahan, 2003). This research also reveals the critical role of intermediaries in the process of pharmaceutical diversion and domestication, which often creates inequalities in access to misoprostol, complicating the narrative of misoprostol as a therapeutic revolution in the prevention of unsafe abortion. This study reminds us that access to misoprostol varies across settings, and while relatively safer than clandestine forms of unsafe abortion, may also be marked by pre-existing social and economic constraints, vulnerabilities and inequities. Therefore, misoprostol is a drug that illustrates and confirms that drugs have a social life. The notion that medicines have a social life is well established in medical anthropology, referring to the fact that medicines are more than their chemical properties and effects in the body; the way they are produced, tested, circulated, used and made meaningful is always shaped by their social and cultural contexts (Van der Geest & Whyte, 1989; Whyte et al., 2002).

## The Social, Legal and Policy Context of Misoprostol in Ouagadougou, Burkina Faso

In 2008, it was estimated that one-third of all pregnancies among women aged 15–49 years in Burkina Faso were unintended. One-third of these unintended pregnancies ended in abortions (Bankole et al., 2014). The incidence of abortion for women of reproductive age in Burkina Faso was estimated at 25/1000 in 2012 (Bankole et al., 2014). That rate is comparable to the level observed in 2008 for the West Africa sub-region (28 per 1000 women aged 15–44 years) (ibid).

In Burkina Faso, induced abortion is socially stigmatized (Drabo, 2013) and legally restricted to cases of rape, incest, foetal malformation or endangerment to the woman's life. According to Burkina Faso's penal code, inducing abortion is punishable by up to 5 years of imprisonment and a fine and, in the case of a woman's death, up to 12 years for a person helping a woman to abort (La voix du Juriste, 2013). Due to the legal restrictions, most women seeking abortion resort to unsafe means to terminate their pregnancy, at significant risk to their health. It is estimated that half of women who induce their abortions alone experience complications, compared with about 2 in 10 women who go to healthcare providers performing illegal abortion (Bankole et al., 2014). The safety of abortion in this context depends on women's social and economic status and the differences between rural and urban areas in terms of cost, accessibility and safety (Bankole et al., 2014). Overall, safe abortion[1] methods are relatively inaccessible throughout Burkina Faso, especially for rural women (ibid). Ninety-seven percent of abortions performed in rural areas are unsafe and poor women in rural areas typically experience the most significant health risks. Seven in 10 women living in rural areas end their pregnancies themselves or use traditional practitioners who are perceived to be discreet.

The government response to unsafe abortion has been limited to implementing a Post-Abortion Care (PAC) policy to treat complications (Ouattara & Storeng, 2014; Storeng & Ouattara, 2014). A range of technological options, including emergency contraception, vacuum aspiration and medical abortion, are used to treat incomplete abortion and prevent unwanted pregnancy in Burkina Faso. Manual vacuum aspiration (MVA) and misoprostol were introduced in the care policy in 1998 and 2014, respectively. In urban areas, private or clinic-based doctors or other healthcare providers, such as midwives and auxiliary midwives, often carry out abortions illegally. Though more costly than those offered by traditional providers, these procedures, including MVA or misoprostol, are considered relatively safe compared to other methods such as the insertion of sticks or sharp objects into the vagina, the consumption or vaginal application of kola, abortifacients like herbal tea, potions and high doses of drugs like anti-malarials, or bleach (Bankole et al., 2014).

## Field Site and Methods

My fieldwork focused on Ouagadougou, a city of 2.7 million (CWF, 2018), which is also Burkina Faso's capital and its administrative and economic centre. In Ouagadougou, women can access abortion care in the public sector only in the circumstances stipulated by law (incest, rape, foetal malformation, health of the mother). However, PAC services are offered in secondary and tertiary healthcare facilities, some primary healthcare facilities in the public sector and in private-care

[1] WHO classifies abortion as safe if it takes place using a safe method and is done by an appropriately trained provider. Less-safe abortions include those done by a trained provider but using an outdated method, and self-induced abortions using a relatively safe method (e.g., misoprostol); least-safe abortions are those done by an untrained person (a provider or the woman herself) using a dangerous method. Both 'less' and 'least' safe abortions are considered unsafe.

facilities (Bodart et al., 2001). Misoprostol can be purchased to treat incomplete abortion and manage post-partum haemorrhage in the city's hundreds of pharmacies (Ministry of Health of Burkina Faso, 2014). Misoprostol also circulates outside the official framework in Ouagadougou, and it is often referred to locally as the 'abortion drug'.

Building on previous experience studying maternal mortality and PAC in Burkina Faso's health sector (Drabo, 2013; Storeng et al., 2013), two periods of ethnographic fieldwork were undertaken between 2015 and 2017 in the city of Ouagadougou. The fieldwork was conducted in the framework of my PhD research focused on the use of contraceptives and abortion drugs. During the first period (October to December 2015), I focused on healthcare professionals' use of misoprostol in nine health facilities, including two University Hospital Centres, four primary healthcare centres, one private medical centre and two private primary care centres. I conducted interviews or had informal discussions with 22 healthcare workers, including gynaecologists, midwives and auxiliary midwives working in maternity care units.

In the second period of fieldwork (March 2016 and February 2017), I focused on women's perspectives and experiences in seeking out an abortion, including medical abortion using misoprostol. I conducted participant observation in streets and market places, interacting regularly with various women and drug vendors. I observed pubs and the streets of Kwame Nkrumah, a main thoroughfare with many hotels, restaurants, pubs frequented by men and women who work as waitresses or sex workers, often referred to collectively as '*les filles de nuits*' (girls of the night). These observations allowed me to start conversations around the issue of abortion and to negotiate in-depth interviews with some of the women, who, because of their work, are at risk of unintended pregnancy, abortion and their consequences (Drabo, 2019; Weldegebreal et al., 2015).

To understand the context of drug sales and the interactions between drug sellers and consumers, I conducted observations and informal discussions with street drug vendors by spending time with them in their market place. During events like movie festivals (FESPACO), the public authorities officially establish a merchant street where traders come to expose their products. Drug vendors participate in these activities by showing and selling their products for 1 week. I stayed in the store of one of the drug vendors who was selling non-western contraceptive methods and other drugs purchased by women. The long hours spent waiting there (3–6 h) gave me the opportunity to have discussions with both the drug vendor and some of his clients (see also Drabo, 2019).

In addition to participant observation, I conducted in-depth interviews with 46 women (in the context of my broader PhD research project) about their reproductive trajectories, perceptions and practices of contraceptive methods and abortion drugs and the decision-making processes and networks involved in the procurement of misoprostol. Healthcare workers assisted me in identifying women who had sought family planning and PAC and were willing to participate. I used my social networks to identify other participants from the general population. This strategy consisted of asking women who were closer to me (neighbours, former classmates and friends) and who agreed to participate in the study. Subsequently, I relied on these women to access other women (friends of friends) who were also willing to participate in the study. Of the 46 women I interviewed, 16 reported that they had undergone induced abortions in the past. These 16 interviews form the basis of the analysis in this paper. Among this group, nine were single women, four were cohabiting with a man, two were married and one was widowed. Seven of these women were working as servers in a pub, three were students, three were petty traders, one was a maid, one a housewife and one a public servant. Five of the women in this group had had more than one abortion. Together, these sixteen women had 23 abortions between 2010 and 2017. Ten of them reported using misoprostol to terminate one or more pregnancy. The other methods women used to terminate their pregnancy included MVA, potassium permanganate, Chinese pills and a recipe made with a plant (see also Drabo, 2019).

### *Data Analysis and Ethical Issues*

I conducted interviews in French, Mooré or Dioula depending on participants' preferences (I speak these three languages fluently). Most interviews were tape-recorded (with the exception of three people who were more comfortable with note-taking) and transcribed verbatim. Interviews lasted between 20 min and 1 h and 30 min. A research assistant transcribed the interviews and those recorded in Mooré or Dioula were translated into French. I did the final editing, checking all the transcripts to ensure accurate transcription and translation. I identified recurrent themes from interview transcripts and observational notes and analysed the texts based on the research question, which was focused on the use of misoprostol.

Quotes used in this chapter to illustrate the findings have been translated from French to English. I obtained ethical approval for the study from the Ethical Committee of Burkina Faso and the Norwegian Centre for Research Data. Informed consent forms were read aloud to the research participants, who provided verbal consent; verbal consent was also the most suitable because of the topic's sensitivity for healthcare providers, drug vendors and women. In addition to receiving informed consent, I assured my participants of my good intentions. For example, I made women understand 'my goal is not to judge but to understand'. This attitude allowed me to establish a climate of trust with participants to make them feel comfortable talking about their reproductive life experiences. I told all participants they could withdraw from the study at any time or choose not to participate in the study. The names of participants cited in the quotes are pseudonyms (see also Drabo, 2019).

## How Health Providers and Drug Vendors Circumvent the Regulation of Misoprostol

There are mechanisms in place in health facilities to prevent misoprostol from being used outside the legal framework for its uses. Interviews with healthcare providers indicate only gynaecologists are authorized to prescribe misoprostol. In the medical centre and hospital, midwives are supposed to use it only under the supervision of a gynaecologist in the treatment of incomplete abortion and in the management of post-partum haemorrhage. In primary healthcare centres, only specially trained midwives are allowed to prescribe misoprostol without the advice of a doctor, and only for PAC. In practice, however, auxiliary midwives often prescribe and use it under the guidance of a midwife. Thus, gynaecologists, midwives and auxiliary midwives are involved in the management of misoprostol depending on the circumstances of care delivery. Furthermore, pharmacists and drug vendors explained that they are required by the Ministry of Health to write down the name of the health facility purchasing the drug, the date and the quantity of the product being purchased, as well as the name and the telephone number of the prescriber and the buyer. These restrictions are intended to avoid misoprostol being re-directed for induced abortion.

In addition to official regulations, health workers involved in the management of the drug in PAC take extra precautions to prevent patients from accessing misoprostol and using it to induce abortion. For example, some healthcare providers confiscate the remaining misoprostol tablets after PAC. A midwife in a district hospital explained: 'We tell them, for example, after prescribing that we cannot leave them with the rest of the product because they can be used to cause an abortion'. Despite regulations that aim to restrict the use of misoprostol to induce abortion, social and institutional factors enable its availability in the health system and individuals' access to it. First, misoprostol has been on the list of essential medicines for clinical use since 2014. Second, there are international and national NGOs working within the field of reproductive health who make misoprostol available in their private clinics and in some public health facilities claiming that they need it for PAC. Task shifting in care delivery allows midwives or auxiliary midwives to perform some of the therapeutic acts that are, on paper, restricted to gynaecologists. As a consequence, most of the healthcare providers working in maternity care units are able to acquire misoprostol and may use it to induce abortions. As a midwife working at the hospital explained: 'We used it for PAC, but there are people who use it to do abortions too. It happens, we have colleagues who do it and I will not give a name'.

In pubs, I observed that some sex workers and servers act as intermediaries between health workers providing abortion services clandestinely and women seeking abortion. Such links are sometimes established during sex workers' health visits and are mutually beneficial in providing sex workers with access to abortions and health workers' access to more clients in need of abortion services. For example, during one of my visits to a pub in Ouagadougou, I met Severine, a 20-year-old woman, who worked as server in the pub and also as a sex worker on the side. Severine told me that a male friend of hers who is a nurse gave her misoprostol tablets for free when she had an unwanted pregnancy and encouraged her to bring other girls who would need abortions to him.

The permissiveness of the drug distribution system in Burkina Faso, which allows individuals to access drugs without showing a prescription, generates conditions that permit illegal abortion (Ouedraogo, 2015). Like many other drugs in low-resource settings, misoprostol circulates as a commodity that can be sold and purchased informally (Van der Geest & Whyte, 1989). Drug vendors play an important role in the illicit distribution of misoprostol, for example, by circumventing the rule to report information about the prescriber and the buyer of misoprostol. A drug vendor in a private pharmacy stated that he sometimes registers fake information in the drug sales record:

> Often it is necessary to have a little imagination: you need the name of a recognized district hospital, it is very easy to write in the notebook. You put a doctor's name that we will never be checked and you write the product and the name of a fake buyer with wrong mobile number and the product is sold.

The same drug vendor explained that circumventing regulations is relatively straightforward; in 21 years of service, he has never been visited by an inspector. Social ties between drug vendors in pharmacies and healthcare workers can also facilitate women's access to misoprostol without a prescription. For example, one healthcare provider who admitted that he offers abortion services at his house explained how he procures misoprostol: 'As I am a health professional, I go with prescriptions to buy. I also know a lot of pharmacists who help me sometimes'.

These examples show the critical importance of intermediaries (health workers, drug sellers, sex workers, friends, etc.) in misoprostol access, though not all women depend on intermediaries to access misoprostol. Some women access misoprostol directly by going to a pharmacy; however, this requires tact and a certain ability to negotiate directly with drug vendors, as well as strong social networks or what Ouedraogo terms an 'abortion managing group' (Ouedraogo, 2015): all the individuals mobilized and involved in the abortion process (seeking out information, individuals, places or products that can assist in providing moral and financial support). In Ouagadougou, drug vendors in pharmacies, health workers and sex workers are among the actors involved in the networks that enable women to access misoprostol. These networks are often characterized by interactions that disappear once misoprostol is accessed. Later on, people involved in the process can contact each other again if the need for an abortion is expressed.

By ignoring the official requirement for a prescription and selling it off-label, drug vendors and health workers can be said to domesticate misoprostol. This domestication involves the diversion of misoprostol for illegal abortion, contrary to the official status assigned to it by Burkina Faso's health policies, and its sale as a commodity that has a negotiable price. These practices are encouraged by women's demands for clandestine abortions and give power to drug vendors and health workers, who can decide who can access the drug according to their rules and logics.

## Intermediaries' Motivations

Some health workers helping a woman to get an abortion take the position that doing so is a matter of the woman's right to health, since doing so can help her avoid the serious social and health consequences of an unwanted pregnancy, whether the consequences of an unsafe abortion or the abandonment of children at birth. For example, one male midwife, who performs abortion illegally, said:

> We have to help. They are women who come to give birth, they tell you vis-à-vis that the guy refused paternity. Sometimes they do not even know the person who is responsible for their pregnancy since they have dealt with two or three people. Some of them will tell you that they were raped. I tell myself that these people need help. There are also some other women who are ashamed because they have a little child. When all these women do not want pregnancy they take odd products to abort and then after they will face many complications. Those who decide to keep the pregnancy will give birth and throw away the baby.

Despite having declared their attitude to help people, individuals who sell misoprostol or practice abortion will do so following some conditions. For example, a drug vendor explained that he and his colleagues prefer requests from women who explain verbally that they need misoprostol, rather than someone who simply holds a piece of paper on which the name of the product is mentioned. In the latter case, drug vendors feel that they should not sell the product because of safety concerns: 'you will see some people who arrive with just a simple piece of paper where it is written misoprostol. You can feel he does not even know what kind of product he is buying. If you give it to them, they may misuse it. So, to avoid problems we refuse to sell'. As for health workers who practice abortion, like the one I met, he helps only people referred to him through his social network; the 'client' has to come through someone he already knows, otherwise she is rejected.

Although misoprostol circulates beyond the clinic and the control of health workers, accessing it is thus not a given and requires negotiation. While health workers and drug vendors may be motivated to provide misoprostol for women on altruistic grounds, others judge the women's need and ability to pay before setting a price or other terms of exchange. In short, buying misoprostol tablets is not just an economic transaction but also a complex process of networks and negotiation, which often involves vendors exerting power over the terms of access to the product.

## Pharmaceutical Diversion of Misoprostol by Women

Pharmaceutical (drug) diversion refers to the transfer of any legally prescribed controlled substance from the individual for whom it was prescribed to another person for any illicit use (Berge et al., 2012; Lovell, 2006). By using this notion, I refer to the way misoprostol, which is meant to be used for official indications such as PAC and the treatment of post-partum haemorrhage, is rather used for acts such as illegal abortions. Through the channel of friends and relatives, drug vendors and healthcare workers, women are able to access misoprostol to induce abortion. Despite the fact that it allows for self-induced abortion, the involvement of abortion providers seems important because they appear as 'skilled' players regarding the use of the drug. Moreover, the involvement of abortion providers in some cases has changed women's access to illegal-induced abortion because it allows abortion providers to perform abortion discreetly (Drabo, 2019). As 23-year-old Awa explained:

> My boyfriend contacted a doctor who gave us an appointment in front of a guest house. My boyfriend paid for the room and then waited outside. I went inside with the doctor who put some white pill inside me...After that I did not see him again. When I arrived home, I started bleeding a bit and it came out.

This example shows how misoprostol enables clandestine abortion providers to work discreetly, by removing the procedure from the healthcare setting where providers may risk prosecution if complications occur. Thus, both women and abortion providers benefit from the discretion misoprostol allows.

In addition to meeting the need for discretion, misoprostol also changes the cost of illegal abortion services. Women report that abortion with misoprostol was relatively affordable, around 8000 XOF (1 USD approximatively equal 580 XOF), compared to abortion induced illegally by MVA, which can cost around 25,000 XOF. Furthermore, the price of misoprostol varies depending on how the product is accessed. It is relatively cheaper when women procure it to have a self-induced abortion than when they pass through a health worker. In the latter case, it is the price of abortion that is fixed and not that of the drug. As one informant told me, 'The price of abortion varies between 25,000 XOF to 200,000 XOF. Last time I was dealing with a former minister. I asked him to pay 200,000 XOF. In addition, with the population it varies from 25,000 XOF to 100,000 XOF'.

The variation of the price of an abortion, which is fixed by the abortion provider based on individual financial resources, suggests that people getting involved in illegal activities like abortion (by asking for the support of abortion providers) could render them susceptible to extortion. Accounts of individuals involved in the provision of abortion services show that although some abortion providers claim to 'help' women, abortion services always come at a price. Misoprostol establishes what Fiske has called an 'instrumental relationship' (Fiske, 1992) between drug vendors, healthcare providers and women (with their supportive person), meaning a relationship characterized by mercantile interest between people involved in a social interaction. This gives rise to negotiation between those who need and those who distribute misoprostol in which the price of the product is adjusted according to the characteristics of the purchaser. For example, the price may be lower or easily negotiated if the purchaser knows the provider or is introduced to them through a friend. Some women I spoke with accessed misoprostol without paying anything because their acquaintances gave them the drug for free, such as 35-year-old Diane, whose partner of 17 years is the father of her two children. After she announced her third pregnancy, her partner asked her to have an abortion and threatened to leave her if she kept the pregnancy. Diane decided to contact one of her friends, a medical doctor, to get misoprostol, who gave it to her free of charge. As she explained:

> When I had my problem, I got the product for free. A friend helped me to get it from another friend. He did not buy it either because they are both health professionals and they mutually support each other. The other could not refuse because he knows that one day he may also need help (not only abortion) from my friend.

In addition to receiving misoprostol free of charge from friends in the medical system, women described how they obtained misoprostol from female friends or relatives who had used it to self-induce abortion. These female friends or relatives gave the remaining pills from the packet they purchased as a gift. One woman confided that though she never had an abortion, her cousin gave her some misoprostol tablets in case she would need it one day. She interrupted the interview to go get the tablets and showed me a blister pack with six tablets missing.

As a gift, misoprostol reinforces the bonds of solidarity, friendship and kinship between women (Gregory, 1982), and means that one woman's abortion can allow that of another woman. Such informal exchanges highlight the agency of women and their role in 'domesticating' misoprostol (that is, how they create a use for the drug that was not intended by regulators) and disrupting the supply chain of misoprostol ordinarily controlled by healthcare workers and drug vendors. This concept of domestication (Childerhose & MacDonald, 2013) emphasizes agency and resourcefulness in the adaptation of technology for one's own ends. However, this adaptation ability is not the case for all women who seek to access misoprostol though informal networks.

## When the Diversion of Misoprostol Reproduces Social Inequities

Although women with strong social networks, including friends and relatives who know healthcare workers or drug sellers, may access misoprostol relatively easily and at little or no cost, other women struggle to obtain the drug. They struggle to find information about where to buy it and the right way to induce abortion. These difficulties in accessing misoprostol push some women to turn to private clinics recognized to provide abortion services at a higher price than they can afford, as highlighted in Francine's story.

Francine, a 23-year-old domestic maid, became pregnant with a 16-year-old boy and decided to terminate the pregnancy. After a week of unsuccessful research, she was finally able to find, through a friend, a private clinic that belongs to an NGO offering abortion services discreetly. Once in the clinic, she paid a consultation fee of 2000 XOF out of her monthly salary of 10,000 XOF. After group family planning counselling, each woman explained their problem to a health worker. Francine told me that she had invented a story in order to convince the health worker to offer her an abortion: 'I told her that the 'author of the pregnancy' (local term to describe the father) had fled and that I had no one to support me. I added that my mother is strict and would banish me from the family'.

After Francine's explanations, the health worker decided to help her. She gave her a piece of paper on which she wrote her name and telephone number and asked Francine to forward it to another health worker (working in the same clinic) who would understand the message. After reading the note, the health worker decided to proceed with the abortion, but first told Francine she needed to do an ultrasound to confirm the pregnancy and its gestation. At a cost of 7500 XOF, the ultrasound was unaffordable for Francine. She left the clinic and returned the following day after she found the necessary money with the support of her uncle (by pretending she was sick). The ultrasound confirmed that she was 2 months pregnant. After the ultrasound, the health worker asked her to do other tests, including serology test, blood type and hepatitis B, which cost 8500 XOF in total.

After the results of these examinations, the health worker gave her four pills, which she drew discreetly from her drawer. She instructed Francine to keep the pills under her tongue for 30 min before swallowing. Then she wrapped another eight tablets in paper and told her to swallow four tablets every 3 h. These tablets cost 15,000 XOF. Francine had no complications after this abortion. As this case illustrates, while Francine's friend directed her to abortion services in a private clinic, even with misoprostol, the cost of the abortion was more than three times Francine's monthly salary.

The experience of Anna, a 30-year-old, exemplifies how accessing abortion means not only incurring unplanned expenses and having trouble accessing abortion services but also experiencing failed abortions, frequenting several different abortion providers and intimidation (Drabo, 2019).

Anna is employed as a hairdresser and earns between 15,000 XOF to 20,000 XOF a week, but supplements her meagre income through sex work. Anna calls her boyfriend a crook and stingy because he cheats people on the internet to get money, but refuses to support her financially when she is in need. She decided to terminate the pregnancy since she was concerned that her boyfriend would take the child to his home country. As she said: "I am not going to struggle to give birth to a child and they will come and take it from me one day". When Anna was one month pregnant, she asked a friend to escort her to a woman who she knew conducted abortions in her home. According to Anna, this abortion provider is not a healthcare worker but she learned how to conduct abortions after working with a healthcare worker.

However, when Anna and her friend arrived at the woman's home, she sent them away, stating that she did not perform abortions. Anna and her friend visited the woman several times over a period of eight days before she finally agreed to help them. She asked them to pay 20,000 XOF, before placing a white product (misoprostol) in Anna's vagina and explaining that once Anna reached home, the fetus would be expelled. Unfortunately, the pregnancy was still intact after a week. After this failed abortion attempt, Anna was afraid to go back to see the woman because their previous meetings were difficult. With the help of the same friend, she decided to go to a clinic known to practice clandestine abortions. Once she reached the clinic, the man who owned the clinic requested that she pay 2000 XOF for the examination. After the examination, he fixed the price of Anna's abortion at 50,000 XOF and gave her an appointment for the same afternoon. Anna did not have enough money but decided to go to the appointment anyways with the intention of negotiating a discount. Once in the clinic, a secretary in the clinic discreetly informed Anna that she knew a place where Anna could have an abortion for less. Anna accepted the offer and was directed to the home of another woman. However, when Anna reached the woman's home, the lady rejected Anna and threatened to call the police. Anna was not able to convince the woman to conduct the abortion until the clinic secretary escorted her. Finally, the woman agreed to perform Anna's abortion in her house using aspiration at a cost of 30,000 XOF.

Although Francine and Anna's experiences differ, they illustrate that, despite the influx of misoprostol, obtaining an abortion in Ouagadougou is a costly and often stressful process. The availability of misoprostol outside the formal healthcare system may not guarantee access nor a successful abortion for less well-resourced and connected women. In addition, given that illegal abortion often obeys the rule of 'no one knows', in case of failure, women do not hold the abortion providers accountable. Instead, they go to official health facilities to get support for treatment if complications occur, or resort to another abortion provider, like in Anna's case.

Furthermore, intermediaries often exercise control over the process of diverting the drug into the hands of women; many women are vulnerable to exploitation by providers of the drug on whom they are dependent. Conversations with women revealed that some women who need to access misoprostol become victims of sexual harassment or abuse from abortion providers. Claudine, a 24-year-old student, explained her experience with one informal abortion provider:

> This man, everybody knows him…He tried to date me and asked for my phone number but I refused. One day I asked for his help because one of my friends wanted to get rid of her pregnancy. He came home and placed the tablet inside…Then he showed us the remaining tablets and told me that my friend must have this last one to finish the abortion. However, that she was not going to get it until he received my telephone number. Since that time, he disturbs me.

In another case, Lisa, a 34-year-old restaurant owner, became friends with a 19-year-old student, who was a regular customer. The student confided in Lisa that she encountered trouble while seeking misoprostol for an abortion. As Lisa explained to me:

> It would have been interesting for you to meet this girl…She suffered a lot because she told me she was pregnant and did not want her parents to know about it. However, she had no money to do the abortion. X [a known abortion provider] helped her to abort using a pill but on the condition of having sex with her…without a condom.

Some women reported that they chose to self-abort in order to avoid harassment, though doing so incurs the risk of inappropriate use of abortion drugs. For instance, Sali, a 21-year-old woman working in a pub, got misoprostol from a friend, who did not tell her how to use it. She took the entire tray at the same time (14 tablets) and she was later admitted to hospital due to dizziness and pelvic pain. Abortion service providers confirmed in interviews that although many women know about misoprostol and that it can be used to induce abortion, few women know the appropriate dosage. This shows how access to misoprostol does not necessarily guarantee a safe abortion.

## Discussion and Conclusion: Safe Access to Safe Abortion

In this chapter, I have shown that understanding access to misoprostol for safe abortion requires going beyond the analysis of formal policies and institutions to study people's actual micro-practices. Despite a legal and regulatory framework that aims to restrict the use of misoprostol for induced abortion, some health workers and drug vendors in pharmacies successfully divert misoprostol for illegal abortions, and some women successfully domesticate it for use in their own homes. The availability of misoprostol outside the formal healthcare system seems to reduce the cost women pay for induced abortion, corroborating findings from other studies (Ngai et al., 2000; Leone et al., 2016; Singh et al., 2018; Moland et al., 2018). Even so, improved access to misoprostol does not necessarily equate with *safe* access to safe abortion (Drabo, 2019).

In fact, much like de Zordo's findings from Brazil (De Zordo, 2016), my study suggests that there is an inequality of access to misoprostol; some women have bargaining power because of their social status and can easily access misoprostol, whereas others cannot. For some women, the route to access is through a network of drug vendors, health workers and sex workers, while others are able to get it directly from private pharmacies or NGO clinics. My findings resonate with a recent study from Ouagadougou showing that misoprostol is used predominantly among women who have attended secondary and post-secondary education and women who have high socioeconomic status (Baxerres et al., 2018).

My findings contribute in several distinct ways to the literature on the topic. First, inequities in access to healthcare innovations are often pictured in terms of dichotomies between urban–rural residence and poverty status (Singh et al., 2018). Meanwhile, my analysis highlights inequities in access to abortion or abortion drugs between people within the same geographical area, as is the case in Ouagadougou. Second, though my study affirms the importance of social networks or 'abortion management groups' in accessing abortion within legally restricted settings like Burkina Faso (Ouedraogo, 2015), the notion of an abortion management group does not fully capture the fact that the management of abortion often occurs through loose, occasional, networks rather than cohesive bounded groups, as I have shown. By circulating misoprostol in their close social networks as a gift, however, even poor women may break the access networks often controlled by health workers and drug vendors and in some instances domesticate the drug for their use at times and places they decide. Finally, my analysis challenges predominant technical definitions of 'safe abortion' that focus on the outcome of the abortion procedure and the professional competence of the operating agent (World Health Organization, 2015). While the diversion and domestication of misoprostol may increase women's access to safe abortion and make it possible to relocate abortion practices to guesthouses and other places, the process is not always conducive to safety. In some cases, the diversion of misoprostol creates conditions that allow the unpleasant treatment or even sexual abuse of vulnerable women. Thus, for some women, the route to accessing a safer abortion, medically speaking, can be unsafe. Access to misoprostol therefore does not necessarily guarantee a safe abortion.

By apprehending misoprostol in its dynamic uses, this study shows how global policies on drugs such as misoprostol can mask social inequalities and power relations around its uses. Actors advocating for safe abortion and policy makers can learn from this Burkinabe example, which shows that a drug like misoprostol, regardless of its properties and its therapeutic effectiveness, cannot alone ensure safe abortion. Indeed, for misoprostol to solve the problem of unsafe abortion globally, women need to be able to access it equitably and safely. However, as long as its use occurs within a legally restrictive context like that of Burkina Faso, the actors and networks that emerge to fill the access gap will not treat all women equally or well, and safe access to safe abortion remains somewhat elusive.

## References

Bankole, A., Hussain, R., Sedgh, G., Rossier, C., Kaboré, I., & Guiella, G. (2014). *Unintended pregnancy and induced abortion in Burkina Faso: Causes and consequences*. Guttmacher Institute.

Baxerres, C., Boko, I., Konkobo, A., Ouattara, F., & Guillaume, A. (2018). Abortion in two francophone African countries: A study of whether women have begun to use misoprostol in Benin and Burkina Faso. *Contraception, 97*(2), 130–136. https://doi.org/10.1016/j.contraception.2017.10.011

Berge, K. H., Dillon, K. R., Sikkink, K. M., Taylor, T. K., & Lanier, W. L. (2012). Diversion of drugs within health care facilities, a multiple-victim crime: Patterns of diversion, scope, consequences, detection, and prevention. *Mayo Clinic Proceedings, 87*(7), 674–682. https://doi.org/10.1016/j.mayocp.2012.03.013

Bodart, C., Servais, G., Mohamed, Y. L., & Schmidt-Ehry, B. (2001). The influence of health sector reform and external assistance in Burkina Faso. *Health Policy and Planning, 16*(1), 74–86. https://doi.org/10.1093/heapol/16.1.74

Childerhose, J. E., & MacDonald, M. E. (2013). Health consumption as work: The home pregnancy test as a domesticated health tool. *Social Science & Medicine, 86*, 1–8. https://doi.org/10.1016/j.socscimed.2013.02.035

De Zordo, S. (2016). The biomedicalisation of illegal abortion: The double life of misoprostol in Brazil. *História, Ciências, Saúde-Manguinhos, 23*(1), 19–36.

Drabo, S. (2013). *Access to Post Abortion Care (PAC) in Burkina Faso: An ethnographic study*. Master's Thesis. University of Oslo.

Drabo, S. (2019). A pill in the lifeworld of women in Burkina Faso: Can misoprostol reframe the meaning of abortion. *International Journal of Environmental Research and Public Health, 16*(22), 4425. https://doi.org/10.3390/ijerph16224425

CIA World Factbook. (2018). *Burkina Faso demographics profile 2018*. https://www.indexmundi.com/burkina_faso/demographics_profile.html. Accessed 28 Apr 2018.

Fernandez, M. M., Coeytaux, F., de León, R. G. P., & Harrison, D. L. (2009). Assessing the global availability of misoprostol. *International Journal of Gynecology & Obstetrics, 105*(2), 180–186. https://doi.org/10.1016/j.ijgo.2008.12.016

Fiske, A. P. (1992). The four elementary forms of sociality: Framework for a unified theory of social relations. *Psychological Review, 99*(4), 689.

Gregory, C. A. (1982). *Gifts and commodities* (Vol. 2). Academic.

Hofmeyr, G. J. (2012). *Obstetric use of misoprostol: Innovations, evidence, controversy and global health perspectives*. University of the Witwatersrand, Faculty of Health Sciences. Thesis (D.Sc.).

La voix du Juriste. (2013). Code penal de 1996.

Leone, T., Coast, E., Parmar, D., & Vwalika, B. (2016). The individual level cost of pregnancy termination in Zambia: A comparison of safe and unsafe abortion. *Health Policy and Planning, 31*(7), 825–833. https://doi.org/10.1093/heapol/czv138

Lovell, A. M. (2006). Addiction markets: The case of high-dose buprenorphine in France. In Petryna, A., Lakoff, A., Kleinman, A. (Eds.), *Global pharmaceuticals: Ethics, markets, practices* (pp. 136–170). Duke University Press.

Ministry of Health of Burkina Faso. (2014). *Liste national des medicaments et consommables medicaux essentiels*. https://www.medbox.org/pdf/5e148832db60a2044c2d5cdc. Accessed 9 Oct 2021.

Moland, K. M., Haukanes, H., Tadele, G., & Blystad, A. (2018). The paradox of access-abortion law, policy and misoprostol. *Tidsskrift for den Norske laegeforening: tidsskrift for praktisk medicin, ny raekke, 137*(2), 1–6. https://doi.org/10.4045/tidsskr.17.0809

Mortimer, J. T., & Shanahan, M. J. (Eds.). (2003). *Handbook of the life course*. Plenum.

Ngai, S. W., Tang, O. S., Chan, Y. M., & Ho, P. C. (2000). Vaginal misoprostol alone for medical abortion up to 9 weeks of gestation: Efficacy and acceptability. *Human Reproduction, 15*(5), 1159–1162. https://doi.org/10.1093/humrep/15.5.1159

Ouattara, F., & Storeng, K. T. (2014). L'avortement volontaire au Burkina Faso: Quand les réponses techniques permettent d'éviter de traiter un problème social. *Autrepart, 70*(2), 109–123.

Ouedraogo, R. (2015). *«L'avortement, ses pratiques et ses soins». une anthropologie des jeunes au prisme des normes sociales et des politiques publiques de santé au Burkina Faso*. Université de Bordeaux.

Potts, M. (2006). Misoprostol in practice. In *Plenary lecture at the international conference on the prevention of post Partum Hemorrhage*. Goa, India.

Singh, S., Remez, L., Sedgh, G., Kwok, L., & Onda, T. (2018). *Abortion worldwide 2017: Uneven Progress and unequal access*. Guttmacher Institute.

Storeng, K. T., & Ouattara, F. (2014). The politics of unsafe abortion in Burkina Faso: The interface of local norms and global public health practice. *Global Public Health, 9*(8), 946–959. http://dx.doi.org/10.1080/17441692.2014.937828

Storeng, K. T., Drabo, S., & Filippi, V. (2013). Too poor to live? A case study of vulnerability and maternal mortality in Burkina Faso. *Global Health Promotion, 20*(1_suppl), 33–38. https://doi.org/10.1177/1757975912462420

Van der Geest, S., & Whyte, S. R. (1989). The charm of medicines: Metaphors and metonyms. *Medical Anthropology Quarterly, 3*(4), 345–367.

Weldegebreal, R., Melaku, Y. A., Alemayehu, M., & Gebrehiwot, T. G. (2015). Unintended pregnancy among female sex workers in Mekelle city, northern Ethiopia: A cross-sectional study. *BMC Public Health, 15*(1), 40. https://doi.org/10.1186/s12889-015-1366-5

Whyte, S. R., Van der Geest, S., & Hardon, A. (2002). *Social lives of medicines*. Cambridge University Press.

Winikoff, B., & Sheldon, W. (2012). Use of medicines changing the face of abortion. *International Perspectives on Sexual and Reproductive Health, 38*(3), 164–166.

World Health Organization. (2006). *The selection and use of essential medicines: Report of the WHO expert committee, 2005 (including the 14th model list of essential medicines)* (Vol. 933).

World Health Organization. (2015). *Health worker roles in providing safe abortion care and post abortion contraception*. https://www.ncbi.nlm.nih.gov/books/NBK316326/. Accessed 9 Oct 2021.

# Chapter 5
# The "Sustainability Doctrine" in Donor-Driven Maternal Health Programs in Tanzania

Meredith G. Marten

## Introduction: Unpacking the Sustainability Doctrine

Each year, offices of the United States' President's Emergency Plan for AIDS Relief (PEPFAR) issue Country Operational Reports (COPs), which outline the "strategic directives" for each country in the following year. In 2008, the peak year of PEPFAR's funding, the 1083-page COP outlined funding plans and objectives for hundreds of implementing agencies in Tanzania. That year, PMTCT was one of the largest focal areas, with US$22 million dedicated to PEPFAR's four-pronged approach: expanding services, increasing mothers' uptake of antiretrovirals, improving follow-up of children and their HIV status, and strengthening monitoring and evaluation. Each PMTCT-related activity undertaken by partner agencies required a one-paragraph sustainability narrative, which described several plans, including developing partnerships with the public sector (integrating PMTCT into maternal and child health services, in particular), prioritizing capacity building through "training, mentoring, and supportive supervision," and empowering community groups to be self-sustaining, resulting in local "ownership" of the interventions by HIV/AIDS committees at ward and village levels (PEPFAR, 2008, p. 123–124).

The demand for a focus on "sustainability" by PEPFAR and other donors comes from decades of concern about the volatility and uncertainty of funding and programmatic practice in donor-dependent countries (Yang et al., 2010). The United States Agency for International Development (USAID), for example, has emphasized sustainability for the past twenty years, defining it as "the ability of host country entities (community, public and/or private) to assume responsibility for programs and/or outcomes without adversely affecting the ability to maintain or continue program objectives or outcomes" (Mehdi, 1999, p. 1). Nevertheless, the sustainability

M. G. Marten (✉)
Department of Anthropology, University of West Florida, Pensacola, FL, USA
e-mail: mmarten@uwf.edu



L. J. Wallace et al. (eds.), *Anthropologies of Global Maternal and Reproductive Health*, Global Maternal and Child Health, https://doi.org/10.1007/978-3-030-84514-8_5

plans in PEPFAR's COP reports did not include predictable and reliable support for implementing interventions over the long-term, or account for varying local contexts, hindering the potential sustainability of programs. Rather, the COP report implied a dependence on either unpaid volunteer work after the program period ended or income generation from an unknown source that would support healthcare worker (HCW) labor, both of which are unlikely in resource-poor environments (Maes, 2012).

These sustainability guidelines illustrate what Swidler and Watkins (2009, p. 1184) argue is the often "manifestly unrealistic" yet frequently replicated "sustainability doctrine" employed by many donors, NGOs, and humanitarian organizations in sub-Saharan Africa. Sustainability has "become a conscious policy of donors" to prioritize programs they believe can be sustained once donor funding ends (Swidler & Watkins, 2009, p. 1184). Health care is therefore principally envisioned and implemented by donors and NGOs in short-term, time-limited, vertical programs (Meinert & Whyte, 2014; see also Basilico et al., 2013), which are often operationalized through the planned use of trainings, dependence on unpaid volunteers, and development of income-generating activities (Swidler & Watkins, 2009), all of which were outlined or alluded to in PEPFAR's (2008) COP. Simultaneously, funding to support the necessary but deficient "staff, stuff, space, and systems" – the building blocks of strong health systems and the backbone of sustainable care (Farmer, 2014, p. 7; WHO, 2007; Yang et al., 2010) – is frequently and pejoratively termed "aid dependency" (UNAIDS, 2012).

A fundamental problem with translating sustainability policies into practice is how imprecise the term "sustainability" is despite its prolific use; as Yang and colleagues note, it "has been neither clearly defined nor consistently applied" (2010, p. 130). This may be strategic, allowing organizations to take on the mantle of sustainability despite outcomes that demonstrably undermine it. In many contexts, sustainability functions as a buzzword, concealing more than it reveals, and importantly, providing legitimacy needed to justify policies and interventions (Cornwall & Brock, 2005). As Sullivan (2016) writes, buzzwords "[envelop] actors mobilizing the terms in moral authority, shielding them from critique" (4). Buzzwords can also take on different meanings depending on context. In the case of "sustainable mining," Kirsch (2010) describes the meaning of sustainability shifting between the sometimes-incompatible goals of environmental conservation, social welfare, and economic development, the "triple bottom line" of sustainable development (Sachs, 2012, p. 2206). Sustainability's slipperiness, Kirsch (2010) writes, allows corporations to adopt the language of their critics: "mining is not sustainable" in the environmental sense becomes "sustainable mining" in the economic development sense if it continually employs a large workforce from a particular region. This shifting meaning can lead to paradoxical outcomes: mining corporations with large workforces and prominent roles in local economies can effectively threaten to leave unless environmental regulations constraining their destructive practices are removed, thus undermining the environmental sustainability of a region.

Discussions and debates about sustainability in global health and how to improve it have been longstanding, and the slipperiness of the term emerges in this history.

As Yang et al. (2010) describe, sustainability became a popular criterion for evaluating health programs decades ago, as part of efforts to address the growing concern about the instability and precariousness of health care in aid-dependent countries. Since the early days of Tanzanian decolonization, for example, donors have been largely resistant to pledging the kinds of financial and technical commitments required to support comprehensive health care and health system strengthening (HSS) (Stirling, 1977). Particularly as public health systems were dismantled in the wake of structural adjustment, the intent of promoting "sustainability" was directly *against* the perpetuation of "unsustainable" vertical programs over the long term. As short-term aid implemented by NGOs ballooned in the 1990s to fill gaps that emerged as public sectors faltered (Pfeiffer et al., 2008), advocates of sustainability tried to address "root causes of health problems rather than to palliate their symptoms" (Yang et al., 2010, p. 129).

The proliferation of overlapping vertical programs and global health initiatives was a consequence of the shift away from post-WWII intergovernmental collaboration coordinated by the World Health Organization (WHO) (Storeng et al., 2019). Instead, in the MDG era "unsustainable" vertical programs multiplied in contexts of neoliberalism, "philanthrocapitalism" (Birn, 2014), and broader efforts to transform "international health" practices structured by and through nation-states to "global health" orientations largely bypassing and transcending them (Adams, 2016; Pfeiffer, 2013; Rees, 2014). As Adams (2016) writes, the shift away from nation-states began with the global economic crises of the 1970s and 1980s, and governments' diminishing capacity to support public health systems. It also derived from a "growing sentiment that national entities often *get in the way* of effective health delivery rather than promoting it" (emphasis in original, p. 5). Non-governmental, humanitarian, and other private sector organizations therefore functioned as the "institutional forms of choice for doing global health work" (Adams, 2016, p. 25). With this shift came an increased dependence on quantitative indicators and cost-effectiveness calculations, rapidly expanding the need for metrics which, Adams (2016) argues, is fundamental to enabling global health initiatives today. The shifting meaning of sustainability in global health contexts mapped on to these broader changes. Rather than indicating support for public sector HSS, in many contexts sustainability has come to primarily mean financing individual NGO-run vertical programs over time, which are more easily measured but less effective in contributing to HSS (Yang et al., 2010; Swidler & Watkins, 2009; Oberth & Whiteside, 2016).

Slow progress in achieving some MDGs – maternal survival in sub-Saharan Africa, in particular – highlighted the shortcomings of this shift in priorities. As Sheikh et al. (2011 p. 3) explain, an "upsurge of interest" in HSS materialized during the MDG era when it became evident that vertical programs could not function effectively with weakened public health systems. This occurred alongside increased emphases on aid harmonization, capacity building, and country ownership as outlined in the 2005 Paris Declaration and the 2008 Accra Agenda for Action (OECD, 2019). Despite these initiatives, in donor-dependent countries like Tanzania, external donors continue to exert undue influence on national agendas and undermine HSS.

Health policies like the sustainability doctrine "are artifices of human creation, embedded in social and political reality and shaped by particular, culturally determined ways of framing problems and solutions" (Sheikh et al., 2011, p. 2). Ethnographic research of how policies are constructed, enacted, prioritized – or rescinded or forgotten – can illuminate the contexts in which they operate, as well as the effects they may have on health systems and population health. In this chapter, I draw on ethnographic findings to describe how sustainability in health has been understood by policymakers and expatriate global health experts and donors in Tanzania, and the ways in which it was undermined by emergent "sustainability doctrine" practices in the MDG era. I illustrate how the sustainability doctrine has been put into practice, and how it has persisted, despite its shortcomings, using examples of donor-prioritized maternal healthcare initiatives in Tanzania rolled out several years apart: prevention of mother-to-child transmission of HIV (PMTCT) and basic emergency obstetric and newborn care (BEmONC) programs in the late 2000s, and more recent (2015) efforts to implement respectful maternity care (RMC) programs.

Considering programs implemented during a period of significant global interest in improving women's health outcomes, I draw out some of their underlying dynamics. I focus on several issues informants identified as crippling efforts to build a strong Tanzanian health system, particularly the internal brain drain of healthcare workers from the public sector to higher-paying NGO jobs, and the prioritization of types of programs donors believed could be sustained after the funding period ended but could simultaneously erode health sector capacity, such as trainings and workshops. I describe how despite widespread acknowledgement of these fundamental issues, international donors still fear a cultivation of "aid dependency," prohibiting many from contributing to long-term health system strengthening (HSS) efforts (McKay, 2017a), and prioritizing short-term interventions. From this, a focus on programs and workshops persists – less effective in part because of their time-limited structure, but also because they fail to account for local circumstances and the challenges that come with implementing vertical programs within weakened health systems. Despite good intentions to solve the unintended consequences of donor volatility, the successive promotion of "sustainable" practices can paradoxically contribute to health system precarity in Tanzania.

## Methods

Research presented in this chapter draws from a larger ethnographic project exploring donor instability, aid withdrawal, and efforts to develop sustainable HIV and maternal health services in Tanzania.

The bulk of fieldwork took place at a large mission hospital in northern Tanzania over the course of 14 months in 2011–2012, and primarily addressed how HIV+ mothers enrolled in PMTCT care maintained their health and that of their families amidst declining program services and funding (see Marten, 2020). During this period, donor-funded health institutions and programs, such as this PMTCT program, experienced high aid volatility following the 2008 global economic crisis. Because of this, I spent an additional three months in Dar es Salaam "studying up" to address how global health and development policymakers and program directors managed this volatility and conceptualized "sustainability" in global health contexts. Findings outlined in this chapter are derived from semi-structured interviews, participant observation, and document review. Sixteen semi-structured interviews were conducted with healthcare workers and policymakers, both in the public sector and at Tanzanian and international NGOs. Six informants were either managing directors or sustainability coordinators at five of the six primary implementing organizations partnered with, and funded in large part by, the US Government's HIV initiative, the President's Emergency Plan for AIDS Relief (PEPFAR). Among the others, four worked for bilateral organizations in departments focused on health or women's rights, two worked for a maternal health project associated with a donor-funded hospital, one directed an international NGO focused on health and development, and one worked as a nurse at a large, private hospital. Only two informants worked in the public sector, a limitation of this research: one held a position at the Tanzanian Ministry of Health, Community Development, Gender, Elderly and Children (hereafter, MoH), and another was a medical school professor. Of these 16 informants, nine were Tanzanian, and of those who worked at NGOs, at least four had previous experience in the public sector. Of the remaining, seven informants were expatriate professionals, four of whom were from the United States. I also draw heavily from long-term key informant interviewing with two of these 16 informants, Tanzanian OB/GYNs I call Esther and Sheila, who have worked in maternal and neonatal health care for decades in the public and private/NGO sectors in Dar es Salaam. Finally, I rely on participant observation in various maternal health and HIV contexts over time in Tanzania, which inform much of my evolving perspective on sustainability and health system strengthening. Ethical clearance for this fieldwork was approved by the University of Florida's IRB and permitted by the Commission for Science and Technology (COSTECH) and the National Institute for Medical Research (NIMR) in Tanzania. All names and other personal identifiers in the chapter have been changed to protect privacy and confidentiality.

## Conceptualizations of "Sustainability" Among Policymakers in the Tanzanian NGO Community

In 2011, three years after the financial crisis, The Global Fund announced it was cancelling Round 11 of its funding, citing donor shortfalls. At the same time, PEPFAR funding stagnated, and numerous bilateral organizations announced rollbacks and changes in aid disbursements. One informant at a large bilateral agency headquartered in Dar es Salaam expressed her concerns about the reductions for health care, telling me "this is a larger scope and scale across multiple countries than I've seen before." Amidst all this, concerns about "aid dependency" and the need for "sustainability" if and when the donors withdrew aid became more urgent (UNAIDS, 2012).

The country director of another bilateral initiative, Isaac, described to me his organization's conundrums with Tanzania's aid dependency. He characterized Tanzania's health sector as "deteriorating" because of its "long history of a culture of dependency." His organization provided critical health services for millions of Tanzanians, and he was doubtful the public health sector could feasibly take it over. Mirroring Adams' (2016, p. 5) observation that many global health actors view governments as "often *get[ting] in the way* of effective health delivery," Isaac continued, "if you want this done you have to do it for them."

In the spring of that year, I endeavored to better understand how sustainability was conceptualized in this context of funding retrenchments and fear of widespread aid exit. I asked informants to explain what they understood sustainability to mean, both in regard to health care and health systems, as well as how their organizations put sustainability into practice. A few participants identified goals for a sustainable health system that closely align with the 17 expansive goals employed by the SDGs (UN, 2017). From this perspective, informants identified sustainability as resting on a foundation of good primary and secondary education, basic health services, roads and infrastructure, electrification, access to safe water, good governance, and a more developed economy that could provide the tax base to fund health care and other social services. For example, when I asked Henry, an expatriate director of an international NGO, what some "best practices" for health sector sustainability might be, he illustrated the need to expand focus beyond the health sector:

> Maybe the 'best practice' would be for all girls to finish Form 6? …I would really overhaul our whole educational system… and work aggressively on rural youth employment, because if all the youth still become hawkers and *boda boda* (motorcycle taxi) drivers on the streets of Dar es Salaam, that is not solving the problem.

Secondly, many of these policymakers and NGO directors identified sustainability as dependent on a robust public health sector. Henry defined it plainly as "the effective running of a health system." To be effective, he said, "it depends on WHO's six building blocks," responsive to the "dynamic nature of public health" and the needs that arise within a population over time. The goal of the WHO Six Building Blocks model (WHO, 2007) is to promote HSS and includes: (1) effective, safe, and quality service delivery; (2) a well-performing health workforce; (3) effective health information systems; (4) equitable access to quality medical products, vaccines, and technologies; (5) a good health financing system; and (6) effective leadership and governance (WHO, 2007).

As Isaac alluded to, financing (block five) is a longstanding challenge. In Tanzania, austerity measures introduced in the mid-1980s reduced public spending on the health system and have been unsuccessful in generating the economic growth and revenue necessary to provide equitable and effective health care for all. Following Tanzania's 1999–2000 Sector Wide Approach (SWAp), the government implemented a series of initiatives to increase revenue, including imposing user fees, improving tax collection, and expanding health insurance schemes (Marten & Sullivan, 2020). Still, in 2018/2019 government spending on the health sector was only 7% of Tanzania's national budget, less than half the 15% Abuja target for health spending (Mamdani et al., 2018).

Informants emphasized that the building blocks that make up strong health systems must all happen in concert, as a critical lack of one component can frustrate improvements in the others (c.f. Farmer, 2014). For instance, the human resources crisis remains a formidable challenge in Tanzania; the country has one of the lowest rates of HCWs (physicians, nurses, and midwives) per capita in the world (WHO, 2015). Financing limitations (block five) constrain necessary human resources expansion (Mamdani et al., 2018), but a lack of functioning equipment (block four) also hinders the effective work of HCWs (blocks one and two) in clinical practice. Henry spoke at length about the extent of the problem that he had witnessed over decades in the Tanzanian health sector:

> There are smart people here in Tanzania...but a key problem is getting those smart people in a working environment where they can use those skills… You can put a well-trained doctor in a national or a regional hospital, but if there is no blood pressure machine, if there are no gloves, if there are no standard operating procedures for delivering babies, if there are no clinical audits for people who died to find out why they died; if all that is [not] done, you can have a perfectly skilled doctor there but they can't operate! You can as well put a nurse there, it's the same thing.

Persistent stock outs of equipment and other logistics in Tanzania's health facilities not only undermine service delivery but also can, according to informants, undermine trust in health workers and health sector institutions. For example, Esther, an OB/GYN and director of an NGO-funded maternal health program, explained how accusations by the public of nurse bribery in hospital labor wards can sometimes stem from misunderstandings about the constraints limited logistics pose to health-care provision. Esther explained that nurses are oftentimes villanized by the public because nurses frequently ask patients for money in order to get supplies that are necessary for their care and which should be free (Citizen, 2005). The persistent lack of supplies, she told me, meant that nurses often had to procure them from private pharmacies. For this reason, a nurse asking a patient for money may in many cases not be evidence of bribery, but in fact could be a result of equipment or medication shortages.

Infrastructural demands are also acute, but as one informant described, donor hesitancy to contribute to building new facilities is implicated in "staff and stuff" shortcomings. In an email interview with Inge, a European maternal health program manager for a Tanzanian NGO, she described how her efforts to develop a strong program and expand hospital services could be stymied:

> Many white elephants have been constructed in Africa and are now not utilised…primary schools without teachers, health centres without staff and supplies, building without utility connections, etc.…donors are afraid that hospitals will not be staffed afterwards and maintenance and operational costs cannot be secured…The human resource crisis in health contributes to this, as donors are afraid that infrastructure is easy to put in place but to man it and to keep it running is another challenge.

## Paradoxical Outcomes from MDG-era Efforts to Build Sustainability: NGO-Driven Brain Drain in the Tanzanian Health Sector

Many healthcare practitioners and policymakers in Tanzania are acutely aware of the problems that arise when efforts to improve maternal health (and health outcomes, more broadly) are unlinked from HSS. Several informants lamented that vertical approaches to HIV care, treatment, and prevention were inadequate, and in interviews, some expressed deep frustration with a failure to learn from previous attempts to improve population health and change accordingly. As George, a Tanzanian NGO Director, explained:

> When TB was a big agenda in the world, we had a kind of vertical [response], it was kind of a reaction to emergency. We thought that we would phase out [vertical programs], because HIV is a problem which would need to be solved by the entire system. But when HIV came, the same thing happened. I don't see that much changes, we don't learn, we don't learn much from what's happened.

During the MDG era in Tanzania, the rapid and widespread implementation of vertical programs contributed to a weakening of the public health sector through various means, but perhaps most significantly through an internal brain drain of Tanzanian HCWs. Aligned with the tenets of the sustainability doctrine, programs were often considered by donors to be more sustainable and "country owned" through the employment of local professionals (c.f. Swidler & Watkins, 2009; Palen et al., 2012), who were simultaneously attracted to the higher wages, benefits, and better working conditions afforded in the offices of international NGOs compared to the overcrowded conditions in public clinics or hospitals (see also Gerein et al., 2006; Ackers et al., 2016). As Bech and colleagues note, since 1978, government health workers have not been able to "live on a government salary without supplementary income" (2013, p. 102–103).

Another director of a Tanzanian NGO, Neema, described to me two principal ways in which the internal brain drain occurs. First, primary care nurses, doctors, and clinical officers were recruited to work in wards and facilities providing disease-specific care, leaving fewer health professionals to provide primary health care. Second was the recruitment of practicing HCWs, particularly MDs, from the public sector to non-practicing "desk jobs" at NGOs, which could include tasks such as developing health policies and guidelines, engaging in program monitoring and evaluation, and working with local government officials to harmonize NGO initiatives with local priorities. Lucia, an MD and professor at the national hospital, and Esther spoke at length with me about the internal brain drain and its effects on the Tanzanian health system, lamenting that the internal brain drain was crippling any effort to create a sustainable system. As Lucia said,

> [Those who leave the public sector] "are not working at (the national hospital), so they're not training new doctors, they're not working in the district hospitals in Dar let alone out in the middle of nowhere. They're working for an NGO, and they're doing paperwork."

As Lucia described, the brain drain leaves its mark on medical schools, too. Despite the current push to educate health workers in Tanzania as part of HSS efforts, overstretched medical school faculty members are seeing some of their most promising colleagues leave for the private sector or abroad, taking with them their years of specialized training. Lucia was concerned for the future of her university when the head of her department retired, because he would not only be leaving himself, but "all the people he has trained are not working in the system," diminishing the chances that his students will be around to train the next generation of doctors.

Additionally, Esther speculated that some international NGOs actively recruited Tanzanian MDs in part to push through their desired changes in treatment guidelines, which they felt would be more palatable to the MoH coming from a Tanzanian and serve as evidence of being "country owned." At one particular US NGO focused on maternal and child health, she said "they've got three OB/GYNs developing treatment guidelines (instead of doing clinical work), and the reason why they are there is because the NGO wants a Tanzanian face to face the Ministry to push the guidelines."

Many things that could help build up strong health systems – cooperating with governments to fund structural gaps identified in their systems, for example (IOM, 2014) – do not fit in with donor conceptualizations of sustainability because of the long-term recurring costs involved. As McKay (2017b) describes, when long-term health systems costs are not supported because they are believed to cultivate dependency, the short-term focus and "ephemeral nature" of donor-funded projects come to dominate health systems, leading to their increasing precarity (474). Further, those projects that are funded can erode the public sector, paradoxically undermining the sustainability of health care that donors and implementers claim to be supporting. One principal strategy for sustainability and capacity building is the widespread implementation of off-site training for HCWs.

## The Sustainability Doctrine in Practice: Basic Emergency Obstetric and Neonatal Care Trainings and Workshops

When I came to Tanzania in early March 2011, Sheila, an OB/GYN with a donor-funded NGO hospital, was just starting to coordinate and plan curricula for a series of Basic Emergency Obstetric and Neonatal Care (BEmONC) workshops for nurses and midwives in the government clinics and hospitals of Dar es Salaam. A goal of the workshops was to provide continuing medical education for safe deliveries and emergency obstetric care to help bring down the high maternal mortality ratio – 454/100,000 – at the time, far from Tanzania's MDG #5 goal of 133/100,000 (URT, 2014; MoHCDGEC, 2016a). Her NGO's hospital coordinated with the District Medical Office and another large, international NGO to run the trainings. I sat in on several days of these trainings, and they resembled others I have observed in Dar. We sat around a conference table, looked at PowerPoint slides, and someone was positioned with a large flip-chart at the front of the room, writing out important notes that we would later tape to the walls. Participants discussed the emergency obstetric care guidelines (Dao, 2012), and nurses from each clinic were responsible for reporting to the group the results of their internal monitoring of progress in meeting the guidelines at their specific facilities.

The daily workshop schedule included tea around 10:00, a large lunch, and then an afternoon snack before breaking for the day. Every participant received a Tsh 120,000 per diem (US$75), enough for a hotel and money to buy dinner. Most people participating in the training live in Dar anyway, Sheila explained, so many ultimately save the money. Per diems have become a critical part of the training culture in Tanzania and are a principal reason people participate; they serve as salary "top ups" and can strengthen patronage ties (see also Swidler & Watkins, 2009). Trainings are conducted for a variety of reasons, perhaps most importantly to serve as continuing professional development and education for Tanzanian HCWs, and fill gaps in pre-service curriculum and quality (Necochea et al., 2015). For donors, trainings like BEmONC are considered sustainable because they align with the "teach a man to fish" objective inherent to the sustainability doctrine – hiring experts to train people (or train trainers who will subsequently train others) involves short-term inputs that will not "breed dependency" but "provide all with the capacity to provide for their own needs" (Swidler & Watkins, 2009, p. 1184). Accordingly, the nurses, midwives, and physicians trained in the BEmONC workshop were expected to train others not in attendance in an in-service capacity. Through this approach, the BEmONC training of trainers was meant to "encourage support systems that aim to create an organisational culture of quality, and ultimately make improvements more sustainable" (Necochea et al., 2015).

By 2012, however, trainings had populated the health system and exacerbated the already dire human resources shortages experienced throughout the country. In many cases, trainings took HCWs out of understaffed clinics and hospitals and placed them in what could end up being a revolving cycle of trainings in various new skills and technologies. For example, in an assessment of 24 health clinics in southern Tanzania, Manzi et al. (2012) discovered that on average, 38% of available staff were out of the clinic or hospital for seminars and long-term trainings.

As Robert, a Tanzanian MD with the MoH, described:

> One of the things which has really affected the health sector is all these trainings…HCWs spend two to three months moving from one training to another…[and] because people have been moving so much, they don't stay [to work] in the hospitals. Sometimes they move from a TB training to an HIV training, and then from there they go to a laboratory HIV training, and then from a laboratory HIV training they go to a pharmaceutical HIV training.

Because per diems for trainings were a supplement that many depended on to top up their salaries, who was chosen to participate contributed to feelings of inequity among HCWs. As Robert continued, "the thing is, you can't train everybody. Now the problem is if you train just a few, the rest who have not been trained will say 'no, I'm not doing it because I've not been trained'." This concern was supported by Sheila's experience, who visited hospitals and clinics for in-service BEmONC training in the maternity wards, in addition to training trainers in BEmONC workshops. She related to me that considerable resentment was created between those who go to trainings, learn the guidelines, and receive per diem, and those who stayed behind to work in the hospital. What shocked her was that some HCWs who stayed behind claimed that the new guidelines for care were "not their guidelines," implying that the guidelines were not their responsibility to carry out, because they were not paid to learn them (see also Magrath & Nichter, 2012). Sheila also said that because she herself was conducting trainings in different hospitals, she could not enforce the new guidelines, since she was not available to supervise practitioners to ensure the new skills were correctly employed. An in-service trainee Sheila encountered in one of the clinics in Dar told her fellow trainees openly that they "only had to perform the new guidelines today" while Sheila was there, "and tomorrow we can go back to doing what we always do" because she would not be around to supervise. This example illustrates how HCW trainings – despite their widely recognized importance – became less effective in building capacity because of the failure to take into account the significant structural gaps in the Tanzanian health system.

In his critique of the training model, Robert explained that he thought the expectations for Tanzanian doctors' performance and professionalism should be much higher. Nevertheless, Robert asserted that compensation for health workers was woefully inadequate, contributing to diminished morale:

> Most of the doctors in Tanzania used to be among the best students. [But now] when you start working, after maybe six or seven years of studies, you are the least paid! All these other students who were mediocre performers [in school] are now making more money... because they are working in another system, like the private sector or a bank.

As NGOs' comparatively higher salaries contributed to significant internal brain drain, practicing staff in the health sector were increasingly overburdened. Over time, the topic of salaries, and perceptions of value tied to salaries, generated many heated conversations and was made particularly contentious when a series of doctors' strikes erupted in 2012, fueled principally by anger over low salaries, few allowances for housing and transport, and stoked by continuing deficiencies in equipment and resources (see also Prince & Otieno, 2014).

The doctors on strike made several demands: a starting salary of Tsh 3.5 million a month (about US$ 2,150) for new doctors (starting salaries at the time were about Tsh 950,000 or about $600), a risk allowance of 30% of their salaries, a housing allowance of 30% of their salaries, health insurance, an increase for on-call allowances, and an allowance of 30% of their salaries for transportation. After a lengthy, antagonistic struggle, the government increased everyone's salaries in the civil service by 20%, of which doctors are a part (TDN, 2012; Maluka & Chitama, 2017).

Doctors' demands for higher salaries and supplemental support for housing and transportation are likely also related to the large population of expatriate international NGO workers who regularly receive all these things (see also Smith, 2007). Working side-by-side with expatriate doctors and NGO workers earning significantly more, with supplemental income for housing and vehicles, seemed to have numerous effects. First, the inflation in housing costs, particularly on the peninsula of Dar es Salaam where the majority of NGO offices were located, frequently prevented Tanzanians from being able to afford nearby housing. These neighborhoods are regularly exempted from scheduled, revolving brownouts; experience less traffic; have more paved roads; and are largely safer. Second, the cost of living was rapidly increasing, with which salaries often did not keep pace (NBS, 2013). Third, many people equated salary with perceived value – which appeared to me to be the most offensive and hurtful to several Tanzanian informants. Esther, who was angered by an argument over her salary with her boss, said that seeing how little she was paid compared with her expatriate colleagues made her "feel black" – which she explained as making her feel undervalued and perceived to be "stupid and silly." Cognizant and too-often reminded of the undercurrents of racism that pervade much of international health efforts, she and Lucia lamented how Tanzanian doctors were perceived by many in the global health community to be "underdeveloped", and that "[living in a] low-resource country means [having] a low-resource mind."

## Persisting Sustainability Doctrine Practices in Tanzania's Respectful Maternity Care Efforts

Numerous lessons learned from the MDG era emerged in anticipation of the UN's new development initiative, the SDGs, which began in 2015 and included a focus on the importance of HSS (UN, 2017). But despite evidence that sustainability doctrine practices like trainings can weaken the health system in Tanzania, some more recent donor-funded RMC interventions often still adhere to its basic tenets: the prioritization of short-term, "feasible," and locally owned programs donors believe may be sustained after donor support ends (URT, 2015).

The paramount importance of HSS for improved maternal health outcomes has been identified and promoted by researchers for decades. In a cross-country analysis, for example, Anand and Barnighausen (2004) found a direct relationship between the ratio of HCWs to population and women's survival in childbirth and that of neonates – as the number of doctors, nurses, and midwives increase, survival increases proportionately. Nevertheless, maternal and reproductive healthcare sectors experience some of the most acute consequences of the human resources limitations in Tanzania (see also Gerein et al., 2006; Shoo et al., 2017), and the labor wards of the major public hospitals of Dar es Salaam are among the places where the lack of "staff, stuff, space and systems" can be most profoundly felt (Farmer, 2014, p. 7). As Esther explained, these hospitals operate at approximately 400% capacity, and on any given day, several women may be found laboring side-by-side in a bed. In efforts to increase institutional births believed to reduce the rate of maternal mortality, the hospitals recently experienced a nearly 34% increase in admissions without the budget line or support to provide quality care for such rapidly increasing numbers (URT, 2015). Further, those most responsible for caring for women – the city's harried labor ward nurses – rush from woman to woman, where

Esther memorably told me "there's a head popping out of a vagina every 20 minutes" (see also Naburi et al., 2017). As one Tanzanian ICU nurse at a private hospital explained to me, conditions in these labor wards are so notoriously bad that nurses are sometimes placed there as "punishment" for underperforming in other wards. Esther described them as akin to "prison islands" with people exchanging tips on how to "get out" and be relocated to other wards. Stories of bribery and corruption among labor ward staff also regularly appear in local newspapers, contributing to corrosive public distrust (Citizen, 2005).

Nevertheless, recent efforts to improve maternal health outcomes still often focus on symptoms of problems rather than the roots – in particular, the widespread and pernicious "disrespect and abuse" of pregnant and laboring women, rather than the critically insufficient "staff, stuff, and space" of Tanzanian labor wards (c.f. Kruk et al., 2018). Despite the uptick in urban institutional births Esther described at Dar hospitals, low rates of institutional births persist nationally, which many attribute to disrespect and abuse encountered in labor wards. This, in turn, is thought to be linked with stagnating maternal mortality rates, which in 2015–2016 was 556/100,000 (see Kujawski et al., 2015; MoHCDGEC, 2016a). A current focus in global maternal health to combat disrespect and abuse is respectful maternity care (RMC), which promotes women's human right to respectful and dignified care (White Ribbon Alliance, 2011).

Similar to earlier HIV and BEmONC programs, RMC interventions primarily involve trainings targeted toward sensitizing HCWs (adapted from the WHO's Health Workers for Change curriculum, Fonn & Xaba, 1996), and birth preparedness education for pregnant women (Ratcliffe et al., 2016a), two interventions that satisfy Swidler and Watkins' (2009) sustainability doctrine mandates. Research suggests, however, that insufficient health system inputs underlie persistent issues of disrespect and abuse (WHO, 2018b). A recent study of RMC in Kigoma region evaluated patient and provider determinants of receipt of RMC based on three dimensions of respectful care: (1) friendliness/comfort/attention; (2) information/consent; and (3) non-abuse/kindness (Dynes et al., 2018). The majority of findings indicated structural and systemic constraints as exacerbating disrespect and abuse. From the provider side, nurses who attended the most births, and those who had the highest number of working hours, were more frequently reported as engaging in disrespectful or abusive actions. Alternatively, Dynes and colleagues note that healthcare providers who had access to multiple kinds of mentoring, and felt fairly compensated for their work, more frequently engaged in respectful maternity care. From the patient side, those who labored with a companion – something frequently not allowed in "bulging" labor wards because of a lack of space – reported more frequently receiving respectful care. The authors recommend strategies to provide more equitable pay, decrease workloads, provide more breaks, and increase mentoring opportunities – all dependent on HSS and long-term, stable funding – as being paramount for decreasing disrespect and abuse (Dynes et al., 2018; see also WHO, 2018b). Indeed, researchers affiliated with Dar's RMC intervention described above note that for dignified care during childbirth to be sustainable, "institutional commitment to providing necessary resources and staff will be needed" (Ratcliffe et al., 2016b, p. 1).

Large-scale efforts to implement RMC in Tanzania were first laid out in a stakeholder meeting in Dar in 2015, convened by the MoH and USAID's Maternal and Child Survival Program, and attended by 47 participants from multiple East African Ministries of Health, Tanzanian regional health offices, bilateral organizations, and NGOs (URT, 2015). Esther was an attendee at the meeting, and voiced her frustration with the continued lack of public sector support, by arguing that supporting staff to manage high workloads and operate effectively within the overcrowded wards was essential. Further, she advised the group that investing in HSS with RMC as a focus area should be prioritized rather than another vertical program. She has since advocated for "caring for carers" as a principal way to improve maternal health outcomes in Dar es Salaam, which include issues like fair pay, more staff, and increasing the space and number of hospitals to accommodate the growing numbers of women. Reflecting on her experience one evening over dinner with me, she rhetorically asserted her objectives, using the same rights-based language that RMC advocates have used: "what about the rights of healthcare workers?"

## Conclusion

A shared framework for HSS was first developed at the WHO's 2005 "Montreux Challenge" when it became evident that strong health systems were essential for effective and sustainable health care (Hafner & Shiffman, 2013; Sheikh et al., 2011). Yet still today, donor policies promoting sustainability can hinder progress toward HSS, one of the "bitter ironies" encountered across PMTCT, BEmONC, and RMC programs described in this chapter (Swidler & Watkins, 2009, p. 1192). In donors' quest to develop more "locally owned," sustainable programs staffed by Tanzanian professionals, an NGO-driven brain drain emerged, shifting HCWs from public to NGO sectors, and from clinical practice to "desk jobs," eroding the pool of practicing health workers. Further, short-term activities like trainings were frequently implemented, which at the same time could undermine the health workforce by enrolling clinicians in a revolving door of trainings. Finally, donors sidestepped opportunities to assist the Tanzanian government in strengthening the public sector (see also Maluka et al., 2018), including supporting policies that would have made their interventions more effective and alleviate some of the pressures on HCWs themselves. In the overburdened labor wards in Dar's largest hospitals, as Dynes et al. (2018) explained, providing more equitable pay, decreasing workloads, increasing mentoring opportunities, and encouraging larger institutional commitments to providing resources and staff are needed, particularly as women are increasingly encouraged to deliver in facilities that are already severely under-resourced (Wendland, 2018).

As outlined in these ethnographic cases, a disconnect between donor rhetoric and action creates an irony of the sustainability doctrine: the cultivation of "aid dependency" is frequently cited as a reason to not pledge long-term, stable resources to

HSS objectives (UNAIDS, 2012), while paradoxically, programs characterized as "sustainable" can undermine them. The harmful consequences of these policies can be significant: as McKay (2017a, b) illustrates in her work in Mozambique, the tradeoff in avoiding "aid dependency" is often the establishment of more precarious systems of care, which can ultimately lead to stagnating or worsening maternal health over the long term.

External donors are not solely responsible for strengthening health systems, of course, and limitations of this work include a gap in information about the Tanzanian government's own efforts and shortcomings in doing so. Despite this, a focus on donor-funded programs illuminates an important question: why do these policies and priorities persist despite widespread acknowledgement of the harm they can do? Through tracking the rhetorical slippage of "sustainability" over time, it can be seen as a buzzword: used to create an appearance of advancing sustainable health care, without significantly challenging the powerful market-based structures of the status quo. While intended to alleviate problems complicated by donor dependency and LMICs' decreasing ability to fund public health services, the sustainability doctrine instead primarily advances neoliberal "global health" orientations, dependent on metrics and accountable to donors more often than to those accessing care (Adams, 2016; Maluka et al., 2018). Sustainability's shifting reference to maintaining a system of short-term, NGO-run programs reinforces the "philanthrocapitalist" model that circumvents nation states in favor of NGOs (Birn, 2014). The lack of support for public care then further entrenches the notion of nation-states' inability to build successful public health systems in resource-poor contexts (Adams, 2016).

The amount of donor funds still available for global health services, and particularly for maternal and child health (MCH) initiatives, provides a window of opportunity to do things more effectively and durably to build up public health sectors (Pfeiffer, 2013). In 2017, US$11.6 billion in DAH was dedicated to MCH, nearly the peak of funding HIV received during the rapid scale up of HIV programming (IHME, 2018). The current SDG development agenda provides further opportunity, emphasizing HSS to achieve SDG #3: "ensure healthy lives and promote well-being for all at all ages" (UN, 2017). Tanzania has embraced the SDG model of harmonization in maternal health contexts, linking not only the multiple domains that can impact maternal health, such as gender-based violence and male engagement in family planning (USAID, 2019a, b), but also better establishing integration of services (MoHCDGEC, 2016b, p. 10).

Donors can support these efforts in part by directing funds to public sector initiatives rather than bypassing them in favor of NGOs (Pfeiffer et al., 2008; Pfeiffer, 2013). This is of particular importance for growing economies like Tanzania's, which is expected to soon transition "beyond aid" (Whiteside et al., 2019), and is in line with the most recent Astana Declaration which affirms "the primary role and responsibility of Governments at all levels in promoting and protecting the right of everyone to the enjoyment of the highest attainable standard of health" (WHO, 2018a). Whether this will come to be in Tanzania or is just another policy on paper remains to be seen – as Henry noted, "We have the most beautiful policies, but they are never put into practice."

## References

Ackers, L., Ioannou, E., & Ackers-Johnson, J. (2016). The impact of delays on maternal and neonatal outcomes in Ugandan public health facilities: The role of absenteeism. *Health Policy and Planning, 31*, 1152–1161. https://doi.org/10.1093/heapol/czw046

Adams, V. (2016). Introduction; Metrics of the global sovereign: Numbers and Stories in Global Health. In V. Adams (Ed.), *Metrics: What counts in global health* (pp. 1–54). Duke University Press.

Anand, S., & Barnighausen, T. (2004). Human resources and health outcomes: Cross-country econometric study. *Lancet., 364*, 1603–1609. https://doi.org/10.1016/S0140-6736(04)17313-3

Basilico, M., Weigel, J., Motgi, A., Bor, J., & Keshavjee, S. (2013). Health for all? Competing theories and geopolitics. In P. Farmer, J. Y. Kim, A. Kleinman, & M. Basilico (Eds.), *Reimagining global health* (pp. 74–110). University of California Press.

Bech, M., Lawi, Y., Massay, D., & Rekdal, O. (2013). Changing Policies and their influence on Government Health Workers in Tanzania, 1967–2009: Perspectives from Rural Mbulu District. *International Journal of African Historical Studies, 46*, 61–103. http://www.jstor.org/stable/24393097

Birn, A. (2014). Philanthrocapitalism, past and present: The Rockefeller Foundation, the Gates Foundation, and the setting(s) of the international/global health agenda. *Hypothesis, 12*, 1–27. https://doi.org/10.5779/hypothesis

The Citizen (Dar es Salaam). (2005, June 11). *Hell hath no fury like a nurse seeking a bribe; nurses who refuse to hear the screaming*.

Cornwall, A., & Brock, K. (2005). What do buzzwords do for development policy? A critical look at 'participation', 'empowerment' and "poverty reduction". *Third World Quarterly, 26*, 1043–1060. https://doi.org/10.1080/01436590500235603

Dao, B. (2012). *Guidelines for in-service training in basic and comprehensive emergency obstetric and newborn care*. Baltimore, MD: Jpheigo Corporation. http://reprolineplus.org/system/files/resources/Guidelines_for_Basic_and_Comprehensive_InService_Final.pdf Accessed 11 October 2021.

Dynes, M. M., Twentyman, E., Kelly, L., Maro, G., Msuya, A. A., Dominico, S., et al. (2018). Patient and provider determinants for receipt of three dimensions of respectful maternity care in Kigoma Region, Tanzania- April-July, 2016. *Reproductive Health, 15*, 1–24. https://doi.org/10.1186/s12978-018-0486-7

Farmer, P. (2014). Diary. *London Review of Books, 36*, 38–39. http://www.lrb.co.uk/v36/n20/paul-farmer/diary. Accessed 23 Oct 2014.

Fonn, S., & Xaba, M. (1996). *Health workers for change: A manual to improve quality of care*. World Health Organization. https://www.who.int/tdr/publications/documents/health-workers.pdf. Accessed 27 Apr 2019

Gerein, N., Green, A., & Pearson, S. (2006). The implications of shortages of health professionals for maternal health in Sub-Saharan Africa. *Reproductive Health Matters, 14*, 40–50. https://doi.org/10.1016/S0968-8080(06)27225-2

Hafner, T., & Shiffman, J. (2013). The emergence of global attention to health systems strengthening. *Health Policy and Planning, 28*, 41–50. https://doi.org/10.1093/heapol/czs023

Institute of Medicine (IOM). (2014). *Investing in Global Health Systems: Sustaining Gains, Transforming Lives*. Washington, DC: The National Academies Press. https://doi.org/10.17226/18940. Accessed 11 October 2021.

Institute for Metrics and Evaluation (IHME). (2018). *Financing global health*. https://vizhub.healthdata.org/fgh/. Accessed 13 Sept 2018.

Kirsch, S. (2010). Sustainable mining. *Dialectical Anthropology, 34*, 87–93. https://doi.org/10.1007/s10624-009-9113-x

Kruk, M. E., Kujawski, S., Mbaruku, G., Ramsey, K., Moyo, W., & Freedman, L. P. (2018). Disrespectful and abusive treatment during facility delivery in Tanzania: A facility and community survey. *Health Policy and Planning, 33*, e26–e33. https://doi.org/10.1093/heapol/czu079

Kujawski, S., Mbaruku, G., Freedman, L. P., Ramsey, K., Moyo, W., & Kruk, M. E. (2015). Association between disrespect and abuse during childbirth and women's confidence in health facilities in Tanzania. *Maternal and Child Health Journal, 19*, 2243–2250. https://doi.org/10.1007/s10995-015-1743-9

Maes, K. (2012). Volunteerism or labor exploitation? Harnessing the volunteer spirit to sustain AIDS treatment programs in urban Ethiopia. *Human Organization, 71*, 54–64. https://doi.org/10.17730/humo.71.1.axm39467485m22w4

Magrath, P., & Nichter, M. (2012). Paying for performance and the social relations of health care provision: An anthropological perspective. *Social Science and Medicine, 75*, 1778–1785. https://doi.org/10.1016/j.socscimed.2012.07.025

Maluka, S., & Chitama, D. (2017). *Primary health care systems (PRIMASYS): Comprehensive case study from United Republic of Tanzania*. Geneva: World Health Organization. https://apps.who.int/iris/rest/bitstreams/1346154/retrieve. Accessed 11 October 2021.

Maluka, S., Chitama, D., Dungumaro, E., Masawe, C., Rao, K., & Shroff, Z. (2018). Contracting-out primary health care services in Tanzania towards UHC: How policy processes and context influence policy design and implementation. *International Journal for Equity in Health, 17*, 1–13. https://doi.org/10.1186/s12939-018-0835-8

Mamdani, M., Kweka, H., Binyaruka, P., Ramesh, M., Kapologwe, N., Hutchinson, E., Bal, D., & Andreoni, A. (2018). *Strengthening accountability for better health outcomes through understanding health-system bottlenecks: Insights from Tanzania* (No. 008), ACE Working Paper. London: Anti-Corruption Evidence (ACE) Research Consortium. https://ace.soas.ac.uk/wp-content/uploads/2018/11/ACE-WorkingPaper008-HealthTanzania-181129.pdf. Accessed 11 October 2021.

Manzi, F., Armstrong Schellenberh, J., Hutton, G., Wyss, K., Mbuya, C., Shirima, K., et al. (2012). Human resources for health care delivery in Tanzania: A multifaceted problem. *Human Resources for Health, 10*. https://doi.org/10.1186/1478-4491-10-3

Marten, M. (2020). Living with HIV as donor aid declines in Tanzania. *Medical Anthropology, 39*, 197–210. https://doi.org/10.1080/01459740.2019.1644334

Marten, M., & Sullivan, N. (2020). Hospital side-hustles: Funding conundrums and perverse incentives in the publicly-funded Tanzanian health sector. *Social Science & Medicine, 244*, 112662. https://doi.org/10.1016/j.socscimed.2019.112662

McKay, R. (2017a). *Medicine in the meantime: The work of care in Mozambique*. Duke University Press.

McKay, R. (2017b). Response to Benton, A., Sangaramoorthy, T., and Kalofonos, I. Temporality and positive living in the age of HIV/AIDS: A multisited ethnography. *Current Anthropology, 58*, 454–476. https://doi.org/10.1086/692825

Mehdi, S. (1999). *Health and Family Planning Indicators: Measuring Sustainability, Vol. II*. US Agency for International Development. https://www.k4health.org/sites/default/files/migrated_toolkit_files/indicators2.pdf. Accessed 6 Sept 2019.

Meinert, L., & Whyte, S. R. (2014). Epidemic projectification: AIDS responses in Uganda as event and process. *Cambridge Journal of Anthropology, 32*, 77–94. https://doi.org/10.3167/ca.2014.320107

MoHCDGEC. (2016a). *Tanzania demographic and health survey and Malaria indicator survey, 2015–2016*. https://dhsprogram.com/pubs/pdf/fr321/fr321.pdf. Accessed 15 Sept 2018.

MoHCDGEC. (2016b). *The National Road Map strategic plan to improve reproductive, maternal, newborn, child, and adolescent health in Tanzania (2016–2020), One Plan II*. https://www.globalfinancingfacility.org/sites/gff_new/files/Tanzania_One_Plan_II.pdf. Accessed 27 Apr 2019.

Naburi, H., Mujinja, P., Kilewo, C., Orsini, N., Bärnighausen, T., Manji, K., et al. (2017). Job satisfaction and turnover intentions among health care staff providing services for prevention of mother-to-child transmission of HIV in Dar es Salaam, Tanzania. *Human Resources for Health, 15*, 1–12. https://doi.org/10.1186/s12960-017-0235-y

National Bureau of Statistics (NBS) of Tanzania. (2013). *Tanzania Consumer Price Index (CPI)*. http://www.tradingeconomics.com/tanzania/consumer-price-index-cpi. Accessed 12 April 2014.

Necochea, E., Tripathi, V., & Gynecology, Y. K. O. (2015). Implementation of the Standards-Based Management and Recognition approach to quality improvement in maternal, newborn, and child health programs in low-resource countries. *International Journal of Gynecology and Obstetrics, 130*, S17–S24. https://doi.org/10.1016/j.ijgo.2015.04.003International

Oberth, G., & Whiteside, A. (2016). What does sustainability mean in the HIV and AIDS response? *African Journal of AIDS Research, 15*, 35–43. https://doi.org/10.2989/16085906.2016.1138976

OECD. (2019). *The Paris declaration and Accra Agenda for action*. http://www.oecd.org/dac/effectiveness/parisdeclarationandaccraagendaforaction.htm. Accessed 9 Feb 2020.

Palen, J., El-Sadr, W., Phoya, A., Imtiaz, R., Einterz, R., Quain, E., et al. (2012). PEPFAR, health system strengthening, and promoting sustainability and country ownership. *Journal of Acquired Immune Deficiency Syndromes, 60*, S113–S119. https://doi.org/10.1097/QAI.0b013e31825d28d7

PEPFAR. (2008). *Tanzania 2008 Country Operational Plan*. https://www.pepfar.gov/documents/organization/113024.pdf. Accessed 10 Jan 2019.

Pfeiffer, J., Johnson, W., Fort, M., Shakow, A., Hagopian, A., Gloyd, S., & Gimbel-Sherr, K. (2008). Strengthening health systems in poor countries: A code of conduct for nongovernmental organizations. *American Journal of Public Health, 98*, 2134–2140. https://doi.org/10.2105/AJPH

Pfeiffer, J. (2013). The struggle for a public sector: PEPFAR in Mozambique. In J. Biehl & A. Petryna (Eds.), *When people come first: Critical studies in global health* (pp. 166–181). Princeton University Press.

Prince, R. J., & Otieno, P. (2014). In the shadowlands of global health: Observations from health workers in Kenya. *Global Public Health, 9*, 927–945. https://doi.org/10.1080/17441692.2014.941897

Ratcliffe, H. L., Sando, D., Lyatuu, G. W., Emil, F., Mwanyika-Sando, M., Chalamilla, G., et al. (2016a). Mitigating disrespect and abuse during childbirth in Tanzania: An exploratory study of the effects of two facility-based interventions in a large public hospital. *Reproductive Health, 13*, 1–13. https://doi.org/10.1186/s12978-016-0187-z

Ratcliffe, H. L., Sando, D., Mwanyika-Sando, M., Chalamilla, G., Langer, A., & McDonald, K. P. (2016b). Applying a participatory approach to the promotion of a culture of respect during childbirth. *Reproductive Health, 13*, 1–7. https://doi.org/10.1186/s12978-016-0186-0

Rees, T. (2014). Humanity/plan: Or, on the "stateless" today (also being an anthropology of global health). *Cultural Anthropology, 29*, 457–478. https://doi.org/10.14506/ca29.3.02

Sachs, J. (2012). From millennium development goals to sustainable development goals. *The Lancet, 379*, 2206–2211. https://doi.org/10.1016/S0140-6736(12)60685-0

Sheikh, K., Gilson, L., Agyepong, I. A., Hanson, K., Ssengooba, F., & Bennett, S. (2011). Building the field of health policy and systems research: Framing the questions. *PLoS Medicine, 8*, 1–6. https://doi.org/10.1371/journal.pmed.1001073.g001

Shoo, R., Mboera, L., Ndeki, S., & Munishi, G. (2017). Stagnating maternal mortality in Tanzania: What went wrong and what can be done. *Tanzania Journal of Health Research, 19*, 1–12. https://doi.org/10.4314/thrb.v19i2.6

Smith, D. (2007). *A culture of corruption: everyday deception and popular discontent in Nigeria*. Princeton University Press.

Stirling, L. (1977). *Tanzanian Doctor*. McGill-Queen's University Press.

Storeng, K. T., Prince, R. J., & Mishra, A. (2019). The politics of health system strengthening. In R. Parker & J. Garcia (Eds.), *Routledge handbook on the politics of global health* (pp. 273–287). Routledge.

Sullivan, N. (2016). Multiple accountabilities: Development cooperation, transparency, and the politics of unknowing in Tanzania's health sector. *Critical Public Health, 27*(2), 1–12. https://doi.org/10.1080/09581596.2016.1264572

Swidler, A., & Watkins, S. C. (2009). "Teach a man to fish": The sustainability doctrine and its social consequences. *World Development, 37*(7), 1182–1196. https://doi.org/10.1016/j.worlddev.2008.11.002

Tanzania Daily News (TDN). (2012, July 2). *Tanzania: Kikwete Bitter with Medics' Strike*. www.allafrica.com/stories/201207021252.html. Accessed 20 July 2013.

UNAIDS. (2012). *AIDS dependency crisis: Sourcing African solutions*. http://www.unaids.org/en/resources/publications/2012/name,67597,en.asp. Accessed 18 Jan 2019.

United Nations. (2017). *Sustainable development knowledge platform, SDG #3*. https://sustainabledevelopment.un.org/sdg3. Accessed 15 Sept 2018.

United Republic of Tanzania (URT). (2014). *Entering 2015 with better MDG scores*. https://www.undp.org/content/dam/undp/library/MDG/english/MDG%20Country%20Reports/MDGR%202014_TZ.pdf. Accessed 1 Oct 2021.

United Republic of Tanzania (URT). (2015). *Respectful maternity care workshop, Meeting report*. https://www.mcsprogram.org/wp-content/uploads/2015/10/MCSP-Tanz-RMC-report_Final.pdf. Accessed 27 Apr 2019.

United States Agency for International Development (USAID). (2019a). *Maternal and child survival program, gender technical brief*. https://www.mcsprogram.org/resource/gender-technical-brief/. Accessed 27 Apr 2019.

United States Agency for International Development (USAID). (2019b). *Boresha Afya – Southern Zone Newsletter*, January 2019. https://www2.deloitte.com/content/dam/Deloitte/tz/Documents/public-sector/Newsletter%20Issue%20%234.pdf. Accessed 27 Apr 2019.

Wendland, C. L. (2018). Who counts? What counts? Place and the limits of perinatal mortality measures. *AMA Journal of Ethics, 20*(3), 278–287. https://doi.org/10.1001/journalofethics.2018.20.3.pfor2-1803

Whiteside, A., Greener, R., & Semini, I. (2019). Planning and sustaining HIV response in the countries of the "risky middle". *African Journal of AIDS Research, 18*(4), 360–369. https://doi.org/10.2989/16085906.2019.1681482

White Ribbon Alliance. (2011). *Respectful maternity care: The universal rights of child-bearing women*. Washington, DC.: 2011. http://www.healthpolicyproject.com/pubs/46_FinalRespectfulCareCharter.pdf

World Health Organization. (2007). *Everybody's business: Strengthening health systems to improve health outcomes, WHO's framework for action*. World Health Organization.

World Health Organization. (2015). *Global Health Observatory data: Health workforce*. http://www.who.int/gho/health_workforce/en/. Accessed 1 Oct 2021.

World Health Organization. (2018a). *Declaration of Astana*. https://www.who.int/docs/default-source/primary-health/declaration/gcphc-declaration.pdf. Accessed 16 Jan 2018.

World Health Organization. (2018b). *WHO recommendation on respectful maternity care during labor and childbirth*. https://extranet.who.int/rhl/topics/preconception-pregnancy-childbirth-and-postpartum-care/care-during-childbirth/who-recommendation-respectful-maternity-care-during-labour-and-childbirth. Accessed 3 Dec 2019.

Yang, A., Farmer, P., & McGahan, A. (2010). "Sustainability" in global health. *Global Public Health, 5*(2), 129–135. https://doi.org/10.1080/17441690903418977

# Part II
# Policy Ambivalence

# Chapter 6
# The Place of Traditional Birth Attendants in Global Maternal Health: Policy Retreat, Ambivalence and Return

**Margaret E. MacDonald**

## A Midwife by Any Other Name

In 2002, the International Confederation of Midwives met for their triennial Congress in Vienna. I attended as a medical anthropologist visiting a field site: mingling with participants, listening to research presentations, learning about how the profession was organised in different countries and hearing about the pleasures and challenges midwives faced in their everyday work. At a panel one afternoon, an Australian midwife gave a paper critical of what was at the time the relatively new World Health Organization (WHO) 'skilled attendant' policy. The WHO had officially abandoned the training of Traditional Birth Attendants (TBAs) as a component of its maternal health policy and turned instead to the goal of ensuring a skilled attendant at every birth. The presentation had the feel of an exposé and murmurs began to ripple throughout the auditorium. During the discussion period, a heated debate broke out. Some midwives hailed the beginning of the end of community-level traditional birth attendants who they saw as ineffective (at best) and dangerous (at worst). Others decried the new policy as an act of selling out 'their sisters' in other parts of the world. Some midwives spoke positively of their experiences training TBAs as part of their work on Safe Motherhood projects while others had come away from such experiences quite unconvinced. An anthropologist in the room weighed in, suggesting the word TBA itself was problematic. 'It's become pejorative' she said. 'If a woman attends another woman in childbirth, she is a midwife'. Canadian, American and New Zealand midwives stood out in their defence of TBAs and their criticism of the official withdrawal of support for them at the level of global policy. Their perspective made sense given the grassroots origins of midwifery as a social movement in these jurisdictions where midwives had often trained

M. E. MacDonald (✉)
Department of Anthropology, York University, Toronto, Ontario, Canada
e-mail: maggie@yorku.ca



L. J. Wallace et al. (eds.), *Anthropologies of Global Maternal and Reproductive Health*, Global Maternal and Child Health, https://doi.org/10.1007/978-3-030-84514-8_6

by apprenticeship, practiced outside the formal healthcare system and had struggled to become recognised as legal and legitimate. Talk soon turned to the role of the International Confederation of Midwives on the issue. 'I would like to see the ICM embrace this workforce as sisters', stated one American midwife present. But the Ghanaian midwife who was moderating the session shook her head and closed the session, saying 'TBAs should be eventually replaced entirely by midwives, even though midwives must try to work with them now out of necessity'.

The next day, an ad hoc group calling itself the Committee to Promote Inclusiveness was struck and a meeting planned with the intention of pressing the ICM to develop a position statement on the TBA question. The ICM was in a difficult position. Midwives' professional standing was dependent on an exclusionary definition that had been developed with the WHO and the Federation International de Gynecologues et Obstetriciens (FIGO) (ICM, 2005). To acknowledge TBAs as their near equivalents was fundamentally at odds with the concept and parameters of a health profession. It was also argued at meetings I attended that such a move would jeopardise the standing of midwifery in the eyes of other health professions and the relatively recent place of the ICM at the table in policy decisions regarding major global maternal health initiatives. Not long after the Vienna Congress, the ICM did make its position clear. In 2004 the ICM signed a joint statement with the WHO and FIGO called 'Making pregnancy safer: the critical role of the skilled attendant'. The statement defines a skilled attendant as 'an accredited health professional – such as a midwife, doctor or nurse – who has been educated and trained to proficiency in the skills needed to manage normal (uncomplicated) pregnancies, childbirth and the immediate postnatal period, and in the identification, management and referral of complications in women and newborns' (2004, p. 1). In this document, TBA training appears in a shaded box as a 'lesson learnt'. The TBA experiment at the level of global maternal health policy appeared to be well and truly finished.

## Introduction

In this chapter, I tell the story of the waxing and waning of the status of the traditional birth attendant in global maternal health policy from the launch of the Safe Motherhood Initiative in 1987 to the present. Once promoted as part of the solution to reducing maternal mortality, the training and integration of TBAs into formal healthcare systems in the global south was deemed a failure and side-lined in the late 1990s in favour of 'ensuring a skilled attendant at every birth' (Starrs, 1997, p. 28). And yet as the opening vignette reveals, the shift in policy was a matter of some debate. In fact, the TBA question – whether and how to effectively engage TBAs in the effort to reduce maternal mortality globally – has been one of the core policy debates in the history of the global maternal health movement and TBAs continue to be regarded with deep ambivalence by many researchers and policy-makers at the national and global levels, not to mention front-line healthcare providers (Campbell et al., 2016; Prata et al., 2011). In the wake of the policy shift, TBAs did not go away, though the programmes to train and support them often did. Non-Governmental Organisations (NGOs) and national health systems focused their efforts elsewhere as funding dried up for such projects and research. And so began an era of policy retreat with regard to TBAs at the global level, which continues in large part today. In major statements and position papers, the training and formal integration of TBAs in the past appears as a policy that did not produce results, advisable only as a stopgap measure or last resort (Starrs, 1997; WHO, 2005). Yet TBAs continue to practice and participate in maternal health projects in many countries with varying degrees of inclusion within formal healthcare systems. In contrast some national-level health ministries have taken strong stances, veering towards outright bans in national level rhetoric, if not in formal policy (Murigi & Ford, 2010; Whitaker, 2012; Rudrum, 2016; Haruna et al., 2019).[1] Thus, the policy retreat at the global level mixed with a diversity of local realities has contributed to widespread policy and practical ambivalence and tension amongst health policy researchers, practitioners and advocates who make up the global maternal health community.

I approach the topic of the TBA question in global maternal health policy from a critical global heath perspective, that is, from a perspective that scrutinises the knowledge, policy and practice of global health with the goal of making visible the broader social, cultural and political context of its making. Joao Biehl's (2007) notion of the 'policy space' captures the complexity of the shifting assemblages of actors and non-neutral interests out of which policymaking emerges: political ideologies, moral investments, professional interests, scientific cultures and new technologies as well as market forces and trade agreements that structure and constrain the flow of money, people, ideas and goods. Critical global health scholarship shares much in common with the health policy and systems research (HPSR) agenda defined by Sheikh and colleagues (Sheikh et al., 2011) in terms of its attention to wider influences and micro processes that shape the multiple levels of policy decisions and practices and sees them as non-neutral (see also Biehl, 2007; Gilson, 2012; Walt et al., 2004). In contrast to HPSR researchers who set out to study policy, anthropologists tend to bump into policy in the field while doing other things; in my case, it was while tracking the emergence of midwifery as a profession on the global stage. Also, anthropologists tend to focus on the local context initially and track policy upwards to its national or global level origins. Amongst the shared goals and perspectives of these critical approaches to the study of global health policy, however, is that knowledge produced by looking critically at the making and practice of policy ought to inform the policymaking process itself.

In this chapter, I focus on four key critiques of the TBA policy shift that illuminate both the limitations of the original TBA intervention that contributed to the shift and broader social, scientific and political context of its making, including:

[1] Sierra Leone, Ghana and Malawi are all jurisdictions in which TBA practice has been banned. In Uganda, the strong anti-TBA stance of the government emphasised in public speeches and documents has not been formally implemented, but the perception of a ban and news reporting around it has been the source of confusion and fear amongst TBAs, birthing women and healthcare providers (Rudrum, 2016).

one, that the evidence cited to underpin the policy shift was weak and inconclusive; two, that the original TBA component itself was flawed in its failure to account for cultural specificity; three, that the political and economic context of the first decade of the Safe Motherhood Initiative (SMI) that constrained its implementation was not taken into account; and four, that the reorganisation of the Safe Motherhood movement at the global level demanded a new humanitarian logic that had no room for the figure of the traditional birth attendant. I present these critiques not only as backdrop for the TBA debates but as a way to illuminate the forces that shape the complex policy space of global maternal health policy.

Some scholars have begun to call for 'the return of the traditional birth attendant' as a partner in the effort to improve maternal health globally (Lane & Garrod, 2016). Meanwhile, a growing number of NGOs are re-engaging TBA-like community health actors as important players in the deployment of new technologies and drugs for maternal health alongside nurses, midwives or physicians or in some cases on their own. In the final section of this chapter, I track the TBA question to the present, observing that the once polarising figure of the TBA has been re-engaged by a set of trends in global health more broadly, including the push for new technological innovations, the rise of evidence-based medicine and advocacy, and the new self-care agenda of the WHO.

## The Traditional Birth Attendant: A Global Health Invention

As early as 1975 the TBA was defined in WHO guidelines as 'a person (usually a woman) who assists the mother at birth, and who initially acquired her skills delivering babies by herself, or by working with other TBAs' (Verderese & Turnbull, 1975, p. 18). UNICEF and other UN agencies, and national ministries of health had been training TBAs for decades and several international and regional technical consultations had been undertaken by the WHO in the 1970s to explore the potential of traditional birth attendants as resources in the domain of maternal health, as a way to extend the reach of limited health services in developing countries (Mangay Maglacas & Simons, 1986; WHO, 1979; WHO, 1985).

The launch of the Safe Motherhood Initiative (SMI) by the World Health Organization, the World Bank and the United Nations Population Fund (UNFPA) in 1987 formalised and extended the training and integration of TBAs throughout the Global South as a component of a larger package of activities including greater access to family planning, the upgrading of perinatal services to approximate western biomedical standards (especially in the area of emergency obstetric care) and making improvements in the scope and quality of education for midwives and TBAs (Starrs, 1987; WHO, 1994). The Safe Motherhood Declaration challenged all nations of the world to halve their maternal mortality figures by the year 2000. The TBA component of the SMI was in keeping with the comprehensive Primary Health Care (PHC) vision of Alma Ata, which had sought to decentralise healthcare services in part by recognising the importance of local knowledge and valorising the participation of local practitioners – including traditional medical practitioners and birth attendants (WHO, 1978). As the practical guidelines for implementing Safe Motherhood programming – a document called the Mother Baby Package – stated, '[i]n countries were TBAs attend a large proportion of home deliveries, training courses can be effective in upgrading their knowledge. Training of TBAs should be seen as a way of bridging the gap until all women and children have access to acceptable, professional health services' (WHO, 1994, p. 15).

Commentaries, reports and discussion papers throughout the late 1980s and early 1990s take a measured but positive approach to TBAs as part of the SMI. A World Bank discussion paper, for example, situates TBAs as potentially effective with training and liaison (1993 p. 15) and goes on to list the tasks and skills envisioned for them: being trained to conduct uncomplicated deliveries, reduce infections, detect complications of pregnancy and make referrals to skilled providers in the formal healthcare system when necessary. Over the next decade, thousands of women throughout the Global South – some with experience attending births and some without – were identified, trained and deployed as TBAs. They were meant to be linked to healthcare facilities and receive collaboration and support from local higher-level healthcare providers.

In 1997, top international reproductive health policymakers, researchers and stakeholders met in Colombo, Sri Lanka for a Technical Consultation on the SMI. After a decade of policy implementation, maternal mortality rates in most impoverished countries remained unchanged. The technical consultation report, The Safe Motherhood Agenda: Priorities for the Next Decade (Starrs, 1997) reflected on the first ten years of the SMI and specified 10 priorities for the next decade of policy development and intervention. Amongst them the priority to 'Ensure skilled attendance at delivery' was identified as the 'single most critical intervention' for safe motherhood (Starrs, 1997, p. 28). As defined in this document, 'A skilled birth attendant can be a midwife, a nurse with additional midwifery education, or a physician with appropriate training and experience, but does not include traditional birth attendants' (Starrs, 1997, p. 29; See also, WHO, 1985). The report from the SMI summarised the scant evidence that existed and concluded that TBAs were 'proven' to be 'not effective' in reducing rates of maternal mortality and that training them was a waste of resources (Starrs, 1997, p. 30). Some responsibility was placed on the TBA component of the original SMI as one of the weak links in the overall programme due to their illiteracy and lack of uptake of scientific knowledge. Historical evidence that improvements in MMR were only realised in other nations with the advent of comprehensive primary healthcare services with professional providers – including emergency obstetric care – was also brought to bear on the decision (Loudon, 1992; de Brouwere et al., 1998).[2]

More nuanced versions of the evidence later emerged. Bergstrom and Goodburn (2001) reported on a small range of studies which showed the limitations of what

[2] For a nuanced discussion of the uses of historical evidence in SMI advocacy, see Behague and Storeng, 2013.

TBAs could do in constrained circumstances as well as how they could be part of successful comprehensive approaches. They also noted the near impossibility of correlating TBA inclusion or exclusion to mortality outcomes given the absence of vital registration systems in most countries at that time. They concluded that TBAs, while still the main caregivers for vast numbers of women, should be given low priority. Likewise, van Lerberghe and De Brouwere, in their analysis of the existing literature, while sympathetic to some of their 'other merits' ultimately discredit TBAs on three counts: their 'resistance (or inability) to change', 'their lack of credibility in the eyes of the health professionals' and 'the *de facto* impossibility to organise effective and affordable supervision' (2000, p. 19). A close look at this statement reveals that all three points have not to do with TBAs but with health providers' attitudes and health systems' weaknesses. Their conclusions nevertheless align with the official position of the technical consultation report.

A new initiative was subsequently launched called 'Making Pregnancy Safer' which explicitly marginalised the TBA component of the SMI in favour of the goal of ensuring a 'skilled attendant at every birth' (WHO, 2004) employing a definition, like the one offered above, which excludes TBAs (Safe Motherhood Interagency Group, 2002). The new initiative also promoted birth in health facilities rather than in the community. In the years following the shift, the narrative of disappointment, failure and lessons learnt on the TBA component of the SMI solidified in both global health policy documents and the research literature on TBAs.[3] For example, in a shaded box entitled 'Traditional birth attendants: another disappointment' in the 2005 *World Health Report*, the authors look back on the TBA component of the SMI with these words: 'The strategy is now increasingly seen as a failure. It will have taken more than 20 years to realise this and the money spent would perhaps in the end have been better used to train professional midwives' (WHO, 2005, p. 70; see also Adegoke & van den Broek, 2009).

## Critical Perspectives on the TBA Policy Shift

As the opening vignette from the ICM reveals, the official end of policy support for the TBA component of the SMI was a matter of deep ambivalence for professional midwives. It continued to be a question for further discussion and debate in the scientific community as well. Anthropologists, midwife-scholars and global health researchers have all been involved in aspects of the debate, four key themes of which I present below: one, that the evidence cited to underpin the policy shift was weak and inconclusive; two, that the original TBA component itself was flawed in its failure to account for cultural specificity; three, that the political and economic context of the first decade of the SMI was not taken into account to explain the

[3] Storeng (2010) and Béhague and Storeng (2013) use the term 'narrative of failure' to refer to the characterisation of the SMI more broadly.

failure of TBAs to reduce maternal mortality; and four, that the reorganisation of the Safe Motherhood movement at the global level demanded a new humanitarian logic that had no room for the figure of the 'traditional' birth attendant.

## *A Question of Evidence*

As I described in the previous section, in the report of the technical meeting held in Colombo, Sri Lanka in 1997 to evaluate the first decade of the SMI, it was argued that the withdrawal of support for TBA training was based on evidence that TBAs had been ineffective in reducing maternal mortality as measured by the lack of reduction in the global maternal mortality ratio (MMR) over the previous ten years (Starrs, 1997; see also Starrs, 2006). Yet research on the effectiveness of training TBAs at that time was quite limited. Studies were varied in focus, and collectively the message they delivered was mixed and inconclusive.

Some scholars reviewing this evidence responded directly to the question of evidence upon which the policy shift was said to be based. For example, midwife scholar Sue Kruske and anthropologist Lesley Barclay published a paper not long after the ICM Congress arguing that the new policy was misguided: first, they argued that a focus on a single indicator – the MMR – was a gross reduction of the idea of effectiveness. Second, they noted that by narrowly focussing on the 'obstetric skills' in the new skilled birth attendant (SBA) definition (which TBAs did not possess) the policy ignored other skills and expertise that they did possess – social and cultural skills, in their words – which they argued did contribute to the less reductionist goal of improving maternal health care (Kruske & Barclay, 2004).

Echoing this observation about the narrowness of the goal, nursing and public health scholar Lynn Sibley and colleagues published a series of summaries and systematic reviews of the evidence concerning TBAs in the early 2000s that added nuance to the understanding of their roles and potential in maternal and child health. A 2004 meta-analysis of studies looked not at whether TBA training reduced maternal mortality *per se*, but as 'a behaviour change strategy to increase women's use of [antenatal care] services provided by skilled health professionals' (Sibley et al., 2004, p. 298). Despite noting variations in how TBAs were trained in the studies they looked at, the authors found significant positive associations between trained TBAs and antenatal care (ANC) attendance, concluding that 'TBAs could play an important role in influencing women's ANC attendance in settings where TBAs are respected, active, and where their activities extend beyond birthing services to include health promotion in the community at large' (2004, p. 303). Sibley & Sipe's 2006 study on the effectiveness of TBA training demonstrated that it was associated with 'moderate to large improvements in behaviours relating to selected intrapartum and postnatal care practices and small but significant decreases in perinatal mortality' (2006, p. 474). They concluded with the argument that TBA training in settings where women do not have access to properly staffed or stocked facilities is an ethical imperative. Other research showed the promise of TBAs as conduits for health promotion (Eades et al., 1993) and referrals (O'Rourke, 1995).

As existing evidence on TBA participation in the SMI was reviewed and synthesised and new studies emerged, a scientific narrative began to emerge that countered the narrative of disappointment, failure and lessons learnt. It called for research that could illuminate the work of TBAs, the content of their training programmes and their relationships with the formal healthcare system with more nuance and specificity. It proposed different questions that looked at how TBAs could increase the use of ANC with skilled providers, for example, rather than trying to demonstrate a direct correlation between TBAs and the reduction of maternal mortality ratios.

In addition to the call for generating new evidence there was a call for a change in perspective. As Sibley, Sipe and Koblinsky wrote: 'There is an urgent need to improve capacity for evaluation and research on the effect of TBA training programs and other factors that influence women's use of ANC' (2004, p. 298). It was, in effect, a call for turning the lens back onto science and policymakers themselves for their failure to understand the roles TBAs played and might play in locally variable maternal healthcare landscapes. Kidney et al. similarly concluded that community-level strategies had yet to be properly evaluated and recommended further study on how interventions involving TBAs actually work in a range of specific contexts (2009, p. 8). The discussion sections of several such studies are careful to refer to the original vision of TBA training and integration within the SMI: that TBAs had been meant to work as points of articulation between communities and a functioning healthcare system – including emergency obstetric care – extending its reach rather than as primary care practitioners responsible for the reduction of the national MMR. This scientific counter narrative, formed in the wake of the policy shift, was that it was *lack* of appropriate evidence that had doomed the TBA component of the SMI.

The fulfilment of this research agenda to look more closely at the work of TBAs in their local contexts in order to build a robust, context-specific evidence base was soon overshadowed, however, by two powerful, inter-related trends in the broader global health research field. First was the rise of evidence-based medicine (EBM), that is, the use of systematically derived clinical evidence to guide clinical practice and the concomitant rise of evidence-based policy-making (EBPM) to guide the selection and implementation of interventions and their evaluation. Second was the demand for more and better metrics to describe and compare in quantitative terms the scope of various global health problems and the interventions used to address them. Both trends were sector wide and had the effect of shifting research focus back towards the evaluation of targeted interventions rather than comprehensive analyses and strengthening of health systems which was roundly acknowledged as the key to ensuring safe motherhood (Storeng, 2010). 'Playing the numbers game' was a calculated advocacy strategy within the global maternal health community to reframe the problem of maternal mortality and its solutions in ways that would appeal to political decision makers and funders (Storeng & Béhague, 2014). Better quantitative data made the sheer magnitude of the problem of maternal mortality globally – and disparities between nations – into numbers that were hard to ignore.

Maternal mortality ratios and related indicators could also be deployed as a tool of accountability against governments (Adams, 2016; Wendland, 2016). The EBM paradigm already had caché in University-based research cultures and the lack of an evidence basis for much of obstetrics in high-income nations prior to this time added to the pressure to demonstrate the evidence basis for interventions into maternal health in global health settings (Campbell & Graham, 2006; Storeng, 2010). By taking up EBM and endorsing the pursuit of better metrics, the global maternal health advocacy community was able to legitimise and secure the profile of the cause on the global stage. In 2000 the reduction of maternal mortality was named as one of the Millennium Development Goals – but that same context, as Storeng and Béhague (2014) have argued lead to the 'technocratic narrowing' of the SMI in terms of the means by which the goal would be accomplished, tending strongly towards quick fixes and vertical interventions rather than comprehensive health systems improvements into which TBA-like providers might fit and where their contributions might be evaluated through research.

## *Flaws in the Original TBA Intervention*

Anthropologists had another critique of the policy shift: they argued that TBAs had not been properly understood in the first place and therefore were not deployed in ways that were appropriate or useful. As the TBA experiment under the auspices of the SMI unfolded, anthropologists researching midwifery and childbirth around the world were in the position to contribute evidence about the roles TBAs were already playing in various settings and what roles they could be expected to play in improving maternal health and reducing suffering and death. On the one hand, anthropologists had documented a vast range of practices and practitioners of birth – and yet they also tended to be in support of the idea of a category of person resembling the TBA. Variously called traditional midwives, parteras, matrones, community midwives, apprentice-trained midwives and many other local names, anthropologists generally sought to illuminate their contributions to maternal and infant health as well as social well-being (Cosminsky, 1977; Jordan, 1989; Laderman, 1983; Sargent, 1989).

Anthropologists were also in a position to contribute descriptive evidence about TBA training programmes and related interventions. Even before the launch of the SMI, Brigitte Jordan, for example, had described ineffective and inappropriate methods used in the training of Maya midwives in the Yucatan: didactic rather than hands-on learning, lack of cultural sensitivity by trainers towards *parteras* and no follow-up (1978). As the SMI got underway a decade later such critiques continued to surface. Carol MacCormack (1989) described how the SMI guidelines for identifying women to be trained as TBAs did not consider factors of ethnicity, caste, language, religion or kinship – which can often figure more significantly than training in the choice of a birth attendant. In my own work I have described the ill-fit between the scope of practice for TBAs imagined by global policy and local realities in Malawi where TBAs were assumed to be in the best position not only to catch babies but also to give prenatal care and contraceptive advice when in fact these tasks were neither traditional nor – in the case of dispensing contraceptive advice – appropriate to their scope of practice. Consequently, they refused to carry them out (MacDonald, 2017). Additionally, scholars noted that government ministries and NGOs often favoured training programmes for TBAs more for economic and political reasons than out of regard for traditional knowledge (Viisainen, 1992) and because trainings could be counted to demonstrate SMI activity regardless of the quality of the training or any outcomes it produced (AbouZahr, 2003). Thus, trainings were implemented in a 'selective' rather than 'comprehensive' way.

Some anthropologists called into question the very notion of a TBA. Stacy Leigh Pigg (1997), for example, noted that in Nepal there was no local equivalent of the TBA; the women who came forward to receive training under SMI programmes had no special clinical experience or expertise with childbirth; rather, they attended births as ritual specialists, while the maternal kin of the birthing women handled the labour and delivery. TBAs in Nepal, Pigg argues, had to be 'invented' to fit SMI activities and ultimately functioned in service of the development paradigm rather than in the lives of women and newborns. Denise Roth Allen observed something similar in Tanzania in Sukuma communities, in which many women gave birth with female relatives or alone and there was no distinct tradition of midwifery. By her reckoning one third of women trained as TBAs by a local SMI project that she studied in the 1990s had never attended a birth before. It is no wonder, she concludes, that local women perceived the newly designated TBAs as risks rather than assets and that the entire scheme failed to produce the results policymakers and programme planners had hoped for (1994, p. 115).

This body of anthropological research speaks to flaws in the original SMI policy and its implementation rather than the failure of TBAs to learn or practice in helpful ways. In sum, anthropological knowledge indicated the variability of birth culture and birth attendants around the world and thus the imperative of policies that could grapple with the particulars of a setting rather than the imposition (however well-intentioned) of an ideal model. What I call the 'universal TBA' (MacDonald, 2017) is an example of Olivier de Sardan et al.'s 'traveling model … developed by international experts and introduced in an almost identical format across numerous countries to improve some aspect of maternal health systems in low-and middle-income countries' (2016, p. 71). When confronted with actual contexts in which these standardised models are supposed to function, their argument continues, it results in 'drifts, distortions, dismemberments and bypasses' (2016, p. 71). The universal TBA, I suggest, also assumes a universal 'third world woman' (Mohanty, 1991) whom we are to assume prefers the TBA for reasons of culture and tradition, rather than as a rational assessment of risks presented by inexperienced and poorly trained birth attendants, on the one hand, and treacherous and costly trips to potentially understocked and understaffed health facilities, on the other.

The irony is that the SMI had tried to acknowledge and incorporate local systems of birth attendance rather than stamp them out. But the local imagined by the SMI was paradoxically too general; the TBA was imagined as a universal type. Not only did the focus on the universal characteristics of traditional birth attendants problematically essentialise roles for both childbearing women and birth attendants in diverse cultural settings, but the invention and implementation of the universal TBA had more insidious consequences as well. Women's inability or unwillingness to conform to roles designated for them by SMI policy was construed as their inability or unwillingness to modernise. A consequence of this traveling model not working to plan was that blame was cast not on the model itself, but on those who were meant to model it. Thus, TBAs came to be seen as obstacles to development – as vestiges of underdevelopment – for their failure to take on these new roles designated for them by SMI policy. In global health the notion of tradition as a 'cultural barrier' to change has often functioned as a stand-in for the decision-making processes of real people in constrained circumstances when their decisions do not resemble a biomedical itinerary. Anthropologist Didier Fassin (2012, p. 172) calls such explanations in humanitarian and development settings 'culturalist' arguments in which social facts are decontextualised and represented as timeless cultural traits – a way of thinking that bears resemblance to colonial ideas about racialised others as unmodern. Such 'static models' of culture also travel throughout health development thinking and policy.

## *The Global Political and Economic Context of the Safe Motherhood Initiative*

The Safe Motherhood Initiative and the activities that it set in motion all took place in steadily worsening economic times, including Structural Adjustment Programs (SAPs) imposed by the World Bank starting in the 1980s that limited the proportion of government spending on health in already debt-ridden nations (Chorev, 2013; Kim et al., 2002; Keshavjee, 2014). This context, in combination with the ascendency of a neoliberal ideology (which I discuss below), undermined the implementation of a comprehensive PHC model and promoted a model of selective primary health care. The result was the promotion of TBA training, without simultaneously developing professionalised midwifery and strengthening health systems to deliver emergency obstetric care. This meant that health infrastructures that were inadequate before the SMI were still inadequate or worse – understaffed, under resourced, without emergency transport or services (Clark, 2016). How could TBAs be expected to 'succeed' in such conditions? The introduction of user fees for primary care services, including maternity care, stemming from the Bamako Initiative may also have encouraged women to continue to seek care from TBAs in the community rather than from trained providers in the formal healthcare system, and to delay referrals (Dzakpasu et al., 2014).

To the extent that politics and economics were understood as factors in the lack of progress in the reduction of the MMR during the first decade of the SMI, it was not in terms of structural violence – Paul Farmer's adaptation of Johan Galtung's term which links the deeply historical and politically created worldwide system of inequality and exploitation to real effects on health today in that it structures basic access to food, clean water and health care (Farmer, 2004; Galtung, 1969; Keshavjee,

2014). Rather, the role of politics was understood in terms of the narrower and more tractable idea of 'political will' to acknowledge the problem of maternal mortality and to prioritise and direct resources to it. Lack of political will certainly was a problem for the Safe Motherhood Initiative during the first decade of its existence (Horton, 2010) and efforts in this area have paid off as the profile of the issue has risen significantly and policy and funding commitments by world leaders and major philanthropic organisations have been greatly scaled up (MacDonald, 2019; Shiffman & Smith, 2007; McDougall, 2016; Storeng, 2010). Thus, the problem of political will was (and has been) more successfully tackled than the problem of politics writ large and historically deep. But without a view (and critical analysis) of the bigger picture it was much easier to conclude that TBAs were simply unable or unwilling to fulfil the roles set out for them by the SMI.

The first decade of the SMI also coincided with the HIV/AIDS pandemic across the global south. Because HIV-infected pregnant women are at increased risk of dying during pregnancy and the postpartum period (Calvert & Ronsmans, 2013; Lathrop et al., 2014), the pandemic took a direct toll on the MMR in many countries. Moreover, caring for HIV/AIDS-affected family members exhausted domestic finances and care networks within families and communities making them less able to direct care and resources to maternal health. The tremendous burden of HIV/AIDS that fell on already weak healthcare systems in turn hampered the care of pregnant and labouring women.

Despite the impact of these forces within communities and on nations struggling to reduce maternal mortality, they did not figure in the dominant narrative of the first decade of the SMI in general, nor on how the TBA component specifically had fared. For example, Barbara Kwast, a Dutch midwife and research scientist in the Maternal and Child Health unit of the WHO in the 1980s and 1990s (1993) mentions briefly the burden of the HIV epidemic on midwives as workers in her keynote address to the 1993 meeting of the ICM in Vancouver but does not address the direct or indirect impact of HIV/AIDS on the lives and deaths of pregnant women. The link between safe motherhood and HIV was sometimes noted (Starrs, 2006) and later commentators chided the global maternal health community for the lack of attention to this relationship (Mataka, 2007), but it did not figure prominently in the analysis of the SMI.

## *A New Humanitarian Logic with no Room for the Figure of the Traditional Birth Attendant*

In the late 1990s, the Safe Motherhood movement underwent an internal reorganisation resulting in a new advocacy coalition and new set of donor partnerships including private corporations, bilateral aid organisations, universities and philanthropic foundations. Known as the Partnership for Safe Motherhood and Newborn Health, this new coalition was an expansion of the Inter Agency Group that had been in place since the launch of the SMI in 1987. The new Partnership diluted the authority of UN agencies, shifting some power to the private sector and made non-profit organisations responsive to a new set of expectations around evidence, programming and evaluation (McDougall, 2016; Storeng & Béhague, 2016). I have already spoken about the shift to the EBM paradigm in global health. In this section, I address how the rise in influence of private sector players through partnerships contributed to a distinct reframing of the problem of maternal mortality and its solutions in what may be described as 'neoliberal terms', that is, when the benefits of health and health care are understood in economic terms such that the goal of health is to enable citizens to optimise human productivity and economic development (Chorev, 2013). In the maternal health sector, the neoliberal turn in global health manifested in what I have called elsewhere the 'economization of maternal survival' (MacDonald, 2019, p. 266). Under this frame, the effort, time and money to address the problem of maternal mortality were argued as worthwhile not in terms of a moral response to human tragedy so much as an investment in the economic potential of women as individuals to contribute to their families, communities and nations (see also Murphy, 2017). Closely related to arguments about the importance of maternal health for economic development was the use of economic cost-effectiveness evidence to show that safe motherhood interventions were a good "global health buy" (Storeng & Behague, 2014, p. 10). As AbouZahr has commented in her review of the history of the SMI, to gain traction at the global level advocates had to tell 'a story of progress' (2001, p. 407). Traditional birth attendants, by their very name, were out of place in this reframing of maternal health as something that would be achieved by the modernisation of social policy and law and the transformation of women's subjectivity. Indeed, they were a barrier to appeals for wider engagement that investing in maternal health was an investment in the future.

Lori McDougall (2016) has observed how the global maternal health community began to cohere around this new shared policy agenda in the early 2000s, manifestly visible in the tag line for the most influential women's health and rights organisation in the world, Women Deliver: 'Invest in Girls and Women. It pays'. Realising the need to appeal to political and policy leaders and private donors in new ways, the global maternal health community was strategic in taking up this 'neoliberal turn' in which individual and collective health would be achieved through economic growth rather than direct government interventions in social, health or education.

Just prior to this reconfiguration into the Partnership, the Inter-Agency Group had undergone another change which also impacted its stance on the TBA question. In 1999 the IAG had expanded to include for the first time two professional associations: the International Confederation of Midwives and the International Federation of Obstetricians and Gynaecologist (FIGO); representatives from both associations had been present at the Technical Consultation in Colombo in 1997 when the policy shift had been made. The vignette with which I opened this chapter reveals the tensions within midwifery as an internationalising profession at this time which played out in the TBA debate. On the one hand, midwives were relative latecomers to the global policy table; despite the fact that they comprise the vast majority of skilled maternity care providers in the world, the midwifery profession had not up to this point been a major global policy player (Varney et al., 2004; MacDonald, 2005). Nor had their skills been recognised as essential to the reduction of maternal mortality in the policy documents of the 1970s and 1980s (Kruske & Barclay, 2004). The struggle for professional legitimacy on the global stage and at the highest level of global policy – a thoroughly biomedical space (Chorev, 2013) – lay in tension with the critique of medicalised childbirth by midwives in many jurisdictions, but especially Canada, the US and New Zealand where midwives had mounted campaigns for direct entry into the profession and advocated the safety of home birth and other non-interventionist approaches which mainstream medicine tended to oppose (Bourgeault, 2006; MacDonald, 2007). This was the landscape of the debate about the inclusiveness of the term midwifery which broke out at the ICM in Vienna in 2002, when some midwives present insisted that all women who attend births are midwives and in contrast to the ICM and national midwifery associations positions which aligned with the high level policy making process and the skilled attendant policy. These changes to the make-up and priorities of the global maternal health advocacy coalitions are part of the broader context of the TBA policy shift.

## Conclusion: The Return of the Traditional Birth Attendant?

Recently there have been calls for the 'return of the traditional birth attendant' in global maternal health, on the grounds that it makes practical and pragmatic sense not only as a last resort or stopgap measure when there is no trained or accessible personnel but also as a permanent feature of maternal health systems (Lane & Garrod, 2016; see also Byrne & Morgan, 2011; Prata et al., 2011). TBA-like providers are being re-positioned by such calls as part of the solution rather than as part of the problem and the range of tasks and roles (re)imagined for them is multiplying. Part of this conversation is being driven by research. The volume and disciplinary diversity of research on TBAs in terms of questions, methods and theoretical perspectives indicates that the evidence to evaluate the work of TBAs as part of health systems has been gaining traction over the last two decades even as TBAs were officially out of favour (See also Blanchard et al., 2019). Byrne and Morgan (2011), for example, have shown through a systematic review of the evidence that appropriate integration of traditional birth attendants within formal health systems as partners to skilled providers actually increases the use of skilled attendance rather than the other way around, as has often been asserted. Miller and Smith (2017) reviewed models by which TBAs can be partnered with skilled providers and attention be paid to local implementation factors required to ensure their success. TBAs did not disappear from communities with the policy shift to the skilled attendant, nor did research about them. Calls for their 'return' speak, in part, to the meaningful, evidence-based reintegration of TBAs into policy at the highest levels.

A key example of this policy return is the 2012 WHO guidelines on optimising health worker roles to improve access to key maternal and newborn health interventions. Known as the OptimizeMNH, these guidelines endeavour to tackle the issues of the global health worker crisis that are hampering improvements in rates of skilled attendance at births globally (WHO, 2012). Drawing on evidence that demonstrates their appropriate and effective utilisation of a number of skills normally reserved for higher level 'skilled' providers, such as the administration of misoprostol at births in the community for the prevention of postpartum haemorrhage, the authors conclude that trained TBAs 'can play an important role in improving maternal and newborn health' (WHO, 2012, p. 9; see also Colvin, 2021).

Does the growing evidence base, and the authority it lends high level guidelines such as the OptimizeMNH, signal the end of policy ambivalence regarding TBAs? Yes and no. TBA bans remain in place in many jurisdictions, and the problems that have long plagued the potentially helpful work of TBAs – lack of meaningful training and integration, lack of respect, lack of remuneration – remain. But perhaps it is fair to say that global level maternal health policy on TBAs is no longer in retreat; it appears that the conversation is changing. For example, the OptimizeMNH guidelines contain a number of noteworthy recommendations and rationales, some of which relate to the critiques I have presented in this chapter. First, the OptimizeMNH document imagines the participation of TBAs not as a stopgap measure until the healthcare worker shortage can be rectified and health facilities everywhere can be adequately staffed and stocked. Rather it recommends changes in the distribution of biomedical authority in a way that makes room for the permanent inclusion of community level health workers who specialise in pregnancy and birth care or accompaniment – whether they are called TBAs or not – to perform an expanding number of skills that can improve and even save the lives of women in pregnancy, childbirth and the postpartum. Second, we see in this document the language of equity in access to health care – an idea that was present in the original SMI that envisioned TBAs as providers who would extend and enable access to maternity care to underserved populations while maintaining safety (2012, p. 2). This idea has been held aloft in some significant corners of the scholarly debate about TBAs where the support and expansion of their roles has been described as an 'ethical imperative' in the absence of other options, and even in the presence of other options (Prata et al., 2011; Lane & Garrod, 2016).

It is also noteworthy that many of the skills being shifted to TBAs in these recommendations are enabled by another significant trend in global health: the new mandate for simple, high-impact and low-cost solutions that can function well in low resource settings. What anthropologist Tom Scott-Smith calls the 'innovation movement' (2016) in global health has given rise to many point-of-use technologies in reproductive and maternal health specifically, including portable hand-held ultrasound machines, anti-shock garments, cell phone apps to track antenatal care or screen for high blood pressure, and prefilled, single-use syringes for the delivery of long-acting reversible contraceptives (LARCs) as well as new protocols that allow for the use of pharmaceuticals such as misoprostol by community-level providers. These developments are notable for the way that they push the normative boundaries of authoritative knowledge and practice in biomedicine – and go hand in hand with the task shifting policies brought by the WHO (2008, 2014, 2015a, b). The case of misoprostol use by community level providers is a prime example of how point of use biomedical technologies can support task shifting (MacDonald, 2020). Another example is the growing use of cell phones by TBAs within local maternal health projects which research is beginning to show can improve antenatal attendance and referrals (Martinez et al., 2018), strengthen healthcare systems (Labrique et al., 2020) and enhance the mutual respect between TBAs and skilled providers (MacDonald & Diallo, 2019) – the lack of which Miller and Smith (2017) identify as an implementation barrier. The role of new technologies is also evident in the new WHO 'self-care' agenda for sexual and reproductive health and rights – launched in June 2019 – which also involves a decentring of the facility and professional health provider as the sole locus of clinical care (WHO, 2019) and the promotion of more evidence-based interventions that can be utilised by community-level providers and women themselves. There is a certain irony that high-tech innovations have been catalysts for the re-engagement of TBA-like providers in the goal of improving maternal health, when in the past it was the perception of their inability or refusal to modernise that helped push them so low on the policy agenda. It is important to note, however, that despite the techno optimism involved in this trend, the balance between safe care and 'self-care' in maternal health will have to be carefully worked out. Relatedly, careful attention to the concomitant scale-up of, and the inter-relationships between, community and facility-based MNCH services is also needed (see McCoy et al., 2010, p. 91).

The policy space of global maternal health in which the TBA is being reimagined and deployed as an asset to global maternal health has been informed and animated by an array of shifting players, evidence and ideas as well as innovations in biomedical and communications technology. Many challenges remain. For example, even as estimates from the WHO suggest that community health workers (CHWs) in maternal health roles fulfil 17 trillion dollars' worth of healthcare service a year, these workers are usually unpaid and often undervalued (Punjabi, 2019; see also Unnithan, 2021). Significant improvements in the delivery of maternal health care still needed in so many locales will not be realised by the return of the TBA, in any form, alone without health systems strengthening, a true reckoning with local context, greater understanding of and respect for women's choices of care giver and place of birth, and equity in access to quality maternal health care everywhere.

## References

AbouZahr, C. (2001). Cautious champions: International agency efforts to get safe motherhood onto the Agenda. *Studies in Health Services Organisation and Policy, 17*, 387–414.

AbouZahr, C. (2003). Safe motherhood a brief history of the global movement 1947–2002. *British Medical Bulletin, 67*, 13–25. https://doi.org/10.1093/bmb/ldg014

Adams, V. (Ed.) (2016). *Metrics. What counts in global health*. Durham, NC: Duke University Press.

Adegoke, A., & van den Broek, N. (2009). Skilled birth attendance-lessons learnt. *BJOG, 116*(Suppl. 1), 33–40. https://doi.org/10.1111/j.1471-0528.1009.02336.x

Allen, D. R. (1994). *Managing motherhood managing risk. Fertility and danger in West Central Tanzania*. University of Michigan Press.

Béhague, D., & Storeng, K. (2013). Pragmatic politics and epistemological diversity: The contested and authoritative uses of historical evidence in the Safe Motherhood Initiative. *Evidence and Policy, 9*(1), 65–85. https://doi.org/10.1111/j.1471-0528.1009.02336.x

Beihl, J. (2007). *Will to live. AIDS therapies and the politics of survival*. Princeton University Press.

Bergstrom, S., & Goodburn, E. (2001). The role of traditional birth attendants in the reduction of maternal mortality. In V. De Brouwere & W. Van Lerberghe (Eds.), *Safe Motherhood Strategies, A Review of the Evidence* (Studies in Health Services Organisation and Policy, 17) (pp. 77–96). ITG Press.

Blanchard, A. K., Prost, A., & Houweling, T. A. J. (2019). Effects of community health worker interventions on socioeconomic inequities in maternal and newborn health in low-income and middle-income countries: A mixed-methods systematic review. *BMJ Global Health, 4*, e001308. https://doi.org/10.1136/bmjgh-2018-001308

Bourgeault, I. L. (2006). *Push! The struggle for Midwifery in Ontario*. McGill-Queens University Press.

Byrne, A., & Morgan, A. (2011). How the integration of traditional birth attendants with formal health systems can increase skilled attendance. *International Journal of Gynecology and Obstetrics, 115*, 127–134. https://doi.org/10.1136/bmjgh-2018-001308

Calvert, C., & Ronsmans, C. (2013). The contribution of HIV to pregnancy-related mortality: A systematic review and meta-analysis. *AIDS, 27*(10), 1631–1639. https://doi.org/10.1097/QAS.0B013e32835fd940

Campbell, O., & Graham, W. (2006). Strategies for reducing maternal mortality. Getting on with what works. *Lancet, 368*, 1284–1289. https://doi.org/10.1016/50140-6736(06)69381-1

Campbell, O. M. R., Calvert, C., Testa, A. et al. (2016). The scale, scope, coverage, and capability of childbirth care. *Lancet, 388*(10056), 2193–2208.

Chorev, N. (2013). Restructuring neoliberalism at the World Health Organization. *Review of International Political Economy, 20*(4), 627–666. https://doi.org/10.1080/09692290.2012.690774

Clark, J. (2016). The global push for institutional childbirths—In unhygienic facilities. *BMJ, 352*, i1473. https://doi.org/10.1136/bmj.i1473

Colvin, C. J. (2021). Making space for qualitative evidence in global maternal and child health policy-making. In L. J. Wallace, M. E. MacDonald, & K. T. Storeng (Eds.), *Anthropologies of global maternal and reproductive health*. Springer.

Cosminsky, S. (1977). Childbirth and Midwifery on a Guatemalan Finca. *Medical Anthropology, 6*(3), 69–04. https://doi.org/10.1080/01459740.1977.9965825

De Brouwere, V., Tonglet, R., & van Lerberghe, W. (1998). Strategies for reducing maternal mortality in developing countries: What can we learn from the history of the industrialized West? *Trop Med Int Health, 3*, 771–782. https://doi.org/10.1046/j.1365-3156.1998.00310.x

Dzakpasu, S., Powell-Jackson, T., & Campbell, O. M. R. (2014). Impact of user fees on maternal health service utilization and related health outcomes: A systematic review. *Health Policy and Planning, 29*(2), 137–150. https://doi.org/10.1093/heapol/czs142

Eades, C. A., Braçe, C., Osei, L., & LaGuiardia, K. D. (1993). Traditional birth and maternal mortality in Ghana. *Social Science and Medicine, 36*, 1503–1507. https://doi.org/10.1016/0277-9536(93)90392-H

Farmer, P. (2004). An anthropology of structural violence. *Current Anthropology, 45*(3), 305–325. https://doi.org/10.1086/382250

Fassin, D. (2012). *Humanitarian Reason. A moral history of the present*. University of California Press.

Galtung, J. (1969). Violence, peace, and peace research. *Journal of Peace Research, 6*, 167–191. https://doi.org/10.1177/002234336900600301

Gilson, L. (Ed.). (2012). *Health policy and systems research. A methodology reader*. The World Health Organization.

Haruna, U., Kansanga, M. M., & Galaa, S. (2019). Examining the unresolved conundrum of Traditional Birth Attendants' involvement in maternal and child health care delivery in Ghana. *Health Care for Women International, 40*(12), 1336–1354.
Horton, R. (2010). Maternal mortality: Surprise, hope, and urgent action. *The Lancet, 375*, 1581–1852. https://doi.org/10.1016/50140-6736(10)60547-8
International Confederation of Midwives. (2005). *International definition of the midwife*. International Confederation of Midwives.
Jordan, B. (1989). Cosmopolitan obstetrics: Some notes on the training of traditional midwives. *Social Science and Medicine, 28*(9), 925–937. https://doi.org/10.1016/0277-9536(89)90317-1
Keshavjee, S. (2014). *Blind Spot. How Neoliberalism infiltrated global health*. University of California Press.
Kidney, E., et al. (2009). Systematic review of effect of community-level interventions to reduce maternal mortality. *BMC Pregnancy Childbirth, 9*, 2. https://doi.org/10.1186/1471-2393-9-2
Kim, J. K., Gershman, J., Irwin, A., & Millen, J. V. (Eds.). (2002). *Dying for growth. Global inequality and the health of the poor*. Common Courage Press.
Kruske, S., & Barclay, L. (2004). Effect of shifting policies on traditional birth attendant training. *Journal of Midwifery and Women's Health, 49*(4), 306–311. https://doi.org/10.1016/jmwh.2004.01.005
Kwast, B. (1993). Safe Motherhood – The first decade. Address to the International Confederation of Midwives Congress. *Midwifery, 9*, 105–123.
Labrique, A., Agarwal, S., Tamrat, T. et al. (2020). WHO Digital Health Guidelines: A milestone for global health. *NPJ Digital Medicine, 3*, 120. https://doi.org/10.1038/s41746-020-00330-2
Laderman, C. (1983). *Wives and Midwives*. University of California Press.
Lane, K., & Garrod, J. (2016). The return of the traditional birth attendant. *Journal of Global Health, 6*(2), 020302. https://doi.org/10.7189/jogh.06.020302
Lathrop, E., Jamieson, D., & Daniel, I. (2014). HIV and maternal mortality. *International Journal of Gynaecology and Obstetrics, 127*(2), 213–215. https://doi.org/10.7189/jogh.06.020302
Loudon, I. (1992). *Death in childbirth: An international study of maternal care and maternal mortality, 1800–1950*. Clarendon Press. https://doi.org/10.1093/acprof:oso/9780198229971.001.0001
MacCormack, C. (1989). Status and training of traditional Midwives. *Social Science and Medicine, 28*(9), 941–943. https://doi.org/10.1016/0277-9536(89)90322-5
MacDonald, M. (2005). *Midwifery on the International stage: The Role of the International Confederation of Midwives in International Reproductive Health Initiatives*. The International Workshop on Comparative Research on the Professions. McMaster University, April 29–30.
MacDonald, M. (2007). *At work in the field of birth: Midwifery narratives of nature, tradition and home*. Vanderbilt University Press.
MacDonald, M. (2017). Why ethnography matters in global health. *Journal of Global Health, 7*(2), 1–4. https://doi.org/10.7189/jogh.07.020302
MacDonald, M. (2019). The Image World of Maternal Mortality: Visual economies of hope and aspiration in global campaigns to reduce maternal mortality. *Humanity: A Journal of Human Rights, Humanitarianism, and Development, 10*(2), 263–285. https://doi.org/10.1353/hum.2019.0013
MacDonald, M. (2020). Misoprostol: The life story of a life-saving drug. *Science, Technology & Human Values*. (1–26). https://doi.org/10.1177/0162243920916781
MacDonald, M., & Diallo, G. S. (2019). Socio cultural contextual factors of an health application to improve maternal health in Senegal. *BMC Reproductive Health, 16*, 141. https://doi.org/10.1186/s12978-019-0800-z2017
Mangay Maglacas, A., & Simons (Eds.). (1986). *The potential of the traditional birth attendant* (WHO Offset publication no. 95). World Health Organization.
Martinez, B., et al. (2018). MHealth intervention to improve the continuum of maternal and perinatal care in rural Guatemala: A pragmatic, randomized controlled feasibility trial. *Reproductive Health, 15*, 120. https://doi.org/10.1186/s12978-018-0554-z

Mataka, E. (2007). Maternal Health and HIV: Bridging the gap. *The Lancet, 370*(9595), 1290–1291. https://doi.org/10.1016/50140-6736(07)61552-9
McCoy, D., et al. (2010). Maternal, neonatal and child health interventions and services: Moving from knowledge of what works to systems that deliver. *International Health, 2*, 87–98. https://doi.org/10.1016/j.inhe.2010.03.005
McDougall, L. (2016). Discourse, ideas and power in global health policy networks: Political attention for maternal and child health in the Millennium Development goals era. *Globalization and Health, 12*, 21. https://doi.org/10.1186/s12992-016-0157-9
Miller, T., & Smith, H. (2017). Establishing partnership with traditional birth attendants for improved maternal and newborn health: A review of factors influencing implementation. *BMC Pregnancy and Childbirth, 17*, 365.
Mohanty, C. T. (1991). Under Western eyes. Feminist scholarship and colonial discourse. In A. Russo & L. Torres (Eds.), *Third World Women and the politics of Feminism* (pp. 51–80). Indiana University Press.
Murigi, S., & Ford, L. (2010). Should Uganda ban traditional birth attendants? *The Guardian*. https://www.theguardian.com/katine/katine-chronicles-blog/2010/mar/30/traditional-birth-attendants-ban. Accessed 29 Apr 2019.
Murphy, M. (2017). *The Economization of Life*. Durham, NC: Duke University Press.
O'Rourke, K. (1995). The effect of hospital staff training on management of obstetrical patients referred by traditional birth attendants. *International Journal of Gynaecology and Obstetrics, 48*(Suppl), S95–S102. https://doi.org/10.1016/0020-7292(95)02324
Olivier de Sardan, J. P., Diarra, A., & Moha, M. (2016). Travelling models and the challenge of pragmatic contexts and practical norms: The case of maternal health. *Health Research Policy and Systems, 15*(Suppl 1), 60. https://doi.org/10.1186/s12961-017-0213-9
Pigg, S. L. (1997). Authority in translation: Finding, knowing and naming traditional birth attendants in Nepal. In R. Davis-Floyd & C. Sargent (Eds.), *Childbirth and authoritative knowledge* (pp. 233–262). University of California Press.
Prata, N., Passano, P., Rowen, T., Bell, S., Walsh, J., & Potts, M. (2011). Where there are (Few) skilled birth attendants. *Journal of Health, Population and Nutrition, 29*(2), 81–89. https://doi.org/10.3329/jhpn.v29i2.7812
Punjabi, R. (2019). Why governments should be paying community health workers. *Time*, (Oct 24).
Rudrum, S. (2016). TBAs in rural Northern Uganda: Policy, practice and ethics. *Health Care for Women International, 37*(2), 250–269. https://doi.org/10.1080/07399332.2015.1020539
Safe Motherhood Interagency Group. (2002). *Skilled care during childbirth*. Family Care International.
Sargent, C. (1989). *Maternity, medicine, and power: Reproductive decisions in Urban Benin*. University of California Press.
Scott-Smith, T. (2016). Humanitarian neophilia: The 'innovation turn' and its implications. *Third World Quarterly, 37*(12), 2229–2251. https://doi.org/10.1080/01436597.2016.1176856
Sheikh, K., Gilson, L., Agyepong, I. A., Hanson, K., Ssengooba, F., & Bennett, S. (2011). Building the field of health policy and systems research: Framing the questions. *PLoS Med, 8*(8), e1001073. https://doi.org/10.1371/journal.pmed.1001073
Shiffman, J., & Smith, S. (2007). Generation of political priority for global health initiatives: A framework and case study of maternal mortality. *The Lancet, 370*, 1370–1379. https://doi.org/10.1016/S0140-6736(07)61579-7
Sibley, L., & Sipe, T. A. (2006). Transition to skilled birth attendance: Is there a future role for trained traditional birth attendants? *Journal of Health Population and Nutrition, 24*(4), 472–478. https://doi.org/10.1016/j.socscimed.2004.02.009
Sibley, L., Sipe, T. A., & Koblinsky, M. (2004). Does traditional birth attendant training improve referral for women with obstetric complications? A review of the evidence. *Social Science and Medicine, 59*(8), 1757–1768. https://doi.org/10.1016/j.socscimed.2004.02.009

Starrs, A. (1987). *Preventing the tragedy of maternal deaths. A report on the international safe motherhood conference*. World Bank, World Health Organization and United Nations Population Fund.
Starrs, A. (1997). *The safe motherhood action Agenda: Priorities for the next decade*. Family Care International and the Inter-Agency Group for Safe Motherhood.
Starrs, A. (2006). Safe motherhood initiative: 20 years and counting. *Lancet, 368*, 1130–1132. https://doi.org/10.1016/S0140-6736(06)69385-9
Storeng, K. (2010). *Safe Motherhood: The making of a global health initiative*. PhD Thesis London School of Hygiene and Tropical Medicine.
Storeng, K., & Béhague, D. (2014). 'Playing the numbers game.' Evidence based advocacy and the technocratic narrowing of the safe motherhood initiative. *Medical Anthropology Quarterly, 28*(2), 260–279. https://doi.org/10.1111/maw.12072
Storeng, K., & Béhague, D. (2016). "Lives in the balance": The politics of integration in the partnership for maternal, newborn and child health. *Health Policy and Planning, 31*, 992–1000. https://doi.org/10.1093/heapol/czw023
Unnithan, M. (2021). Conflicted reproductive governance: The co-existence of rights-based approaches and Coercion in India's family planning policies. In L. J. Wallace, M. E. MacDonald, & K. T. Storeng (Eds.), *Anthropologies of global maternal and reproductive health*. Springer.
Van Lerberghe, W., & De Brouwere, V. (2000). Of blind alleys and things that have worked: History's lessons on reducing maternal mortality. *Studies in Health Services Organisation and Policy, 17*, 7–34.
Varney, H., Kriebs, J. M., & Gegor, C. L. (Eds.) (2004). *Varney's Midwifery*. Fourth Edition. Jones and Bartlett Publishers.
Verderese, M., & Turnbull, L. (1975). *The traditional birth attendant in maternal and child health and family planning: A guide to her training and utilization*. World Health Organization.
Viisainen, K. (1992). *Nicaraguan Midwives: The integration of indigenous practitioners into official health care*. University of Helsinki Institute of Development Studies.
Walt, G., Lush, L., & Ogden, J. (2004). International organisations in transfer of infectious diseases: Iterative loops of adoption, adaptation, and marketing. *Governance: International Journal of Policy, Administration, and Institutions, 17*(2), 189–210. https://doi.org/10.1110/j.1468-0491.2004.00243.x
Wendland, C. (2016). Estimating Death. A close reading of maternal mortality metrics in Malawi. In V. Adams (Ed.) *Metrics. What counts in global health* (p. 57–81). Duke University Press.
Whitaker, K. (2012). Is Sierra Leone right to ban traditional birth attendants? *The Guardian*. https://www.theguardian.com/global-development/poverty-matters/2012/jan/17/traditional-birth-attendants-sierra-leone). Accessed 29 Apr 2019.
World Health Organization. (1978). *Alma Ata Declaration*. WHO.
World Health Organization. (1979). *Traditional birth attendants: A field guide to their training, evaluation and articulation with health services* (WHO offset publication 44). WHO.
World Health Organization. (1985). *Report of the consultation on approaches for policy development for traditional health practitioners, including traditional birth attendants*. WHO.
World Health Organization. (1994). *Mother-baby package. Implementing safe motherhood in countries, a practical guide* (Maternal Health and Safe Motherhood Program. Division of Family Health). WHO.
World Health Organization. (2004). *Making pregnancy safer: The critical role of the skilled attendant. A joint statement by WHO, ICM and FIGO*. WHO.
World Health Organization. (2005). *The World Health Report: Making every mother and every child count*. WHO.
World Health Organization. (2008). *Task Shifting. Rational redistribution of task among health workforce teams. Global Recommendations and Guidelines*. WHO.
World Health Organization. (2012). *WHO Recommendations – Optimize MNH: Optimizing health worker roles for maternal and newborn health interventions through task shifting*. WHO. http://apps.who.int/iris/bitstream/10665/77764/1/9789241504843_eng.pdf. Accessed 25 May 2015

World Health Organization. (2014). *Using auxiliary nurse midwives to improve access to key maternal newborn health interventions*. WHO.

World Health Organization. (2015a). *WHO recommendation on partnership with traditional birth attendants (TBAs)*. WHO.

World Health Organization. (2015b). *WHO recommendations on health promotion interventions for maternal and newborn health*. WHO. https://www.ncbi.nlm.nih.gov/books/NBK304983/. Accessed 20 Apr 2017.

World Health Organization. (2019). *Self-Care Agenda*, launching June 24 2019. https://www.bmj.com/selfcare-srhr. Accessed 7 June 2019.

# Chapter 7
# Conflicted Reproductive Governance: The Co-existence of Rights-Based Approaches and Coercion in India's Family Planning Policies

**Maya Unnithan**

## Introduction

The late 1990s saw a shift in the implementation of Indian health and population policies from a focus on fertility control in its Family Planning programme towards a rights-based and choice- and participation-oriented Reproductive Health approach. On the ground, in everyday contexts of service provision, this meant an abolition of 'targets' (numbers of women to be sterilised monthly and annually) set by the state for community health workers. On the face of it, the adoption of a 'target-free approach' relaxed state surveillance of poor pregnant women and released health workers from the burden of achieving a set number of cases over a specified period, a regulatory mechanism through which they were held to account (Ramasubban & Jejheebhoy, 2000; Visaria, 2000). Instead of actively pursuing tubectomy cases, staff at health centres and sub-centres were to focus instead on the provision of a choice of contraceptive options, offering reversible methods (condoms, pills, intra-uterine devices) alongside sterilisation. Popularly known in health policy parlance as the 'cafeteria approach' to contraception (GOI, 2007), the practice came to symbolise the significant shift from a population to a people-centred policy approach to maternal and reproductive health.

In this chapter I examine the processes, contradictions and outcomes that accompanied such a critical and important shift in population policy and what this reveals about the dynamics of reproductive governance in India. I build on the concept of reproductive governance as the 'subject making powers of moral regimes directed towards reproductive behaviours and practices' (Morgan & Roberts, 2012, p. 244) in the context of the Indian state's long embrace of rights-based, empowerment approaches in its development practice. Drawing on ethnographic work on maternal

M. Unnithan (✉)
Department of Anthropology, University of Sussex, Sussex, UK
e-mail: M.unnithan@sussex.ac.uk

 
L. J. Wallace et al. (eds.), *Anthropologies of Global Maternal and Reproductive Health*, Global Maternal and Child Health, https://doi.org/10.1007/978-3-030-84514-8_7

and reproductive health in the state of Rajasthan in Northwest India from 1998 to the present, and more recently with policy makers, health professionals and NGOs, I suggest that the discourse of rights in the area of maternal and reproductive health speaks more to processes of State empowerment than to enhancing reproductive autonomy among claimants on-the-ground. Participatory forms of policymaking and rights discourse have instead helped to transform the State itself into an 'activist' institution in terms of its modus operandi and rights advocacy work (Biehl, 2004; Unnithan, 2019; Unnithan & Heitmeyer, 2014).[1]

The main policy focus in the chapter is India's axiomatic National Population Policy (NPP) of 2000 (GOI, 2000), which is examined alongside a set of reproductive and child health policies in India (RCH-I and RCH-II) implemented between 1997 and 2005, and the policy of Safe Motherhood (*Janani Suraksha*) actioned under the National Rural Heath Mission (NRHM) of 2005. Drawing on intersectional, feminist and Foucauldian analysis in the domain of population governance (Greenhalgh, 2005; Morgan & Roberts, 2012; Ram, 2001; Das, 2015; De Zordo, 2012; Dean, 2001; Gupta, 2001), I suggest that the simultaneous promotion of two conflicting approaches to governance within the same NPP policy may stem from a broader dilemma that faces modern states 'doing' development (Hanson & Stepputat, 2001). It may also stem from a more particular concern of well-being and reproductive choice in policymaking at the end of the second millennium in India.

Policy in an anthropological sense is regarded as a field that is constituted by performative social practices of regulation which are both created by and 'create particular social and cultural worlds' (Shore et al., 2011). These have a 'domaining effect' and are agentive in that they shift action (Wright, 2011, p. 27). I also regard policy through an affective lens and a Critical Medical Anthropology (or CMA) approach to health policy. Such an approach regards policy formation and enforcement 'as reflecting simultaneously the compromise between, as well as the balancing of power among, conflicted forces (social groups with different and opposed interests)' (Singer & Castro, 2004, p. xiv).

Policymaking as a *contextual* practice is developed in the chapter through the policy perspectives of community health workers, health professionals (doctors, clinicians, public health specialists) and policy makers (bureaucrats, prominent civil society actors, lawyers and politicians). Policy guidelines and programme reports have enabled analysis of the embedded hierarchies and power at play in practices of health governance. Analysis of these documents reveals a *return* to previous coercive (in terms of restricted choice) family planning policies, even as the language of human rights frames the overall approach. The only difference is that the language of coercion is more implicit and less overt than in the previous family planning policies of the 1970s, a pre-rights-based policy era. I use the term 'coercive' to mean 'choice restrictive' in the sense that policies which may or may not intend to be coercive are those where, in practice, choice is restricted (also see Brunson, 2019;

[1] I use the word 'state' to denote regional states in India, and the term 'State' to mean the central authority ruling a sovereign territory.

Senderowicz, 2019). I also suggest that contraceptive coercion, as Senderowicz argues, 'sits on a spectrum and need not involve overt force or violence but can also result from more quotidian limits to free, full and informed choice' (2019, p. 1).

Despite current, ostensible state withdrawal from an explicit promotion of sterilisation (especially tubectomies for women), it is a practice that is promoted on the ground with some poorer women and couples who have met their childbearing aspirations continuing to use the method. However, I argue that the reasons for this uptake are very different from those which policy makers envision. Examining the factors underlying the local reproductive behaviour that shapes health worker practices as well as some women's preference for tubectomies provides key insight into the exercise of reproductive choice as simultaneously supporting and resisting government control. These observations lead me to suggest that the substitution of an existing bio-politics of population control with a bio-politics of the 'self', aimed at enhancing individual choice and personal autonomy (de Zordo, 2012) is not as clear-cut as imagined by policy makers in India (Unnithan, 2019).

## A Note on Methods

The chapter is an outcome of discussions and reflection on several previous periods of ethnographic work. During the first period (1998–1999), I gathered data on the reproductive journeys of over 50 members of a peri-urban Muslim community and urban *basti* dwellers in Jaipur city, with a further focus on emotion and agency in contraceptive practices and recourse to sterilisation (2000–2006). Between 2009 and 2012, I participated in collaborative research with members of 34 civil society groups in Rajasthan. This included consultation with over 55 individuals from a range of policy-engaged civil society organisations (henceforth CSO) members and state and regional health and family planning policy members working on promoting (and challenging) rights-based maternal and reproductive health policies (Unnithan et al., 2010). During a further period of fieldwork in 2015 and with local field assistance, I conducted semi-structured interviews and life-histories with 12 newly formed Accredited Social Health Activist (ASHA) health workers in Jaipur district. The chapter also draws on my analysis of national and regional health and family welfare policy documents (GOI, 2000, 2006, 2007). Recent informal discussion (2017–2019) with members of civil liberty, legal professional and rights-based organisations as well as university academics has also informed the ideas in this chapter.

In the next section, I elaborate on the conceptual approaches which underpin the observations made in this chapter. The section following that explains the policy rationale underlying the simultaneous roll out of conflicting reproductive objectives within the latest Indian family planning policy. The final sections explore the effects of these policies in-situ through the work of local health workers and the conflicted governance practices of the Indian State.

## *The Anthropology of the State and Reproductive Governance*

Anthropological analysis of the cultural processes through which the state is 'instantiated' and experienced has shown how it is an entity which is less coherent and more fragmentary than imagined (Sharma & Gupta, 2006, p. 11). With the increasing pervasiveness of rights-based advocacy in global health, CSO members who have established expertise of operationalising rights-based ideas and language in their maternal and reproductive health programmes have become increasingly valued in national level policy working groups. This has led to the co-construction of the rights-based parts of State policy documents by policy makers, bureaucrats and members of leading CSOs.

Conceptualising the state as a 'dispersed ensemble of institutional practices and techniques of governance' (Hanson & Stepputat, 2001, p. 14) and governmentality as 'beyond the state' (Foucault, 1998; Dean, 2001; Gupta, 2001), offers two profound insights when applied to the processes of reproductive health policymaking in India. First, it suggests the potential for multiple practices of State policymaking to co-exist, and second, to realise that the co-creation of policy occurs across different state and non-state actors. Hanson and Stepputat (2001) trace the simultaneous execution of competing policies to the increasingly challenging conditions under which modern states function: where their authority is constantly being called into question through global markets, separatist movements and ethnic conflicts, on the one hand, but equally where the state is being framed as indispensable to global efforts, for instance, to deliver development programmes effectively or promote a human rights culture and through which new modalities of governance emerge. As I argue later, this is clearly the case in India's population policy, which is situated between two conflicting discourses of population management: The first is governed by a demographic rationale that advocates strict State regulation of fertility. The second has a rights-based rationale that promotes individual reproductive choice and bodily autonomy. The Indian population policy is at the same time a technique of *reproductive* governance, which Morgan and Roberts regard as:

> ...the mechanisms through which different historical configurations of actors – such as state, religious, and international financial institutions, NGOs, and social movements – use legislative controls, economic inducements, moral injunctions, direct coercion, and ethical incitements to produce, monitor, and control reproductive behaviours and population practices (2012, p. 241).

Anthropological scholarship on reproduction, in addition, provides critical understanding of family planning policies as part of broader processes, especially those concerned with State projects of modernity and citizen-making. It is useful to delineate three kinds of narratives and related concepts that emerge within this approach which are resonant with policymaking around family planning in India. First, a dominant narrative identified in anthropological studies of family planning policymaking in high population, 'developing' country contexts is about 'becoming modern' and achieving economic growth through curtailing demographic expansion (a rationale driven by the classic demographic transition theory; Greenhalgh, 1995).

Anti-natal State population policies in India and China, for example, are primarily framed through a narrative of progress whereby modern citizens are produced (Greenhalgh, 2005; Chen, 2011; Anagost, 1995; Van Hollen, 2003; Ram, 2001). Such policies work by attributing value to specific kinds of populations (rural, poor and so on) whose members become subjects to be modernised. They also objectify women by defining them primarily through their reproduction (Ram, 2001; Brunson, 2016). However, individuals within specific social groups/classes, including women community health workers such as the ASHA (Accredited Social Health Activist) described in this chapter, differ in the extent to which they partake in such projects deemed to be of national importance (also Anagost, 1995; Kanaaneh, 2002; Mishra, 2014). People do not necessarily follow state directives or take up family planning incentives without paying heed to their own agendas for social reproduction (Kanaaneh, 2002; Varley, 2012).

A second important narrative in anthropological work on family planning is of the pervasiveness of neoliberalism and market economics within health policy discourse. This economic thinking in public health policy is reflected best in India in the embrace of privatisation as an effective mechanism in the delivery of public health care (Qadeer & Viswanathan, 2004; Roalkvam, 2014, among others). Private services may often be popular precisely because they are presented as caring not coercive (Chen, 2011). Indian population policies, as Qadeer and Viswanathan (2004) argue, have supported the privatisation of public health care guided by the principle that private care is more cost-effective, efficient and of better quality compared to public services. Policymakers consider state provision of monetary incentives and linked penalties (such as the exclusion from standing from political office) linked to contraceptive uptake as an effective means to regulate family size (the 'small family norm'; Das & Uppal, 2012).

A third perspective in the anthropological literature on family planning is that of morality, affect and the role that emotions such as desire and fear play in the internalisation (in a Foucauldian sense) of the missives of family planning programmes, both by the health workers tasked with implementing the policies and those targeted by them. More broadly, these perspectives speak to (a lack of) power and notions of stratified reproduction – where the fertility of some individuals and classes is more highly valued than others (Ginsburg & Rapp, 1995; Unnithan, 2019).

Next, I analyse how each of these perspectives is also critical to framing Indian family planning policies before returning to examine their embodiment within health-worker practices.

## *India's Family Planning and Underlying Policy Rationale*

India is hailed in global health policy and planning circles as the first country to have instituted a family planning programme in 1952 and has several policy documents and draft policy statements setting out its population programmes, especially between 1976 and 2000. The Indian National Population Policy (NPP) 2000 (GOI,

2000), the final and most comprehensive policy to date, is a landmark document which is connected to policy thinking about family planning. Here, I examine the policy framework approved by parliament in 1999, developed over the previous decade alongside critiques of earlier reproductive health programmes and policies in the run up to the International Conference on Population and Development in Cairo in 1994, and its projection forward into the rights-based policies of the National Health Mission in 2005.

The Indian National Population Policy (NPP) 2000 provides a policy framework for advancing the goals and strategies from 2000 to 2010 (and now till 2026) suggesting that family planning be carried out to the '*extent necessary*' for reducing birth rates to stabilise population at a level consistent with the requirement of the national economy and replacement levels of the 'Total Fertility Rate' or 'TFR' (GOI, 2000, p. 2; emphasis added).[2] At the same time, the NPP is distinctive from previous policy statements on family planning in its use of the language of choice and consent and the explicit removal of the aggressive pursuit of family planning 'targets'. In its opening statement, the NPP affirms the commitment of the government towards the twin goals of a '*voluntary and informed choice and consent of citizens* while availing of reproductive healthcare services, and the *continuation of a target-free approach* in administering family planning services' (NPP 2002 ibid.; emphasis added), explicitly referring to the removal of sterilisation targets for health workers. I use the word 'target' in the specific context of sterilisation as it was referred to in policy documents and in conversations with health workers.

The policy is set out with three time-bound objectives in mind: (i) an immediate goal of addressing unmet needs for contraception[3]; (ii) a medium term objective of bringing the TFR down to replacement levels by 2010; and (iii) a longer term goal of stabilising population growth by 2045 at a level consistent with the requirements of sustainable economic growth, social development and environmental protection. It was deemed imperative that the small family norm be adopted by the reproductive age group 'without delay or exception' given that 45% of the population increase was due to births of over 2 children per family.

The NPP recognised three causes for the high fertility rates: first an 'unmet need for contraception' as approximately half of the population in their reproductive years were not protected; second high levels of infant mortality, which it was deemed increased the desire for having more children (referred to as 'wanted fertility'); third, the high numbers of marriages taking place under 18 years (and births with intervals of less than 24 months) was another factor which was regarded as contributing to high levels of fertility.

As it is set out, the policy demonstrates a desire to reduce population numbers in order to enhance the benefits of economic growth, but equally shows concern for the

[2] The Total Fertility Rate or TFR is defined in the document as the average number of children born to a woman during her lifetime.

[3] The 'unmet need for contraception' is a problematic metric which in the context of global health discourse often serves to exclude health subjectivities and everyday experiences (Storeng & Béhague, 2017; Das, 2015; Unnithan, 2019).

welfare (health and well-being) of the population, especially mothers and children in a context of high maternal and child mortality. The underlying family planning policy rationale in India, as in other high population, high mortality settings, is driven by the public health perspective of maternal risk. Here, risk is conceptualised as the risk to the life of the mother and accompanied by statistics which demonstrate that contraceptive use has the potential to reduce maternal deaths (also Storeng & Béhague, 2017; Brunson, 2019). The World Health Organization (WHO), for example, suggests that in 2017, contraceptive use prevented approximately 308 million unintended pregnancies in developing countries and the need for unsafe abortion. Public health literature underscores the significance of using reversible methods in contexts where birth intervals (spacing) between children are less than 3 years as mothers and infants are more prone to a higher risk of death in this instance (WHO ibid).

Thus, pursuing a family planning policy becomes an example of a practice of 'good government' by which the State not only exercises authority over its citizens but also sees itself as fostering their health and happiness – much in the same way as Gupta notes for the *anganwadi* creche programmes focused on improving child nutrition (2001, p. 66). India's attention to the welfare of its population is an example of 'governmentality' (in Foucault's sense), where modes of government are not necessarily parts of state apparatus (Gupta, 2001, p. 67). It is the 'welfare' aspect, conceived as health benefits that the spacing of children confers on married women, which has provided the underlying rationale for Family Planning since the start of official health planning in the 1950s. This logic can be traced back to the concerns of the colonial state and medical establishments about high levels of maternal mortality and the health of poor Indian women who were most prone through malnutrition and anaemia to maternal complications (Arnold, 2006; Hodges, 2006). It was thought that poor women's health would improve substantially when their fertility was controlled. The provision of contraceptives would empower poor women to practice spacing and would bring them relief from constant childbearing and related physical exhaustion.

Ideas about 'fertility control as beneficial to women's health' emerge within the colonial period and take hold within the closing years of the British rule as set out by the Bhore committee report of 1946 which was regarded as the first health 'policy' in terms of its recommendations (Government of India & Ministry of Health and Family Welfare, n.d.). Some of this early thinking around fertility and women's health is evident in India's first family planning programmes from 1952 onwards (Jeffrey & Jeffrey, 1997). It is, as feminists have argued, a population control approach that views women as 'potential contraceptors' or 'producers of too many babies' rather than as individuals whose health is of inherent…' value (Lane, 1994, p. 1303). The instrumentalist view of women as reproducing machines was taken to task in the deliberations on the rights approach to reproductive health at the International Conference on Population and Development at Cairo in 1994 (UNFPA, 2004, 2008) to which India was signatory and to which the NPP policy is formulated in response.

A key strategy outlined in India's National Planning Policy 2000 for making the State more accountable to women's welfare was a devolution away from responsibility of individual states for delivering family welfare programmes. Instead, political and health functionaries and structures at the village level (namely *panchayats* or village councils and sub- and primary health centres) would deliver such programmes. Decentralisation intended to 'strengthen, energise and make accountable' the first points of contact in the health system (2002, p. 7). Two further strategies were notable: (i) to collaborate with NGOs in the private sector (especially where government interventions were deemed to be insufficient) in a complementary manner, and (ii) to bring in legislation which would support the process. It was with the latter in mind that the 42nd constitutional amendment Act 1976 was enacted in 2000, freezing the number of parliamentary seats until 2026 so that state governments could 'effectively and fearlessly pursue the agenda for population stabilisation' (2002, p. 16).

The 'strategic themes' as laid out earlier in the NPP 2000 were accompanied by a set of motivational measures for the adoption of a small family norm. No similar measures are mentioned to ensure the exercise of rights-based choices. For example, village councils and their leaders were rewarded and honoured for 'exemplary performance' in universalising the small family norm. Poorer couples, who were the focus of the programme, gained health insurance and cash benefits if they had only two children and chose to go in for sterilisation (GOI, NPP, 2000). Community health workers were valorised for their motivational work in the uptake of family planning and institutional deliveries. Before we turn to explore how local ASHA health workers embodied their motivational work in the next section, it is important to track the narrative of choice and reproductive rights within family planning policymaking.

## Tracking Rights-Based Ideas in Family Planning

Modern Indian health-planning history from the 1950s, as we saw earlier, begins with an emphasis on population control and contraception as urgent and invested with national importance. With the seductive notion that 'contraception was the best form of development', individual rights and choices with regard to childbearing quickly came to be regarded as secondary to the 'human rights of the nation' (public address of Congress Prime Minister Indira Gandhi on Indian's family planning programme; Dhanraj, *Something like a War* 2011(1991)). Following the family planning atrocities committed during her political reign, the mid to late 1980s in India became a time of popular dissent against the failure of the state more broadly, but also against the failure to meet women's reproductive rights and related health needs. Activists and feminist organisations particularly highlighted the malpractices and unethical conduct of health workers, who were subjected to sterilisation targets to carry out coercive birth control strategies (Ramasubban & Jejheebhoy, 2000; Visaria, 2000). The critiques of India's family planning programme by women's organisations, health activists and feminist scholars (see, for example, Visaria,

2000; Ramasubban & Jejheebhoy, 2000; Ram, 2001; Rao, 1999; Chatterjee & Riley, 2001; Qadeer & Vishwanathan, 2004) subsequently drove the policy focus on reproductive rights and women's health at the Cairo conference on Population and Development.

In its rights-based language and target-free approach, the NPP was very much influenced by the Reproductive Health approach adopted at the International Conference on Population and Development (ICPD) held in Cairo in 1994, to which India was a signatory. Population stabilisation as agreed at ICPD 1994 could be met naturally and not as a matter of control or coercion if people's needs for family planning and reproductive health services along with basic health and education needs were met (Muttreja, 2019). Post-Cairo, India ostensibly adopted a rights-based approach in its Indian health policy documents, and a 'target-free' approach in its family planning programme. However, we find a continued emphasis in the NPP and in the new Reproductive and Child Health (RCH) programmes described later on the pursuit of aggressive family planning methods of irreversible means of contraception (sterilisation) rather than a choice of reversible forms of contraception (pills, condoms, IUD). The state, as scholar-activists note, preferred to mobilise targets to enforce reproductive control (Rao, 1999; Visaria, 2000) and to practice coercive population control even as it supported a policy of reproductive health rights. The fact that international aid was tied to demographic performance and the uptake of contraceptives was identified by these activists as a key factor in shaping the approach of the Indian state (Rao, 1999; Qadeer & Vishwanathan, 2004).

Between 1997 and 2003 in a post-Cairo reproductive health context, the Ministry of Health and Family Welfare (MoHFW) launched its new RCH-I programme in which a comprehensive and integrated reproductive service approach was devised to act as a corrective to the overly family planning (i.e., contraception-orientated) character of primary healthcare services. A new Reproductive Health approach was set out as being about a decentralised, comprehensive, non-vertical, integrated focus on the 'quality of care' and in which there would be no family planning 'targets' (cases of sterilisations) set for health workers at the primary and sub-centre levels such as the Auxiliary Nurse Midwife (ANM).

However, on-the-ground ANMs were expected to continue to push family planning in their work above all else. This was further reflected in the RCH policy documents discussed next. In 1998, the role of the ANM became limited to family planning, immunisation and 'superficial healthcare' (Mavlankar et al., 2010).

When the Reproductive and Child Health (RCH) programmes, RCHI (1997–2002) and RCH II (2003–2005) (programmes which predated the National Rural Health programmes of 2005) were rolled out, it was stated that their 'strategic orientation' was to be consistent with the Millennium Development Goals, the National Population Policy (2000–2010), the tenth five-year plan (2002–2007), the National Health Policy 2002 and the Vision 2020 document. The programmes would therefore promote a combined focus on reducing the maternal mortality ratio, the infant mortality rate and the total fertility rate. At the same time, the programmes would promote 'couple protection' (term used for contraceptive uptake) through the provision of a range of contraceptive options from condoms and intrauterine devices

(IUDs) to the pill. The RCH documents referred to the provision of this range of contraceptives as the 'cafeteria approach' to family planning and were set out as offering reproductive choice to women and couples.

## *The Policy Rationale for a Return to Sterilisation*

According to principle 6 of the RCH II planning document: 'the programme would include *voluntary and informed choices* in administering family planning services (there will be) clear tasks for service providers to provide quality services to meet unmet needs of family planning and spacing methods in desirable quantities' (my emphasis). The word 'right' appears in 3 of the 9 RCH II programme principles: principle 3: the poorest have the *right* (my emphasis) to get full value for the money being spent by the government or by themselves; principle 5: female children have an equal *right* to health, emergency medical aid and to live with human dignity and in principle 6: promoting contraceptive choice, as alluded to earlier. The same paragraph continues to state an overriding concern with population growth especially in the 'lagging' states (referring to the poor economic growth in the five states of Bihar, Madhya Pradesh, Odisha, Rajasthan and Uttar Pradesh), where it was estimated it would take over 26 years to achieve the replacement level fertility rate of 2.1. In these economically 'lagging' states, financial incentives (referred to as 'compensation') were to be provided to clients (term used in the document) to enhance contraceptive uptake. Cash incentives were provided to encourage uptake of contraceptive services. These ranged from approximately INR 600/– for tubectomies and INR 650/– for vasectomies, with a heftier sum of INR 5000/– including access to medical termination services offered in case of failures.

There are thus clear policy measures to return to state-promoted sterilisation (and the preference for an irreversible form of contraception) in Rajasthan despite the contraceptive choice espoused in national policy documents. In this sense, the RCH II plan, like the National Population Plan, reaffirmed the State's commitment to 'promote vigorously the small family norm to achieve replacement levels of TFR' (GOI MoHFW, 2000). The continued focus on sterilisation which Das and Uppal (2012) suggest demonstrates not just a continuing anxiety of the state around 'population explosion' but more fundamentally a lack of understanding of the actual dynamics of population growth. India has an increasingly 'young' population which they emphasise requires provision of spacing rather than the terminal methods of contraception entailed in sterilisation. The predominance of sterilisation as a method provided by the State ironically leads to a greater spurt in population growth, precisely because younger couples rush to complete their families (ibid.).

Other, neoliberal forms of argument were also mustered in the policy document to legitimise the case for a return to sterilisation. An argument that gained currency in Indian health policy circles was that female sterilisation or tubal ligation (and as described in the health planning documents) was both a popular and cost-effective choice with little surgical time involved, as requiring inexpensive equipment especially with the recent mini laparotomy (key hole sterilisation) method employed. As the client could be discharged 2–4 h after the surgery and without need for post-operative hospital-based care, it placed a minimum burden on institutional resources (Unnithan, 2019). The popularity of this method among planners was backed by statistics showing that sterilisation was the preferred option for 34% of currently married women (in 1998–99).[4] Accordingly, it was argued that sterilisation procedures were to be made available and provision was to be expanded in the future from the existing programme into 2005–2010 to all the community health centres and primary health centres in the country (and not just the five 'lagging' states). Each location would be provided additional funds for an operating theatre and to hire a medical officer trained in sterilisation. The government set up incentive packages to attract clinics in the private sector to provide family planning services especially sterilisation (promising fixed payments for clients served by the private facility as well as access to public facilities on a fee sharing basis (RCH II planning document)).

From a close reading of the state planning documents, I suggest that the continued emphasis on sterilisation signals a deeper neoliberal rationale in operation. As most other contraceptive methods are resource intensive and expensive to provide, policy makers do not regard them as cost-effective. For instance, the copper T intrauterine device requires administering and counselling by a trained paramedic.

It also requires monitoring over the period of its use. Sterilisation by comparison requires 'little surgical time, involves minimal discomfort and the client is discharged 2–4 hours after surgery' (GOI, 2007, p. 87). The use of reversible methods (IUDs, condoms and pills) is also regarded as a 'riskier' (including cost-wise) option for the state than sterilisation as it entails the possibility that women could 'change their minds' and discontinue use which would be difficult and expensive to monitor (RCH PIP ibid). As a result, the very contraceptive methods which provided women with the most choice were also those regarded as most 'unreliable' by health planners. As a result, even though the planning documents espoused a 'cafeteria' approach to contraceptive choice, only one method (sterilisation) was available. Even when the options of the Copper T or condoms were available at primary health centres, it was sterilisation that was continuously promoted as the most reliable method by community health workers during the post RCH policies from 2005 as evidenced during my later field research discussed in the next section.

The renewed emphasis on sterilisation targets and camps in the family planning program was accompanied by the introduction of new metrics of 'Expected Levels of Achievement' (or ELA) as Iyengar and Iyengar (2000) note, to evaluate health-worker performance. But as the authors suggest this is commonly perceived as the new phrase for 'targets' in the clinical context of Rajasthan where they work.

---

[4] The group of currently married women is not broken down by age, which I have found to be an important factor in determining whether to go in for reversible or irreversible forms of contraception.

## Embodying Conflicted Governance: ASHA Health-Worker Perceptions and Practices

In 2005, the Indian government launched its flagship National Rural Health Mission (NRHM), its most ambitious restructuring of health delivery systems, in line with a rights-based approach to deliver on the Millennium Development Goals (GOI, 2006). There was major financial investment in promoting safe childbirth under the NRHM and a new category of health worker, the Accredited Social Health Activist (ASHA), was created under its *Janani Suraksha Yojana* (JSY) or safe motherhood programme in addition to the Auxiliary Nurse Midwife (ANM). By 2015, over 300,000 ASHA had been selected and this was further advanced to approximately 825,000 women working as ASHA nationally (NHSRC, GOI, 2011).

The appointment of the ASHA health worker was in keeping with the vision of an 'integrated development' approach and the 'multi-purpose' nature of health work expected from her. The ASHA appointed were tasked with improving the health status of their communities through: (i) 'securing people's access to health services; (ii) improving health practices and behaviours; and (iii) providing essential and feasible healthcare provision' (GOI & NHSRC, 2011). The primary work assigned to the ASHA was 'to act as a health motivator and educator for women in the villages' (referred to by the women health workers I met as *motivator ka kaam*, or 'motivation work') and to identify and accompany pregnant women to hospital. In terms of the role of the ASHA in the JSY safe motherhood programme, the NRHM guidelines state her to be an 'honorary volunteer' who was to 'escort' women for institutional deliveries and work closely with the Auxiliary Nurse Midwife (ANM) as her helper (NHSRC, GOI, 2011, p. 2).

In 2009, the first ASHA were appointed in Rajasthan and along with a research team I conducted interviews with both ASHA and ANM at joint meetings of the Village Health and Sanitation Committees (VHSC) led by nodal Civil Society Organisations working closely with the state (Unnithan & Heitmeyer, 2014). A major activity which the ASHA undertook along with the Auxiliary Nurse Midwife (ANM) was to promote family planning especially the use of reversible methods of contraception (IUD, condoms and hormonal pills). Both ASHA and ANM provided contraceptives and raised awareness of their use, with the ASHA conducting home visits while the ANM remained in the health centre. Promotion of contraceptives was a component of a whole host of other activities which were part of an ASHA's everyday schedule of home visits to pregnant women and children under 5 years. ASHA activities included referral to government facilities for a pregnancy complication, sharing knowledge of best breastfeeding practices, prevention of diarrhoea, promoting immunisation for infants and undertaking sputum tests for the identification of TB. The diverse work of the ASHA was reflected in the diverse content of the bag each ASHA carried, which apart from an identity card had a drug kit filled with a range of items from ORS rehydration salts to paracetamol to contraceptives and betadine. ASHA were also expected to motivate women to give birth in state-accredited hospital settings.

In 2015, I interviewed 12 ASHA from nine villages in the Sanganer sub-division (*tehsil*) of Jaipur district. These were women who were between 23 and 45 years old and had educational qualifications ranging from eighth class pass (the minimum requirement for the job) to MA and BEd. I was told that their 'motivation work' (*motivation ka kaam*) involved regular visits to all the village households (typically 200 in number) and involved discussions on contraceptive use with pregnant, lactating and young mothers identified and a use of persuasive arguments and convincing tactics, including to ensure these women would go through with their children's immunisation plans and follow this through by bringing their children to the state-run creche (Anganwadi) centre which also provided nutritious food handouts. The work of motivation was itself based on a lot of preparatory 'field-based' work (*field ka kaam*) which included monthly household surveys (an average of 10 households per day) as part of providing a detailed socioeconomic and maternal health related profile of the village (*gaon ki bhumika*). As one ASHA put it, 'the whole burden of maternal health work has come to rest on us'. This was an observation made especially in comparison with the work of the ANM, a permanent member of the safe motherhood programme with a salary of 30,000–40,000 rupees (approximately 500–600 USD) a month in 2015 compared with the honorary position of the ASHA. Apart from a small salary of 1600 rupees (approximately 30 USD) per month, women who were recruited as ASHAs would get cash-based incentives linked to their performance (ANM could also access this if they accompanied women to hospital). As Renu,[5] an ASHA speaking for the rest of the focus group, explained,

> Apart from my salary of 1600/- [paid by the Women and Child development department into my bank account online], I receive Rs 300/- online for registration of women and 3 antenatal check-ups. I then get 300/- whenever I accompany a pregnant mother to a government hospital. I also receive 100/- for every child vaccinated against measles and 50/- for a DPT booster administered. If I get a woman to undertake sterilisation after 2 children, I will get 1200/-, other wise 200/- for women who go in for sterilisation after 3 children.

There was an overall sense among the ASHA I talked to of a highly imbalanced and unjust remuneration between ASHA and ANMs as well as a lack of recognition (*pehchan*) of their work as ASHA compared with the ANM.

Apart from a nominal salary, hierarchised cash incentives (with more money for convincing women of lower birth orders to undertake sterilisation) have contributed to a culture of competitiveness between the ASHA and ANM where each strives to accompany the labouring woman for birth or sterilisation. Renu said each ASHA was in competition with her ANM around the 'targets' they had to fulfil but that they often lost out on being remunerated as the ANM was their superior and supervised their work. The women whom Renu motivated in the village could not be registered by her if they decide to receive immunisation, undergo sterilisation or give birth in hospitals because the ANM says unless they receive care from the ASHA at the

---

[5] All names and other personal identifiers in the chapter have been changed to protect privacy and confidentiality.

primary health sub-centre, they will not be registered as part of the ASHA's quota. This seemed to be an unofficial regulation imposed by the ANM as it was not stated in the policy documents. Renu and other ASHAs that I spoke to suggested that this was a big issue because it caused their performance, and subsequently, their remuneration to be poor. Renu said 'the big madam (supervisor) at Goner asks me what is the reason my *target* is so low' and 'what can I say to her'? Renu explained to me that the ASHA are set a target of motivating 12–13 pregnant women a month for antenatal care (vaccines and tablets) and hospital delivery. I am surprised by the use of the word 'target' previously used to indicate numbers of women who were motivated to undertake sterilisation in the 1970s when the word gained a negative connotation given the coercion associated with state policy and the evaluation of ANM performance at the time. In March 1998, I had interviewed Sushma, the Malayali ANM who had been posted to work in the regional primary health sub-centre in the Goner area of Jaipur district. She only talked to me about the significance of the family planning work and the targets she was assigned. Sushma specified that her target for 1998 was 53 cases, higher than in the previous year when it had been 35 cases which she had exceeded. When I pointed out that at the central level at the time there was a huge push for expunging family planning targets, she said the only change she had experienced was that *'cases didn't bring in money anymore'* (i.e., no cash incentives were attached to this kind of work anymore but they were still expected to meet the sterilisation numbers). In more current ASHA practice, its use indicates how the category 'target' (rephrased as 'Expected Levels of Achievement' or ELA; Iyengar & Iyengar, 2000) has not only regained a monetary connotation but more so become an overall metric of ASHA performance, proliferating as a technique of reproductive governance.

It was striking to observe, for instance, that the ASHA health workers had a contraceptive bias towards sterilisation similar to others in her community (a fact little recognised in various ASHA training literature). This bias is strongly driven by a pressure to fulfil 'targets' set by the state as Donnelly (2013) has also found in her study in Udaipur district in Rajasthan. In addition, I have suggested that the ASHAs' inclination to reinforce the benefits of sterilisation rather than other forms of reversible methods is also largely because, she herself is convinced of the harmful nature of the copper-T (intrauterine device) and Mala N (hormonal contraceptive pills) based on her own experiences and observations in her community (most ASHA have undergone sterilisation or use condoms). I was repeatedly told by ASHA about the safety of sterilisation procedures compared to IUD insertions or hormonal pill regimes. Ethnographic insights from 1998 and through 2010 on contraceptive practice in peri-urban Jaipur especially among older Hindu and Muslim women showed recourse to sterilisation among a certain demographic of women (older) who had achieved a desired family size (three to four children with at least one son) (Unnithan-Kumar, 2010). Given the choice, the practice of sterilisation was regarded as safe and favoured above intrauterine devices by this generation of women mainly because it required least intervention and follow-up by health workers. Here we find 'safety' conceptualised as protection from the inexperience of health workers. It was not so much that fears of sterilisation were not present as indeed the many stories of botched operations confirmed (Sarojini et al., 2015), but rather it was more the case that tubectomies were regarded as the *least risky* option.

Similarly, users perceived reversible forms of contraception without the back up of appropriate counselling and paramedic support as 'unreliable' (Iyengar & Iyengar, 2000). These observations reinforce the statistics from the latest demographic survey which show that while 40% of women do not use any contraceptive method, 8.7%, 2.4% and 1.2% go in for the condom, pill and intrauterine device, respectively, compared to 41% of women who use sterilisation (IIPS, 2017). According to my respondents in peri-urban Jaipur district, intrauterine devices get lost in the upper abdomen where they were believed to get 'stuck', hurting their partners during sex (fieldwork conversations with Unnithan, 2019). Contraceptive pills were also less popular as they required both regularity and commitment, difficult to sustain by women who experienced heat and dizziness which they perceived as dangerous side effects. Condoms were regarded as equally problematic and shameful as they involved openly alluding to intercourse and talking about sex between spouses. A combination of ASHA experience and state directives to fulfil targets thus combines to influence their focus on sterilisation promotion practices on-the-ground, in line with the remuneration incentive which they receive for this. A senior NGO worker commenting on the embeddedness of the ASHA within her community values and beliefs suggested to me the misplaced expectation of health planners about the effectiveness of the ASHA, 'when she cannot even contest the authority of her mother-in-law': *asha apne saas ka virodh jub nahi kar sakti to kis ghar mein ja ke ladegi?* (when the ASHA cannot challenge her own mother-in-law then in which house can she go and fight for change?). Similar observations on the social context in which the ASHA in Rajasthan work have also been made by other scholars (Roalkvam, 2014, Mishra, 2014, for example). Given the difficult social negotiations with powerful members in the community, family and household, the ASHA often also promoted family and indigenous ideas and practices to do with childbearing. In their role in promoting state directives on reproductive health policies, ASHA more so than the ANM who did not belong to the communities she served, was at once an agent of and subject to State policy processes, *and* of her community's ideologies, preferences and practices related to childbirth and reproductive care. The ASHA were subject to the fulfilment of contraceptive and other 'targets' to do with safe motherhood as stipulated by State policy and programmes. They were also subject to control by ANMs over the process of achieving their targets. Their work promoted contraceptive choice and rights as stipulated by the state but was also constrained in offering 'restricted choice' according to their community experiences which regarded sterilisation as the least risky option for reproductive control. In this sense the ASHA embodies and symbolises conflicted reproductive governance in India.

## Concluding Discussion: Contrariness as Effective Policy

Indian family planning policies reflect a State entangled within the desire to promote the liberal rights-based values of informed consent, choice and participation on the one hand, and the wish to be guided by economic principles and a demographic rationale based on fertility regulation and population management, on the other hand. The resulting conflicting policies embody what Ram describes as a condition of the State being caught between two distinct guiding principles of liberalism and developmentalism. These principles become manifest in dual processes whereby they are both reiterated by the state and simultaneously subject to erosion (Ram, 2001, p. 85).

Family planning has been a focus throughout Indian health planning and policy since its inception as a postcolonial, modern nation state. However, as I have discussed in this chapter, its policy approach changed, from a focus on compulsory, non-reversible sterilisation to an ostensibly rights-based voluntary approach. This was a result of the Cairo deliberations where Indian feminists and health activists took the state to task for the atrocities committed through a coercive promotion of sterilisation (especially tubectomies), which, they observed, openly denied the human rights of bodily autonomy of its citizens (mainly poor women). Following the 'turn to rights' and the Indian State's pledge to promote informed choice and comprehensive counselling with regard to contraceptive methods, there was a policy swing towards *reversible* contraceptive methods. Under the National Rural Health Mission (NRHM), in 2005 the Government of India also promoted incentivised institutional birth alongside financially rewarded *voluntary* family planning programmes. The creation of a new category of health worker, the ASHA to work under instruction of the ANM is emblematic of the state's twin policy. Both workers are required to undertake the dual responsibility of promoting 'safe delivery' as well as 'voluntary' family planning. On the ground, this translates into the delivery of a 'package of services', which promote child immunisation, institutional delivery as well as contraceptive choice.

Ethnographic observations of the work of health workers and a review of the policies from 1998 to 2015 have shown, however, that contraceptive targets have remained a powerful regulator of health-worker practices. Public health workers continue to be bound in terms of their job security to measures of Expected Levels of Achievement (ELA targets; Iyengar & Iyengar, 2000) in their family planning work. The ELA incorporate the achievement of a certain expected 'target' number of family planning cases (Visaria, 2000). A 'target'-based approach has thus continued to dominate the outlook of health workers even as health provision takes on a new, rights-based form and language (personal communication with CSO directors and policy makers K. Iyengar, A. Das, V. Ramachandran; also see Visaria, 2000; Das & Uppal, 2012).

Ethnographic work with the ASHA workers discussed in the chapter further suggests that the nuanced, rights-based framing and language of civil society organisations which influenced the RCH policies has been lost in the processes of implementation. With a lack of further translation and connection with the life-worlds of local health workers, these notions contend with the perceptions that local health workers have of what is expected of them by their communities and the State. There have been similar processes at work in the pre-rights policy era of the 'Women's Development Programme' (WDP) in Rajasthan in the 1980s (Unnithan & Srivastava, 1997) where the ideas of empowerment instilled by feminist activist groups were challenged by the village-level functionaries whose basis of engagement was to procure permanent employment contracts rather than action rights-based change. These observations suggest that overtly rights-based policy approaches adopted by the State have not necessarily permeated beyond the programme documents to engage community health workers in the ways imagined within policy-CSO-academic discourse on rights (Unnithan & Pigg, 2014). As a policy frame, a rights-based approach to family planning may thus be failing as a regulatory technique of reproductive governance as Morgan and Roberts (2012) define it. For a State keen to exercise reproductive control, the pursuit of contrary family planning agendas may be an effective strategy after all.

## References

Anagost, A. (1995). A surfiet of bodies: Population and the rationality of the state in Post Mao China. In F. Ginsburg & R. Rapp (Eds.), *Conceiving the new world order* (pp. 22–41). University of California Press.

Arnold, D. (2006). Official attitudes to population, birth control and reproductive health in India, 1921-1946. In S. Hodges (Ed.), *Reproductive health in India: History, politics, controversies* (New perspectives in South Asian history, No. 13, pp. 22–51). Orient Longman.

Biehl, J. (2004). The activist state: Global pharmaceuticals, AIDS and citizenship in Brazil. *Social Text, 80*(22), 105–132.

Brunson, J. (2016). *Planning families in Nepal: Global and local projects of reproduction*. Rutgers University Press.

Brunson, J. (2019). Tool of economic development, metric of global health: Promoting planned families and economized life in Nepal. *Social Science & Medicine, 254*(112298). https://doi.org/10.1016/j.socscimed.2019.05.003

Chen, J. (2011). Globalising, reproducing and civilising rural subjects: Population control policy and constructions of rural identity in China. In C. Browner & C. Sargeant (Eds.), *Reproduction, globalisation and the state: New theoretical and ethnographic perspectives*. Duke University Press. https://doi.org/10.1215/9780822393948-004

Chhatterjee, N., & Riley, N. (2001). Planning and Indian modernity: The gendered politics of fertility control. *Signs, 26*(3), 811–845.

Das, V. (2015). *Affliction: Health, disease and poverty*. Fordham University Press.

Das, A., & Uppal, L. (2012). *Family planning in India: A need to review our current approaches*. Publication of the National Coalition against the Two Child Norm and Coercive Population Policies. [document made available by authors].

De Zordo, S. (2012). Programming the body, planning reproduction, governing life: The '(ir-) rationality' of family planning and the embodiment of social inequalities in Salvador da Bahia (Brazil). *Anthropology & Medicine, 19*(2), 207–223. https://doi.org/10.1080/13648470.2012.675049

Dean, M. (2001). 'Demonic societies': Liberalism, biopolitics and sovereignty. In T. Blom Hanson & F. Stepputat (Eds.), *States of imagination: Ethnographic explorations of the postcolonial state* (pp. 41–65). Duke University Press.

Dhanraj, D. 2011 (1991). *Something like a war – YouTube*. www.youtube.com/watch?v=J4vaELkhjhs

Donnelly, K. (2013). *Accredited social heath activists' knowledge, attitudes and practices regarding family planning in Southern Rajasthan*. ARTH, Udaipur: Draft report.

Foucault, M. 1998 (1976). *The history of sexuality: 1. The will to knowledge*. Penguin Books.

Ginsburg, F., & Rapp, R. (1995). *Conceiving the new world order: The global politics of reproduction*. University of California Press.

GOI, Government of India. (2000). *National Population Policy*. Ministry of Health and Family Welfare. https://www.nhp.gov.in/national-population-policy-2000_pg. Accessed 10 Oct 2010.

GOI, Government of India. (2007). *Document 2: The principles and evidence base for state RCH II Programme Implementation Plans* (PIPs). http://www.xiss.ac.in/RCH/Others/RCHII.pdf. Accessed 9 Aug 2014.

GOI, Government of India. *National Health Portal, Bhore Committee Report 1946*. https://www.nhp.gov.in/bhore-committee-1946_pg. Accessed 11 June 2020.

GOI, Government of India, Ministry of Health and Family Welfare. (2006). *National rural health Mission: Draft report of the reconstituted task group on public–private partnership under the NRHM*. https://nhm.gov.in/images/pdf/guidelines/nrhm-guidelines/ppp_task_force_report_draft.pdf. Accessed 5 June 2012.

GOI, Government of India, Ministry of Health and Family Welfare. (n.d.). *National rural health mission*. http://www.mohfw.nic.in/NRHM/Documents/Mission_Document.pdf. Accessed 11 Nov 2010.

Greenhalgh, S. (1995). Anthropology theorizes reproduction: Integrating practice, political-economic and feminist perspectives. In S. Greenhalgh (Ed.), *Situating fertility: Anthropological and demographic enquiry* (pp. 1–3). Cambridge University Press.

Greenhalgh, S. (2005). Globalisation and population governance in China. In A. Ong & S. J. Collier (Eds.), *Global assemblages: Technology, politics, and ethics as anthropological problems* (pp. 354–372). Blackwell.

Gupta, A. (2001). Governing population: The integrated child development services program in India. In T. Blom Hanson & F. Stepputat (Eds.), *States of imagination: Ethnographic explorations of the postcolonial state* (pp. 65–67). Duke University Press.

Hanson, T. B., & Stepputat, F. (Eds.). (2001). *States of imagination: Ethnographic explorations of the postcolonial state*. Duke University Press.

Hodges, S. (2006). *Reproductive health in India: History, politics, controversies. New perspectives in South Asian history No. 13*. Orient Longman.

International Institute for Population Sciences (IIPS) and ICF. (2017). *National Family Health Survey (NFHS-4), India, 2015–16: Rajasthan*. IIPS. https://dhsprogram.com/what-we-do/survey/survey-display-355.cfm. Accessed 22 July 2020.

Iyengar, K., & Iyengar, S. (2000). The Copper T 380A IUD: A ten year alternative to female sterilisation. *Reproductive Health Matters, 18*(16), 125–133. https://doi.org/10.1016/S0968-8080(00)90194-0

Jeffrey, R., & Jeffrey, P. (1997). *Population, gender and politics: Demographic change in rural India*. Cambridge University Press.

Kanaaneh, R. (2002). *Birthing the Nation: Strategies of Palestinian Women in Israel*. California.

Lane, S. (1994). From population control to reproductive health: An emerging policy agenda. *Social Science and Medicine, 39*(9), 1303–1304. https://doi.org/10.1016/0277-9536(94)90362-X

Mavalanker, D., Vora, K., & Sharma, B. (2010). The midwifery role of the auxiliary nurse midwife. In K. Sheikh & A. George (Eds.), *Health providers in India: On the front-lines of change* (pp. 38–57). Routledge.

Mishra, A. (2014). 'Trust and teamwork matter': Community healthworkers' experiences in integrated service delivery in India. *Global Public Health, 9*(8), 960–974. https://doi.org/10.1080/17441692.2014.934877

Morgan, L., & Roberts, E. (2012). Reproductive governance in Latin America. *Anthropology & Medicine, 19*(2), 241–254. https://doi.org/10.1080/13648470.2012.675046

Muttreja, P. (2019, November). ICPD@25: India must prioritise reproductive rights. *The Hindustan Times*.

NHSRC, National Health Systems Resource Centre, GOI. (2011). *ASHA programme: ASHA Resource Centre Strengthening*. Policy and Guidelines | National Health Systems Resource Centre, MoHFW, Government of India. www.nhsrcindia.org/catgory-detail/policy-and-guidelines/MTc=

Qadeer, I., & Viswanathan, N. (2004). How healthy are health and population policies? The Indian experience. In A. Castro & M. Singer (Eds.), *Unhealthy health policies: A critical anthropological examination* (pp. 145–163). Altamira Press.

Ram, K. (2001). Rationalising fecund bodies: Family planning policy and the modern Indian nation state. In M. Jolly & K. Ram (Eds.), *Borders of being: Citizenship, fertility and sexuality in Asia and the Pacific*. University of Michigan Press.

Ramasubban, R., & Jejheebhoy, S. (Eds.). (2000). *Women's reproductive health in India*. Rawat.

Rao, M. (Ed.). (1999). *Disinvesting in health: The World Bank's prescriptions for health*. Sage.

Roalkvam, S. (2014). Health governance in India: Citizenship as situated practice. *Global Public Health, 9*(8), 910–926. https://doi.org/10.1080/17441692.2014.941900

Sarojini, N., Sri, S. B., Ambhore, V., & Venkatachalam, D. (2015). Bilaspur sterilisation deaths: Evidence of oppressive population control policy. *Indian Journal of Medical Ethics, 12*(1), 2–5.

Senderowicz, L. (2019). 'I was obliged to accept': A qualitative exploration of contraceptive coercion. *Social Science and Medicine, 239C*, 112531. https://doi.org/10.1016/j.socscimed.2019.112531

Sharma, A., & Gupta, A. (2006). Introduction: Re-thinking theories of the state in an age of globalisation. In A.Sharma & A. Gupta (Eds.), *The Anthropology of the State: A Reader* (pp. 1–43). Blackwell Publishing.

Shore, C., Wright, S., & Pero, D. J. (Eds.). (2011). *Policy worlds: Anthropology and the analysis of contemporary power*. Berghahn.

Singer, M., & Castro, A. (2004). Anthropology and health policy: A critical perspective. In A. Castro & M. Singer (Eds.), *Unhealthy health policies: A critical anthropological examination* (pp. xi–xx). Altamira Press.

Storeng, K., & Béhague, D. (2017). 'Guilty until proven innocent': The contested use of maternal mortality indicators in global health. *Critical Public Health, 27*(2), 163–176. http://dx.doi.org/10.1080/09581596.2016.1259459

Unnithan, M. (2019). *Fertility, health and reproductive politics: Re-imagining rights in India*. Routledge. https://doi.org/10.1111/dech.12135

Unnithan, M., & Heitmeyer, C. (2014). Challenges in 'translating' human rights: Perceptions and practices of civil society actors in Western India. *Development and Change, 45*(6), 1361–1384.

Unnithan, M., & Pigg, S. L. (2014). Sexual and reproductive health rights and justice – Tracking the relationship. *Culture, Health and Sexuality, 16*(9–10), 1181–1245. https://doi.org/10.1080/13691058.2014.945774

Unnithan, M., & Srivastava, K. (1997). Gender politics, development and women's agency in Rajasthan. In R. D. Grillo & R. L. Stirrat (Eds.), *Discourses of development* (pp. 157–182). Berg.

Unnithan, M., Heitmeyer, C., & Kachhawa, P. (2010). *Thinking through rights-based development in health: Institutional approaches to social inequality and gender violence in reproductive, maternal and sexual health* (All India consultation and dissemination workshop report, Institute of Development Studies, Jaipur, April 9th–10th 2010). TTC Centre.

UNFPA. (2004). *State of the world population 2004: The Cairo Consensus at ten: Population, reproductive health and the global effort to end poverty*. https://www.unfpa.org/sites/default/files/pub-pdf/swp04_eng.pdf. Accessed 11Oct 2021.

UNFPA. (2008). *State of the world population: Reaching common ground: Culture, gender and human rights*.https://resourcecentre.savethechildren.net/node/1278/pdf/1278.pdf. Accessed 11 Oct 2021.

Unnithan-Kumar, M. (2010). Female selective abortion beyond 'Culture': Gender inequality and family making in a globalising India. *Culture, Health and Sexuality, 12*(2),153–166. https://doi.org/10.1080/13691050902825290

Van Hollen, C. (2003). *Birth on the threshold: Childbirth and modernity in South India*. University of California Press.

Varley, E. (2012). Islamic logics, reproductive rationalities: Family planning in northern Pakistan. *Anthropology & Medicine, 19*(2), 189–206. https://doi.org/10.1080/13648470.2012.675044

Visaria, L. (2000). From contraceptive targets to informed choice. In R. Ramasubban & S. Jejheebhoy (Eds.), *Women's reproductive health in India* (pp. 331–383). Rawat.

Wright, S. (2011). Studying policies, methods, paradigms, perspectives – Introduction. In C. Shore, S. Wright, & D. Pero (Eds.), *Policy worlds: Anthropology and the analysis of contemporary power* (pp. 27–32). Berghahn.

# Part III
# Contesting Authoritative Knowledge and Practice

# Chapter 8
# Regulating Midwives: Foreclosing Alternatives in the Policymaking Process in West Java, Indonesia

**Priscilla Magrath**

## Introduction

Promotion of "skilled birth attendants" (SBAs) in global maternal health policy raises the question of how policymakers should respond to lay midwives, termed "traditional birth attendants" (TBAs). TBAs are widely reported to be both popular and needed, especially in low-resource settings where licensed midwives may be unavailable (Rudrum, 2016; Niehof, 2014). Nevertheless, in many countries TBAs have been banned from attending births on the basis that their practices are dangerous (Rishworth et al., 2016; Guerra-Reyes, 2019). In marked contrast, Indonesia's policy of partnership between licensed midwives, termed *bidan*, and lay midwives, termed *dukun bayi*, offers formal recognition of the *dukun bayi's* role as a partner to the *bidan*. In this chapter I trace the development of a district regulation that gave legal force to the national partnership policy. I investigate how and why officials at Lahanbesar[1] district health office in West Java prioritized the regulation on partnership between *dukun bayi* and *bidan* as an important means of addressing maternal death. How did Lahanbesar's partnership regulation gain prominence within the local policy agenda despite multiple challenges to successful partnership including a weak enabling environment[2] for skilled attendance, particularly, weak referral

[1] Lahanbesar is a pseudonym. All names and other personal identifiers in the chapter have been changed to protect privacy and confidentiality.

[2] The World Health Organization lists six building blocks of health systems that comprise the enabling environment: service delivery; health workforce; information; medical products, vaccines and technologies; financing; and leadership and governance. However, it is the interactions and

P. Magrath (✉)
Department of Health Promotion Sciences, Mel and Enid Zuckerman College of Public Health, University of Arizona, Tucson, AZ, USA
e-mail: pmagrath@arizona.edu



L. J. Wallace et al. (eds.), *Anthropologies of Global Maternal and Reproductive Health*, Global Maternal and Child Health, https://doi.org/10.1007/978-3-030-84514-8_8

pathways and under-resourced obstetric care units in district hospitals (Agarwal et al., 2019; Makowiecka et al., 2008)?

My analysis draws on Shore and Wright's (1997) elucidation of policymaking as a process of foreclosing alternatives. They define policy as sets of principles, rules, or guidelines that outline a course of action. Policies are prescriptive and normative and appear as technical instruments for improving efficiency and effectiveness. Yet the policymaking process is political and ideological. Problems are presented in ways that limit consideration of a broad range of options, such that one solution emerges as the obvious or only feasible option (Nichter, 2008). Similarly, the district regulation on partnership between *bidan* and *dukun bayi* was presented by certain district health officials as the fastest means to reduce maternal mortality. Attention was thereby diverted away from other ongoing approaches to reducing maternal mortality, such as improving the performance of health facilities and referral systems. Analysis of the policymaking process reveals how particular logics used by district policymakers foreclosed alternatives. These logics included framing the practices of the *dukun bayi* (known in West Java as *paraji*) as a key cause of maternal death and presenting the partnership regulation as the only means for addressing the *paraji* problem. I argue that the development of Lahanbesar's district regulation on Partnership between *bidan* and *paraji* (dukun) was influenced by three larger policy contexts: the Millennium Development Goals that generated increased pressure to address maternal mortality (MDG 5); a global focus on skilled birth attendance as a means to achieve this goal; and the decentralization of health services in Indonesia from 1999 that increased accountability for maternal health outcomes at the district level.

## Methodology

### *Site Selection*

This chapter was part of a larger dissertation project examining health decentralization in Indonesia (Magrath, 2016). This included 10 months of research in 2012–2013 in Lahanbesar district, West Java; this place was selected because I had done research there for a World Bank project in 2000 and wished to track changes in health governance over time. Lahanbesar is located approximately midway between Indonesia's capital city, Jakarta, and West Java's provincial capital, Bandung. The main road linking these two cities passes through the northern part of Lahanbesar and factories located along the road provide wage employment, especially for women. The south of the district is relatively remote and poor with less access to wage employment.

---

coordination between these building blocks that is critical to ensuring adequate maternal health care, including effective referral systems, and comprehensive obstetric care at health facilities.

Lahanbesar was originally selected due to high maternal and infant mortality statistics and the enduring popularity of TBAs known in the local Sundanese language as *paraji.* One of the largest districts in Indonesia, in 2012 it had a population of 2.3 million inhabiting 363 villages. There were three district government hospitals and several private hospitals and clinics, although specialists, including obstetrician gynecologists, rotated between hospitals/clinics and were not always available; 58 *puskesmas* (sub-district health centers providing outreach and clinical services by a doctor or nurse from 7 am to noon Monday to Saturday); and 3281 *posyandu* (neighborhood health posts organized by health volunteers, held monthly, attended by *bidan* and providing prenatal care, vaccinations, and growth monitoring). There were 628 *bidan,* the majority employed by government but many simultaneously running private practices (2.7/10,000 population compared with national average of 2/10,000 reported by Achadi et al. (2007)). There were over 2071 *paraji* (9/10,000 population). Many of the *bidan* have been working in the district for years or even decades, although *bidan* sent to remote villages tend to be the least experienced. Not all *bidan* speak the local language and they are frequently relocated. By contrast, *paraji* tend to remain in the same community for life.

Study sites were selected with the aim of tracing health policies from the district health office down to communities, and included the district health office, two health centers, and two villages, one village served by each health center. Eight additional health centers were visited while accompanying health personnel on monitoring visits.

## Methods

Methods included participant observation; semi-structured interviews; focus group discussions; and document analysis conducted between June 2012 and April 2013. I carried out semi-structured interviews with key decision makers at the district office and staff at the health centers, and informal conversations with health volunteers, *paraji* and mothers (Table 8.1).

My key informants were the head of health services and one of her staff, both of whom had been village *bidan*, and the head of health promotion, Pak[3] Yudi and two of his staff; the two case study health center heads; and two village *bidan* for the selected villages. Up to 12 interviews were conducted with each key informant over the course of the research.

Participant observation included over 100 days accompanying district health officials at their offices, on field trips and at 30 meetings and events; 30 days at case study health centers observing outpatient and obstetric services, interviewing staff, accompanying *bidan,* and attending 12 *posyandu.* I stayed in one village for 6 days accompanying and interviewing families and made frequent visits to families in the

[3] Pak, short for Bapak (father), is a term of respect for older men.

**Table 8.1** Number of interviews, types of interlocutor, and topics covered

| Research site and position | Number of interviews | Topics |
|---|---|---|
| **District health office:** | | Job description and duties, views on decentralization, maternal health policy, and causes of maternal death |
| Head | 1 | |
| Deputy | 1 | |
| Department heads | 7 | |
| Section heads | 15 | |
| Junior staff | 10 | |
| TOTAL: | **34** | |
| **Health center:** | | |
| Heads | 10 | |
| Doctors | 5 | |
| Other staff | 30 | |
| TOTAL: | **45** | |
| **Health center/ village** | | Job description and duties, experiences of partnership with *paraji* |
| *Bidan* (SBA) | 14 | |
| *Kader* (volunteers) | 43 | Duties, experiences, *paraji* |
| *Paraji* (TBA) | 5 | Work, views on partnership with *bidan* |
| TOTAL: | **62** | |
| **Parents/patients:** | | Childbirth experiences, views on *paraji*, *bidan* and partnership |
| Women | 85 | |
| Men | 17 | |
| Total | 102 | |

**Table 8.2** Number of focus group discussions, participants, and topics

| Participants | Number of focus groups | Topics |
|---|---|---|
| Community | 2 | Health seeking, childbirth attendance |
| Health volunteers | 2 | Maternal and child health policies |
| District Health Office including: | | Research findings on decentralization and maternal health policy |
| Department heads | 1 | |
| Section heads | 2 | |
| TOTAL | 7 | |

second village which was near my residence. Focus group discussions (FGD) were conducted with community groups, health volunteers and district office staff (Table 8.2).

I consulted statistical data, laws, policy documents, health promotion materials, and annual reports from the district health office, health centers, and village offices. I used *Bahasa Indonesia,* the official national language, spoken by most of my interlocutors. Occasionally Sundanese was used, and an Indonesian speaker translated for me. I took notes on a laptop and most interviews and focus groups were audio-recorded with permission. I used MAXQDA software for data analysis. The research was approved by the Indonesian Ministry for Research and Technology, *RISTEK*, and ethical clearance was obtained from University of Arizona IRB.

## The Promotion of "Skilled Birth Attendants" in Global Health Policy

Promotion of "skilled birth attendants" (SBAs) has been a component of global maternal health policy at least since the safe motherhood initiative was launched in 1987. An SBA is defined as an "accredited health professional – such as a midwife, doctor or nurse – who has been educated and trained to proficiency in the skills needed to manage normal (uncomplicated) pregnancies, childbirth and the immediate postnatal period, and in the identification, management and referral of complications in women and newborns" (WHO, 2004, p. 24). The policy focus on SBAs is based on statistical evidence suggesting that birth outcomes improve when SBAs are present (Freedman, 2003). The pivotal role of SBAs increased with the inclusion of the percent of births attended by SBAs as an indicator under Millennium Development Goal (MDG) 5 – "reducing by three quarters the maternal mortality ratio" (MMR) by 2000 (UNDP, 2003, p. 12).

The hidden text in the promotion of SBAs is the presence of lay midwives, known in public health discourse as Traditional Birth Attendants (TBAs), who use systems of knowledge about pregnancy and birth that predate Western biomedicine and generally acquire skills through apprenticeship to another TBA. The World Health Organization (WHO) defines TBAs as "traditional, independent (of the health system), nonformally trained and community-based providers of care during pregnancy, childbirth and the post-natal period" (WHO, 2004, p. 8). However, anthropologists have documented great diversity in the social roles, training, and scope of practice of "traditional birth attendants" around the world (Pigg, 1997; Hay, 2015).

The expectation of global health policymakers is that SBAs will eventually replace TBAs (Hildebrand, 2017). Yet TBAs continue to assist women in the provision of maternity care, particularly in low-resource settings, where the essential inputs for quality maternity care, such as trained health workers, well-resourced health facilities, and a robust referral system, are often limited (Rudrum, 2016; Niehof, 2014; Rishworth et al., 2016). Even where SBAs are available TBAs remain popular due to the continuous and comprehensive care they often provide before, during, and after childbirth. This may include emotional support, religious and culturally important rituals, massage, and assistance with household chores. TBAs are often more easily available in remote and resource poor settings and their services are perceived to be more affordable (Hay, 2015; Titaley et al., 2010; Guerra-Reyes, 2019).

From the medical and policy perspective, the skills and services of TBAs are undervalued (Hildebrand, 2012; Bennett, 2017), and they are often blamed for high maternal and infant mortality ratios (MMR and IMR) due to perceived dangerous practices or the failure to refer emergency cases to medical services (Rishworth et al., 2016; Niehof, 2014). Global policies have shifted since the 1960s when the WHO encouraged training of TBAs in hygienic practices, identification of danger signs, and referral on the assumption that TBAs would often be the only person called to attend a birth. As the number of formally trained midwives has increased, new global guidelines discourage birth attendance by unsupervised TBAs since, even after training, they are not considered to be "skilled birth attendants." Instead, health policymakers are encouraged to provide TBAs with roles that link them to SBAs and formal health services (WHO, 2004). Such roles include encouraging women to use biomedical antenatal, postnatal, and birthing services, and providing companionship, interpretation, massage, and drinks to women during and after childbirth. In some cases, TBAs are even allowed to manage uncomplicated births (Miller & Smith, 2017).

The overall effect of these policies has been to reduce the professional independence of TBAs. In many countries TBAs practices are regulated, with adverse consequences for their social status and for maternal health (Niehof, 2014; Rudrum, 2016; Rishworth et al., 2016; Guerra-Reyes, 2019). In Ghana, where there is a ban on TBAs practicing alone, they are torn between providing needed care and complying with the law. The shortage of SBAs results in some women giving birth by the roadside on the way to a distant health facility (Rishworth et al., 2016). In Peru, an inter-cultural birthing policy involves integrating "traditional" birthing practices through training SBAs in vertical birth. Yet TBAs (termed *parteras*) are excluded from this process and prohibited from attending home births (Guerra-Reyes, 2019). Given the ongoing role that TBAs play in maternity care, it is important to understand how policies relating to TBAs are developed at the local level and how they impact the care that TBAs are able to provide.

## *Maternal Health Policy in the Context of Decentralization in Indonesia*

In Indonesia efforts to shift birthing practices away from use of TBAs, known in the Indonesian language as *dukun bayi*, predate contemporary global policy. The Dutch colonial government that introduced Western scientific medicine into Indonesia in the nineteenth century framed *dukun bayi* as dangerous to mothers' health. They initiated trainings in hygienic practices that were continued after independence by Indonesia's first two presidents Soekarno (1945–1967) and Suharto (1967–1998) (Stein, 2007). Suharto complemented training of *dukun bayi* with deployment of formally trained and licensed midwives, known as *bidan*. These *bidan* became part of the health workforce that was needed to manage an expanded public health infrastructure including district level hospitals, sub-district health centers (*puskesmas*), and village level monthly health posts (*posyandu*). The *bidan* program was rapidly expanded following the global conference on safe motherhood held in Kenya in 1987 that called attention to high MMR globally, including in Indonesia where it was estimated at 446 deaths per 100,000 births in 1990. Indonesia compared unfavorably with other nations in the region, for example, MMR was 152 in the Philippines, 79 in Malaysia, and 40 in Thailand (WHO et al., 2015). The high MMR in Indonesia was not only a health and humanitarian concern but also a source of national shame (Achmad, 1999).

The high proportion of mothers giving birth with *dukun bayi*, estimated at two thirds of births in 1991, was perceived to be a significant factor contributing to maternal mortality in Indonesia (Shiffman, 2003). In response, the *bidan di desa* (village midwife) program was launched in 1989 with financial assistance from the World Bank and UNICEF, with the goal that every village would have a resident *bidan*. Initially, nurses were given 1-year training in midwifery at a government or private university. In 1998 this was replaced by 3-year midwifery training for high school graduates (Heywood & Harahap, 2009). Indonesia's *bidan de desa* program was part of a broader set of strategies to improve maternal health that included expansion of 24-h obstetric care facilities located at *puskesmas* and financial assistance to mothers giving birth through government health insurance programs. *Jamkesmas*, health insurance for the poor, initiated in 2008 was supplemented by *Jampersal* (2011–2014) that covered the cost of childbirth attended by a skilled birth attendant at a health facility (Magrath, 2016).[4] In combination, these policies contributed to substantial gains in maternal health. In 1990, 79% of births occurred at home, 65% of them with no skilled attendant (NPFPB & MoH, 1991). By 2017, 74% of births were delivered at health facilities and 91% of mothers used a skilled attendant (NPFPB & MoH, 2017). While Indonesia fell short of meeting its MDG 5 target, by 2015 maternal mortality had declined by 31% from 1990 levels to 305 deaths per 100,000 live births (Badan Pusat Statisk, 2015). Although these gains are considerable, national averages mask wide regional variation (Hay, 2015). Indonesia has 262 million inhabitants with more than 300 ethnic groups spread over 17,744 islands (Agustina et al., 2019).

As the number of *bidan* increased over time, relationships between *bidan* and *dukun bayi* evolved. Initially, *bidan* were encouraged to train *dukun bayi*, thereby supporting their independent practices. *Dukun bayi* were provided with birthing kits including scissors, aluminum pans, and baby weighing scales (Hildebrand, 2012). By 2000, many villages had *bidan* and it became mandatory for every birth to be attended by an SBA. In line with WHO policy at the time, training programs for *dukun bayi* were phased out. Instead, they were encouraged to work as partners with *bidan*, under a national Policy on Partnership between *bidan* and *dukun bayi* that was formalized in 2007 (Titaley et al., 2010). Under the partnership *dukun bayi* are

[4] From 2014 Jampersal and Jamkesmas were integrated into the national health insurance program, Jaminan Kesehatan Nasional.

incorporated into the health system with a defined role that apparently reconciles the popularity of the *dukun bayi* with concerns over the safety of her practices. According to the implementation manual for Partnership between *Bidan* and *Dukun Bayi* (Indonesia Ministry of Health, n.d., p. 9–10), *dukun* are to encourage pregnant mothers to use ante-natal, birthing, and post-natal services of the *bidan*; accompany mothers to these services and assist the *bidan*; carry out local religious or traditional rituals beneficial to health; educate mothers about pregnancy, danger signs, nutrition, birth planning, family planning, and breast feeding; and make home visits after the birth. *Bidan* are supposed to provide guidance to *dukun* and give them a share of their income from birth attendance (ibid p. 16). Although the manual describes the *dukun* as no less important than *bidan* (ibid p.6), the description of their roles is asymmetrical with *dukun* expected to give up independent practices to assist the *bidan*. This reinforces longstanding inequities in the social status and valuation of the two types of midwives from the perspective of the formal health system. Even though *dukun bayi* are highly regarded in their communities they are not always respected by *bidan* and other health professionals (Hildebrand, 2012).

Despite the clear and detailed guidelines, there has been wide variation in the implementation of the Policy on Partnership for *Bidan* and *Dukun Bayi* across Indonesia. Responsibility for implementing the policy falls on districts, according to decentralization laws, implemented in Indonesia from 1999. Decentralization, the devolution of authority from central to lower levels of government (Manor, 1999), offers increased scope for policy entrepreneurship as policymakers innovate in adapting national policies to fit local agendas (Pisani et al., 2016). This tends to increase regional variation in policy implementation and health outcomes (Agustina et al., 2019). For example, in Nusa Tenggara Barat (NTB) district officials have not enforced the partnership policy strictly. *Bidan* prefer not to partner with *dukun* arguing the policy is not applicable in their region. They claim mothers will be confused if they involve the *dukun* and they want to send a clear message that the *bidan* is best (Hildebrand & Magrath, 2016). In contrast, in West Java, the policy has been supported by provincial and district health officials. In Lahanbesar district, the government passed a district regulation in 2013 to strengthen partnership through provision of a budget to pay *dukun bayi* for each birth attended in partnership with *bidan*, and legally enforceable sanctions if they fail to partner.

## *The Development of the District Regulation on Partnership Between* **Bidan, Paraji,** *and* **Kader***: Policy Entrepreneurship, the Use of Evidence, and the Role of Numbers*

The key policy entrepreneur in the development of the district regulation on Partnership was Pak Yudi, a charismatic and ebullient individual, who was the head of Health Promotion, one of four departments in the District Health Office. His department was responsible for communicating health policy to the public, encouraging community participation in health policy and services, improving access to services through health insurance, and dealing with complaints from the public. Pak Yudi regarded regulation of *paraji* as one of the responsibilities of his department. He argued that many maternal and infant deaths occurred at the hands of *paraji*. While acknowledging that *paraji* were popular because they performed important cultural and spiritual roles, he maintained it was necessary to regulate their practices to ensure safer births. He argued the impact of the national policy on partnership was limited because it did not have legal force, hence the need to legalize the policy through a district regulation.

Over a period of 2 years from 2011 to 2013, Pak Yudi applied his entrepreneurial skills toward building support for his initiative. As head of Health Promotion, Pak Yudi had developed an extensive social network including NGOs, the media, businesspeople, and politicians. His office saw a steady stream of visitors and Pak Yudi used his connections to promote the regulation through a series of meetings and media engagements (see, for example, Ruslan, 2013).

In the following sections I provide ethnographic details of the policy-making process followed by Pak Yudi, focusing on three key components: building an evidence base, developing the text of the regulation, and presenting the regulation to key stakeholders from the district parliament. I highlight the ways evidence was used to narrow the options for accelerated efforts to address maternal death so that the regulation emerged as the best and most obvious solution.

## *Building the Evidence Base: Partnership Pilots and* Paraji *Perspectives*

Pak Yudi gathered two sources of evidence to support his case for the partnership regulation: assessments of existing cases of legalization of the partnership policy; and research on *paraji* perspectives on the partnership policy. Two cases of legalization were examined, the first in Takalar District, South Sulawesi province, implemented in 2007 in nine sub-districts covering 83 villages. Reported births with *bidan* increased to 94% and maternal deaths fell from eight cases in 2007 to zero in 2009 and 2010. The second was a pilot within Lahanbesar district enforcing partnership in 23 villages in Cikakak sub-district in 2007 that had increased the percentage of births with *bidan* to 95%. During this second pilot *paraji* were paid Rp 50,000 (US$ 5) and *kader* were paid Rp 25,000 (US$ 2.5) for each birth attended in partnership.

The research with *paraji* was conducted by a member of Pak Yudi's staff, Bu[5] Irni, who invited *paraji* to participate in group interviews. Recordings from interviews conducted in three sub-districts give a consistent picture. The *paraji* all say that partnership with *bidan* is better than before because now the *bidan* takes the

[5] Bu, short for Ibu (mother), is a term of respect for older women.

responsibility. According to one *paraji* "after birth, if there is heavy bleeding or the placenta hasn't come out yet, I don't have to worry." Another stated she had taken five mothers to hospital, indicating her commitment to partnership.

In one interview two *paraji* were asked about the income they received. One *paraji* stated that she sometimes received Rp 20,000–30,000 (US$ 2–3) from the *bidan*, and about Rp 150,000 (US$ 15) from the mother. The *bidan* would say "here is something to buy soap," thereby presenting it as a gift. According to Sundanese culture this made it easier to receive because it suggested a social rather than a purely economic transaction. The implication is that the partnership is an ongoing social relationship of care not motivated purely by economic gain. This distinction is reflected in the *paraji's* explanation: "I wouldn't want it to look as though I was profit seeking." Hildebrand (2017) offers an extended analysis of how social relations of maternal care are understood as forms of gift giving by *bidan*, *dukun bayi*, and mothers in rural Indonesia. Asked if they knew mothers reluctant to give birth at the health center, one answered "many in the villages," saying mothers feared their bodies would be exposed, contrary to Islamic guidelines on modesty (*aurat*). The second *paraji* quoted a mother saying, "I don't want any fuss."

Concerns with partnership did not emerge from these interviews, perhaps because *paraji* accepting an invitation to meet with district health officials were those who supported the partnership policy. Voicing criticism would have been unlikely since the power dynamic placed a district official in a superior social position to a *paraji*. Criticism is valued negatively in Sundanese culture, similar to Javanese culture (Berman, 1998).

## Alternative Views on Partnership: Perspectives of Mothers, *Paraji* and *Bidan*

I elicited a wider range of views from interviews with *paraji* and mothers in their homes, in the absence of government officials. Three positions on partnership emerged: *paraji* who supported partnership, those who complied reluctantly, and those who avoided partnership. Mak[6] Lestari's views are similar to those of *paraji* interviewed by Bu Irni. She stated: "now it is better because there is no burden, the *bidan* takes the tension, it's much better now." Ma Halimah partnered reluctantly. She had worked with five different *bidan*, reflecting the high turnover for *bidan*. She preferred it before partnership when she could practice on her own. She explained: "If the baby comes quickly and I don't report I am scolded."

Mak Uma exemplifies the avoidance of partnership. She said "it was better before, now we have to go to the *bidan*, that's the government recommendation. But I follow the mother, if she wants to go with the *bidan*, go ahead, if she wants to come with me, that's fine too." Mak Uma had attended to a mother 8 days previously. "I went to her house, she didn't use a *bidan*, she said she didn't want to. I took my kit

[6] Mak is a term of respect used for *paraji*.

and, there was no problem, I gave her massage three days after the birth, then seven days, I'll continue up to 40 days." Mak Uma did not understand why she was not supposed to practice independently. "I already finished my training, they gave me a plaque" she pointed to the sign outside her door stating she was practicing under the auspices of the district health office. She showed me the kit she had received in the 1990s, including scissors and aluminum pans. Although Mak Uma claimed she often worked with *bidan*, local *bidan* claimed she did not partner with them and that she discouraged mothers from using *bidan*.

Interviews with mothers who used the *paraji's* services reveal how partnership works in practice. Three low-income mothers resided close to Mak Lestari who regularly partnered with the local *bidan*, Bidan Canti. One mother had given birth to her four children at home with only a *paraji*, in another village. She said, "it's easier with the *paraji*, you just have to call one person, you don't have to go anywhere." Asked what advice she would give her 22-year-old daughter she responded, "if there is no problem, the *paraji*, but if it is a difficult birth then she would need to go to hospital." She thought the *paraji* would refer her to hospital if necessary. The second mother always had difficult births and preferred "medis," a medical birth. Two of her children were born with *Mak Lestari* in partnership with local *bidan*; the other two were born in the hospital due to complications. She explained that since Mak Lestari lived close to Bidan Canti, they always came together, whoever was called first. The third mother had her first two children with *paraji* in another village. She gave birth to her third child with Mak Lestari and Bidan Canti and was happy with the partnership.

Different stories emerged from Mak Uma's clients. I met three mothers who had recently given birth with Mak Uma and two who were planning to, while attending a *posyandu*. One mother explained her baby was born at 2:00 am; they lived far from the road and the baby came fast. She had used a *bidan* during her pregnancy. Another mother stated, "with the *bidan* you will definitely be cut," although Bidan Wawan, attending the *posyandu* explained cutting (episiotomy) was only done if necessary. One of the expectant mothers explained: "I'm afraid the baby will come too fast." She feared engaging with the *bidan* anticipating that the *bidan* would emphasize the risks of childbirth. As Bidan Wawan explained, in Sundanese culture pregnant mothers should avoid hearing negative things.

## What Makes for a Successful Partnership Between *Bidan* and *Paraji*?

These cases suggest that successful partnerships between *bidan* and *paraji* depend on the quality of relationships between mothers, *paraji* and *bidan*. With Mak Lestari and Bidan Canti's good relationship, mothers follow partnership, but in the absence of such relationships, as with Mak Uma, mothers receive conflicting advice from the *paraji* and the *bidan*.

*Bidan* acknowledged that there are often tensions in relationships between *bidan* and *paraji*. Some expressed concern that legal enforcement of partnership could strain their relationships with *paraji* further, as *paraji* and mothers would become intimidated, fearing sanctions. One *bidan* related a case of "shock treatment" when a health center head had called the police to visit a *paraji* so that she would become afraid to practice alone.

A senior *bidan* thought *bidan* lacked communication skills needed to work effectively with *paraji* and mothers, while another confided that the quality of *bidan* training had declined due to the focus on rapid deployment. Furthermore, the least experienced *bidan* are deployed in remote areas where utilization of health services is low. I encountered this during a *Jampersal* (health insurance for childbirth) monitoring visit and it is also consistent with Makowiecka et al. (2008).

*Bidan* related additional concerns about the health system. They referred mothers to district hospitals not knowing whether there would be an obstetrician gynecologist, or necessary medical supplies. Sometimes they accompanied mothers to several hospitals with the risk of death due to delayed medical interventions increasing at each referral. Under-resourced hospitals also featured in mothers' stories. One mother had delivered at the district hospital and noticed babies in the ICU unit sharing oxygen tubes. Subsequently she learned several of the infants died. The shortage of ICU units was confirmed by the Hospital Services Department head whom I subsequently interviewed. It was also said that health insurance was increasing demand on already inadequate resources. These concerns are consistent with the literature on maternal health in Indonesia that links high maternal mortality to weaknesses in the enabling environment for skilled attendance. Agarwal et al. (2019) refer to the low standard of emergency obstetric care in hospitals while Makowiecka et al. (2008) raise concerns over the quality of training and care provided by village *bidan*. Both emphasize inadequacies in referral systems.

My data reveal gaps between the assumptions of policymakers and the lived experiences of *paraji*, mothers, and *bidan* in relation to the partnership policy. When I presented my findings to Pak Yudi, he insisted that the regulation on partnership was the fastest way to address maternal death. Furthermore, *paraji* would benefit as they would no longer be blamed for poor birth outcomes and they would be paid whenever they partnered. Yet my conversations with *paraji*, mothers, and *bidan* revealed broader concerns relating to respect for *paraji* and professional support for *bidan*. These concerns prompt consideration of alternatives to legal enforcement of partnership, such as building more reciprocal partnerships based on mutual respect and trust and strengthening the enabling environment for skilled attendance through developing transportation and referral systems[7] and increasing resources at health centers.

Reciprocal partnerships were envisaged in an AusAid (Australian) program implemented in 1995–1998 that advocated: "practices of partnership that are truly collaborative, and not hierarchical" (Hull et al., 1998, p. 36). A DfID–AusAID–MoH partnership initiative launched in several districts in 2007 included formal recognition, payment, and technical training for *dukun bayi*. Monthly meetings of

[7] USAID funded Expanding Maternal and Neonatal Survival (EMAS) project initiated in 2011 aims to improve referral systems, but was not operational in Lahanbesar at the time of the research.

*dukun* and *bidan* at *puskesmas* were used to strengthen partnerships (UNICEF, 2010). Bennett (2017) goes further, suggesting a two-way relationship, with *bidan* learning from *dukun* about patient-centered care. The national policy on partnership provides a framework for the development of such programs. Lahanbesar's district regulation instead focuses on providing financial incentives and sanctions to encourage *paraji* to comply with the partnership policy. Less emphasis was placed on improving the quality of relationships through training of *paraji* or *bidan.*

## *Formulating the Text of the Regulation*

The development of the text of the regulation represents another element in Pak Yudi's strategy of policy promotion. He organized a series of meetings between district health staff and legal advisors, with participation from *bidan* and *paraji.* I attended some of these meetings and observed how the text of the national policy implementation manual was modified to accommodate the goals of the district regulation. Comparing the two documents, both share the objective of improving mothers' access to quality midwifery services, encouraging *dukun bayi/paraji* to become partners to the *bidan*, and shifting mothers' behaviors toward accessing services via partnership. The district regulation adds *kader* (health volunteers) into the partnership, reflecting the important role that they play as intermediaries between *bidan*, mothers, and *paraji* in West Java. Aside from this difference, the same definition of partnership is used in both documents:

> Partnership between *bidan*, *dukun bayi* (and *kader*) in providing health services to women and children is a form of cooperation between *bidan* and *dukun bayi* that is mutually beneficial and based on principles of openness, equity and trust in an effort to ensure the safety of mothers and babies (Indonesia Ministry of Health, n.d., p. 4; Lahanbesar District, 2013, p. 5, author translation).

Both documents describe specific roles for *bidan* and *paraji.* Within the district regulation, the respective roles are detailed using the legal language of rights, duties, and sanctions (Lahanbesar District, 2013). The duties of the *paraji* include informing the *bidan* if a mother is pregnant or about to give birth, and encouraging the family to use the *bidan's* ante-natal, birthing, and family planning services. Whereas the duties of the *paraji* are entirely framed in relation to the *bidan*, the term '*paraji*' is not even mentioned among the duties of the *bidan*, suggesting an asymmetry in the partnership that is also reflected in the national policy. Sanctions specified in the regulation for both *paraji* and *bidan* include verbal or written warnings for failure to partner. In addition, the regulation provides a legal framework under which village officials may develop their own village laws, including additional sanctions such as fines for non-compliance. The district regulation was circulated within district government offices and went through several drafts before it was submitted to the district Parliament.

## *The District Parliamentary Meeting*

Pak Yudi's entrepreneurial efforts culminated in a meeting with parliamentary commissioners responsible for legislation on health, held on February 4, 2013 at which the case for the regulation on partnership was presented. The meeting was attended by six members of the parliamentary commission, several staff from the district health office, two *bidan*, and two *paraji*. Key speakers included Dr. Nia, head of the district health office, Pak Yudi, head of health promotion, and Bu Tia, head of the district *bidan* association. I detected three themes emerging from the speeches and ensuing discussions: first, the urgency of the problem of maternal death as mothers and infants should not be dying; second, the focus on *paraji* as a cause of maternal death, and third, the need for a partnership regulation as a mechanism for dealing with the problem of the *paraji* because the alternative, competition with the *bidan*, would not work. The sequential presentation of these three themes served to foreclose a broader discussion of the causes of and possible solutions to maternal death.

### Theme 1: Mothers and Infants Should Not Be Dying

Dr. Nia stated that the purpose of the partnership regulation was to address the high infant and maternal mortality rate in the district. Whereas neonatal deaths had fallen from 551 in 2009 to 369 in 2012, maternal deaths had been rising from 33 in 2005 to 70 in 2011 and 77 in 2012. According to theory, Dr. Nia explained, maternal deaths should fall as births at health facilities rise, but in this district the reported incidence had risen, despite increased deployment of *bidan* and a rise in the proportion of births at facilities. One reason, she argued, was improved reporting, since it is *bidan* who report maternal deaths. Nevertheless, she emphasized further action was needed to address the high rates of maternal death.

Drawing on district-level administrative data, Dr. Nia then explained the causes of maternal deaths in the district, including bleeding, pre-eclampsia, and other sickness such as TB. She also discussed indirect causes such as inadequate health services and delays in accessing services, a veiled reference to the communities' preference for home births with *paraji*. Dr. Nia stated dramatically that 25 of the 77 maternal deaths in 2012, or 32.47%, were associated with births attended by a *paraji* with no *bidan* present. She ended by presenting results of the partnership pilot carried out in Cicaklak sub-district of Lahanbesar district: "We implemented a trial, regulating partnership in 23 villages in 2007/8 and as a result 95% of births were attended by *bidan* and maternal deaths fell."

### Theme 2: *Paraji* Are of the Past, Not the Future

Following Dr. Nia's speech, Pak Yudi, head of health promotion, commented that the main problem was that the public still choose the *paraji* over the *bidan*. The head of the *bidan* association took up this theme stating that although there were

628 members of her organization, the ratio of *bidan* to *paraji* was 1:5. "We have to clarify the limits of their work. We have to ensure that there won't be additional numbers of *paraji*." Here we have a new nuance. Not only are *paraji* presented as in need of regulation through a partnership that clarifies the limits of their work, the sheer numbers of *paraji* are presented as a threat that also needs to be contained. Partnership now appears as a temporary stage, as an ideal future with no *paraji* is anticipated.

Several members of the Commission defended the *paraji,* one stating "we don't want to eliminate *paraji* as they have done in some areas. We need to protect the rights of both *paraji* and *bidan*." Another argued *paraji* were community leaders who mobilized the public while a third added "they are people who are needed." Yet despite this defense, they also acknowledged that individual *paraji* performed dangerous practices, suggesting a degree of ambiguity toward the *paraji.*

Although the commissioners' plea to protect the rights of *paraji* could be interpreted as referring to their collective rights to exist as *paraji*, the response from the district health officials highlighted government programs offering the children of *paraji* the chance to train as *bidan.* According to Dr. Nia, 50 children of *paraji* had entered the program and had become government contract *bidan* earning a good salary. She explained the examinations and licensing required of *bidan*, a theme taken up by the head of health services, who added that *bidan* also receive on the job training. She added that *paraji* are invited to meetings, but many do not come. "There are difficult *paraji* and their arrogance leads to deaths at the hospital (from late referral)." In this way she presented *bidan* as governable in contrast with the *paraji*, some of whom appear ungovernable.

### Theme 3: Competition Between *Bidan* and *Paraji* Will Not Work

Pak Yudi, head of health promotion, who had done most to bring the regulation into being, then argued that since *paraji* were more popular and more populous than *bidan* "we need partnership so that they don't compete." With a ratio of five *paraji* to every *bidan* "if they compete the *bidan* will not win." This is an appealing argument in a cultural context where competition is seen as potentially destructive and is generally avoided in the interests of promoting harmony (Berman, 1998). Pak Yudi painted the roles of *paraji* and *bidan* as complementary with *paraji* providing cultural and spiritual roles and *bidan* providing *medis*, the medical role. But "*paraji* do not know how to sew tears after a birth, and some place money on the newly cut umbilical cord." He added "in one month 7 infants died."

This dramatic statement acted as a catalyst for the head of the commission who responded, with a conciliatory chuckle, saying "if there were 7 deaths in one month, why have we not done this earlier?" He agreed to push forward the regulation as fast as possible but added that guidance was needed for all parties and that the *paraji* should not lose their rights. The specific rights of *paraji* were not elaborated by the commissioners, however, in marked contrast to the well-defined rights for all parties outlined in the regulation. Shortly after the meeting, the regulation was passed and became effective mid-2013.

## Discussion

> the definition of alternatives is the supreme instrument of power (Schattschneider, 1960)

I left Indonesia just before the district regulation on Partnership between *Bidan*, *Paraji*, and *Kader* was passed in 2013, and was unable to monitor the impact of the regulation first hand. There have been no formal evaluations of the program to date, but informal WhatsApp conversations with several *bidan* suggest it did strengthen the partnership policy in Lahanbesar district, although payments to *paraji* dwindled once Pak Yudi was transferred to a different position. There have also been improvements in resource allocations to the district hospital, improving the enabling environment for *bidan* and *paraji* (Personal Communication, district hospital program manager 2019).

Despite the limitations of time, my account does shed light on the policymaking process that led to the passing of the district regulation on partnership. As predicted by Shore and Wright (1997) this involved foreclosing alternatives. During the process of building the evidence base and presenting arguments to law makers and other stakeholders, the regulation on partnership was presented not only as beneficial to all parties involved, but also as the fastest means to address maternal death. This diverted attention away from alternatives such as provision of more resources to health centers; improving referral systems; training *bidan* in communication skills; or deployment of more experienced *bidan* in remote areas.

Analysis of the presentations made during the parliamentary meeting illustrates how certain logics were used to present partnership as the optimal option for addressing maternal death. First, the problem of maternal death is given a sense of urgency through Dr. Nia's presentation of the rising number of deaths from 33 in 2005 to 70 in 2011 and 77 in 2012. Although this dramatic increase may have been partly an effect of improved reporting, as Dr. Nia pointed out, it operated strategically to strengthen Dr. Nia's message which was that according to theory, deaths of mothers and infants should be falling, not rising, given the increase in the number of *bidan* attended births. The unacceptably high numbers provided a moral injunction to act, paving the way for the second step in the logic, the framing of the *paraji* as the cause of unacceptably high numbers of maternal deaths. Reflecting global framings of SBAs as the solution to MMR this involves bracketing off shortcomings in the referral system and in the services provided by *bidan* and hospitals and instead shining the spotlight on incidents involving *paraji*, even though this represented only 32% of all cases of maternal death in 2012. Notably, the data provided did not allow for a comparison of the relative risks of birth with *paraji* and *bidan*. By omitting this information attention was focused on the *paraji* as the cause and therefore the obvious target for intervention.

The third step involved presenting legalization of the existing partnership between *bidan* and *paraji* as the only mechanism for dealing with *paraji*. The possibility of a more equal partnership encouraging *bidan* to learn from the skills and experience of the *paraji* as well as vice versa is not entertained. The *paraji* is included within the partnership to avoid a negative outcome – competition with the *bidan* – rather than because her services are valued by government. The logical steps used in these speeches are represented schematically in Fig. 8.1.

At play here is a manifestation of power described by Lukes (2005) as the capacity to evade conflict by omitting issues from the agenda. Tensions in the relationship between *bidan* and *paraji* were not acknowledged or addressed in the regulation. These tensions remain latent through health promotion messages that frame partnership as mutually beneficial and as fulfilling the rights of all parties involved (Magrath, 2019).

Three factors in the broader policy environment help explain why district health officials in Lahanbesar foregrounded the regulation of *paraji*. First, global policy on TBAs has evolved from recommending training of TBAs in the 1990s, to a sidelining of TBAs from the early 2000s, as SBAs have become more available. Discussions of global maternal health policy sometimes fail even to mention TBAs, despite their continuing presence and popularity in many parts of the world (for example, Agarwal et al., 2019). The expectation, voiced by Bu Ika in the parliamentary meeting, that *paraji* will soon disappear, is entirely consistent with the expectation of global policymakers at the time, although ideas of incorporation and partnership are re-emerging (Miller & Smith, 2017).

The Millennium Development Goals present a second factor in the global policy context that influenced the development of the partnership regulation. Percent births attended by SBAs is one of two key indicators for goal 5 to reduce maternal mortality, reflecting the prominent role given to skilled attendance as a solution to maternal death. Pressure to achieve the MDGs creates a domino effect at each level of the health system, and in the context of decentralization in Indonesia, particularly at the district level.

This brings us to the third factor, the national policy context of decentralization. Decentralization shifted lines of management and authority such that district officials are now more accountable to their district parliament and the public for health outcomes. Pak Yudi and his colleagues therefore needed to demonstrate competency in addressing the issue of maternal deaths. Their options for doing so were, however, limited by the amount of decision space actually granted to districts under decentralization in Indonesia (Heywood & Harahap, 2009; Trisnantoro, 2009).

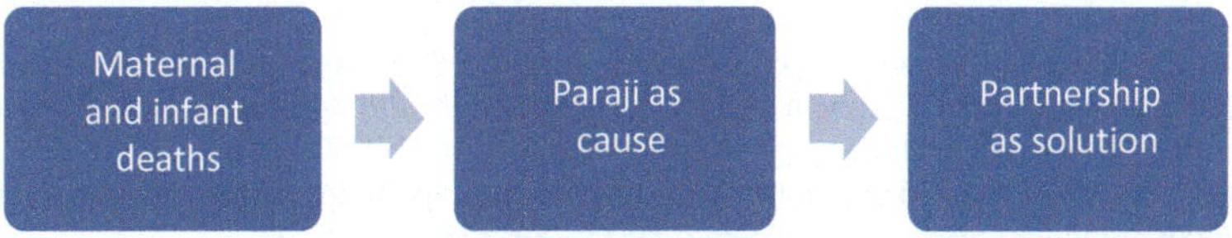


**Fig. 8.1** Schematic logic of foreclosing alternatives to address maternal and infant death

Decision space is defined as the capacity for officials at a given level of government to make decisions over a range of functions, including finance, administration, management, and policymaking (Bossert, 2014; Roman et al., 2017).

Some have argued that decentralization in Indonesia has been incomplete due to the limited decision space accorded to districts where central government has retained control over most forms of taxation (Fane, 2003). Thus, districts rely heavily on block grants from central government. Heywood and Harahap (2009) estimated that districts in Java rely on central government for up to 90% of their budget and that much of this is spent on salaries of permanent civil servants and programs mandated by central government, giving district health offices discretion over less than 25% of the budget. Whereas Pisani et al. (2016) refer to increased scope for policy entrepreneurship under decentralization in Indonesia, this is more evident in policy spheres such as health promotion that require limited funding. For districts in West Java with little discretion over spending of central government block grants, the capacity for innovative investments in infrastructure or human resources required to improve maternal health is limited. In this context, developing a regulation on partnership was a realistic option requiring a small amount of funding to compensate the *paraji* who joined the partnership.

## References


Achadi, E., Scott, S., Pambudi, E. S., Makowiecka, K., Marshall, T., Adisasmita, A., & Ronsmans, C. (2007). Midwifery provision and uptake of maternity care in Indonesia. *Tropical Medicine and International Health, 12*(12), 1490–1497. https://doi.org/10.1111/j.1365-3156.2007.01957.x

Achmad, J. (1999). *Hollow Development: The Politics of Health in Suharto's Indonesia*. PT Gramedia Pustaka Utama.

Agarwal, K., Lilly, K., & Jeffry, S. (2019). Innovative approaches to enhancing maternal and newborn survival: Indonesia's experience in an era of global commitments to reducing mortality. *International Journal of Gynecology and Obstetrics, 144*, 1–6. https://doi.org/10.1002/ijgo.12729

Agustina, R., Dartanto, T., Sitompul, R., Susiloretni, K. A., Suparmi, A., et al. (2019). Universal health coverage in Indonesia: Concept, progress, and challenges. *The Lancet, 393*(10166), 75–102. https://doi.org/10.1016/S0140-6736(18)31647-7

Badan Pusat Statistik. (2015). *Indonesia – 2015 Intercensal Population Survey*. Retrieved from https://microdata.bps.go.id/mikrodata/index.php/catalog/715/related_citations. Accessed 10 May 2020.

Bennett, L. R. (2017). Indigenous healing knowledge and infertility in Indonesia: Learning about cultural safety from Sasak midwives. *Medical Anthropology: Cross Cultural Studies in Health and Illness, 36*(2), 111–124. https://doi.org/10.1080/01459740.2016.1142990

Berman, L. (1998). *Speaking through the silence: Narratives, social conventions, and power in Java*. Oxford University Press.

Bossert, T. J. (2014). Decentralization of health systems: Challenges and global issues of the twenty-first century. In K. Regmi (Ed.), *Decentralizing health services: A global perspective* (pp. 199–207). Springer. https://doi.org/10.1007/978-1-4614-9071-5_12

Fane, G. (2003). Change and continuity in Indonesia's new fiscal decentralization arrangements. *Bulletin of Indonesian Economic Studies, 39*(1), 159–176.

Freedman, L. (2003). Strategic advocacy and maternal mortality: Moving targets and the Millennium Development Goals. *Gender and Development, 11*(1), 97–108. https://doi.org/10.1080/741954259

Guerra-Reyes, L. (2019). *Changing birth in the Andes: Culture policy and safe motherhood in Peru*. Vanderbilt University Press.

Hay, M. C. (2015). Maternal mortality in Indonesia: Anthropological perspectives on why mother death defies simple solutions. In D. A. Schwartz (Ed.), *Maternal mortality: Risk factors, anthropological perspectives, prevalence in developing countries and preventive strategies for pregnancy-related deaths* (pp. 339–371). Nova Science Publishers, Inc.

Heywood, P., & Harahap, N. (2009). Human resources for health at the *kabupaten* level in Indonesia: The smoke and mirrors of decentralization. *Human Resources for Health, 7*(6). https://doi.org/10.1186/1478-4491-7-6

Hildebrand, V. M. (2012). Scissors as symbols: Disputed ownership of the tools of biomedical obstetrics in rural Indonesia. *Culture, Medicine and Psychiatry, 36*(3), 557–570.

Hildebrand, V. M. (2017) Gift giving, reciprocity and exchange. In M. Ettorre, E. Annandale, V. M. Hildebrand, A. Porroche-Escudero, & B. K. Rothman (Eds.), *Health, culture and society* (pp. 179–211). https://doi.org/10.1007/978-3-319-60786-3

Hildebrand, V. M. & Magrath, P. (2016). In policy's shadow: Right to reproductive health in Indonesia. In *Paper presented at the Annual Meeting of the American Anthropological Association*, Minneapolis, November 16–20.

Hull, T. H., Rusman, R., & Hayes, A. (1998). *Village midwives and the improvement of maternal and infant health in NTT and NTB*. Australian National University.

Indonesia Ministry of Health. (n.d.). *Pedoman pelaksanaan kemitraan bidan dan dukun*. Ministry of Health.

Lahanbesar District. (2013). *Peraturan tentang kemitraan bidan, paraji dan kader kesehatan*.

Lukes, S. (2005). *Power: A radical view* (2nd ed.). Palgrave Macmillan.

Magrath, P. (2016). *Moral landscapes of health governance in West Java, Indonesia*. PhD dissertation. University of Arizona.

Magrath, P. (2019). Right to health: A buzzword in health policy in Indonesia. *Medical Anthropology: Cross Cultural Studies in Health and Illness, 38*(6), 464–447. https://doi.org/10.1080/01459740.2019.1604701

Makowiecka, K., Achadi, E., Izati, Y., & Ronsmans, C. (2008). Midwifery provision in two districts in Indonesia: How well are rural areas served? *Health Policy and Planning, 23*(1), 67–75.

Manor, J. (1999). *The political economy of democratic decentralization*. The World Bank.

Miller, T., & Smith, H. (2017). Establishing partnership with traditional birth attendants for improved maternal and newborn health: A review of factors influencing implementation. *BMC Pregnancy and Childbirth, 17*(365). https://doi.org/10.1186/s12884-017-1534-y

National Population and Family Planning Board (NPFPB) & Ministry of Health (MoH), Indonesia. (1991). *Indonesian Demographic and Health Survey 1991*. https://dhsprogram.com/what-we-do/survey/survey-display-35.cfm. Accessed 10 May 2020.

National Population and Family Planning Board (NPFPB) & Ministry of Health (MoH), Indonesia. (2017). *Indonesian Demographic and Health Survey 2017*. https://dhsprogram.com/publications/publication-fr342-dhs-final-reports.cfm. Accessed 10 May 2020.

Nichter, M. (2008). *Global health: Why cultural perception, social representations, and biopolitics matter*. University of Arizona Press.

Niehof, A. (2014). Traditional birth attendants and the problem of maternal mortality in Indonesia. *Pacific Affairs, 87*(4), 693–715. https://doi.org/10.5509/2014874693

Pigg, S. L. (1997). Authority in translation: Finding, knowing, naming, and training "traditional birth attendants" in Nepal. In R. E. Davis-Floyd & C. F. Sargent (Eds.), *Childbirth and authoritative knowledge: Cross-cultural perspectives* (pp. 233–262). University of California Press.

Pisani, E., Kok, M. O., & Nugroho, K. (2016). Indonesia's road to universal health coverage: A political journey. *Health Policy and Planning, 32*(2), 267–276. https://doi.org/10.1093/heapol/czw120

Rishworth, A., Dixon, J., Luginaah, I., Mkandawire, P., & Tampah Prince, C. (2016). "I was on the way to the hospital but delivered in the bush": Maternal health in Ghana's Upper West Region in the context of a traditional birth attendants' ban. *Social Science and Medicine, 148*, 8–17. https://doi.org/10.1016/j.socscimed.2015.11.018

Roman, T. E., Cleary, S., & McIntyre, D. (2017). Exploring the functioning of decision space: A review of the available health systems literature. *International Journal of Health Policy and Management, 6*(7), 365–376.

Rudrum, S. (2016). Institutional ethnography research in global south settings: The role of texts. *International Journal of Qualitative Methods,* 1–8. https://doi.org/10.1177/1609406916637088

Ruslan, H. (2013, March 17). Sukabumi gagas perda kemitraan bidan dan paraji. *Republika.* https://www.republika.co.id/berita/nasional/jawa-barat-nasional/13/03/17/mjtbzf-sukabumi-gagas-perda-kemitraan-bidan-dan-paraji

Schattschneider, E. E. (1960). *The semisovereign people: A realist's view of democracy in America.* Holt, Rinehart and Winston.

Shiffman, J. (2003). Generating political will for safe motherhood in Indonesia. *Social Science and Medicine, 56*(6), 1197–1207.

Shore, C., & Wright, S. (1997). Policy: A new field of anthropology. In C. Shore & S. Wright (Eds.), *Anthropology of policy: Critical perspectives on governance and power* (pp. 3–39). Routledge.

Stein, E. (2007). Midwives, Islamic morality and village biopower in post-Suharto Indonesia. *Body & Society, 13*(3), 55–77. https://doi.org/10.1177/1357034X07082252.

Titaley, C. R., Hunter, C. L., Dibley, M. J., & Heywood, P. (2010). Why do some women still prefer traditional birth attendants and home delivery? A qualitative study on delivery care services in West Java Province, Indonesia. *BMC Pregnancy and Childbirth, 10*, 43–53.

Trisnantoro, L. (2009). *Pelaksanaan desentralisasi kesehatan di Indonesia 2000–2007: Mengkaji pengalaman dan skenario masa depan* (2nd ed.). BPFE-Yogyakarta.

UNICEF. (2010). *Programme experiences in Indonesia: Documentation collection.* https://www.medbox.org/document/programme-experiences-in-indonesia-documentation-collection#GO. Accessed 10 May 2020.

United Nations Development Program (NDP). (2003). *Indicators for monitoring the Millennium Development Goals: Definitions, rationale, concepts and sources.* United Nations https://www.undp.org/content/dam/aplaws/publication/en/publications/poverty-reduction/poverty-website/indicators-for-monitoring-the-mdgs/Indicators_for_Monitoring_the_MDGs.pdf. Accessed 9 Feb 2019.

WHO. (2004). *Making pregnancy safer: The critical role of the skilled attendant: A joint statement by WHO, ICM and FIGO.* World Health Organization.

WHO, UNICEF, UNFPA, World Bank Group, United Nations Population Division. (2015). *Maternal mortality 1990–2015, Indonesia.* World Health Organization.

# Chapter 9
# Making Space for Qualitative Evidence in Global Maternal and Child Health Policymaking

**Christopher J. Colvin**

## Introduction

The success of health interventions often hinges on complex processes of implementation, the impact of sociopolitical and cultural contexts, resource constraints and opportunity costs, and issues of equity and accountability. Qualitative research offers critical insights for understanding these issues. "Qualitative evidence syntheses" (or QES)—modeled on quantitative systematic reviews—have recently emerged as an important vehicle for integrating insights from qualitative evidence into global health policy.

However, it is challenging to integrate QES into policymaking in ways that are both *acceptable* to the often-conservative health policy world and *consonant* with social science's distinctive methodologies and paradigms. Based on my experiences participating in and observing numerous guideline working group meetings and interviews with key informants, this chapter offers an auto-ethnographic account of an effort to integrate QES into the World Health Organization's global OptimizeMNH guidelines for task shifting in maternal and newborn health (MNH).

"Global guidelines," like those developed by the World Health Organization (WHO) and other major international health institutions, are a critical component of global health policy. They synthesize evidence on key policy questions and set norms and standards for health decision-making and practice by "assist[ing] providers, recipients and other stakeholders to make informed decisions about appropriate health interventions" (WHO, 2003). WHO guidelines, in particular, carry significant authority in global public health and have an outsize influence on health decision-making across a wide range of contexts (Ruger & Yach, 2009).

C. J. Colvin (✉)
Department of Public Health Sciences, University of Virginia, Charlottesville, VA, USA
e-mail: cjc5r@virginia.edu



L. J. Wallace et al. (eds.), *Anthropologies of Global Maternal and Reproductive Health*, Global Maternal and Child Health, https://doi.org/10.1007/978-3-030-84514-8_9

As a technology for consolidating the latest knowledge and best practices, and for setting policy norms and standards, guidelines are a recent development, emerging only in the last three decades (Bhaumik, 2017). The birth of the health policy guideline was closely tied to the rise of "evidence-based medicine" (or EBM). EBM has become the hegemonic framework in contemporary biomedicine and health policymaking for legitimizing knowledge claims. At the methodological heart of EBM and "evidence-based policy-making" (EBPM) is the systematic review, which involves the identification, collation, and synthesis of all the available (quantitative) evidence on the safety, efficacy, and cost-effectiveness of health interventions (Mykhalovskiy & Weir, 2004).

Guidelines are typically developed in response to specific policy and practice questions that, in turn, reflect knowledge gaps or contentious debates within the field. Systematic reviews are meant to provide independent, "evidence-based" answers to these questions as well as guidance on policy options and preferences. During the first few decades of EBM—from the mid-1970s to the early 2000s—the preferred form of evidence in systematic reviews was the randomized controlled trial (RCT), a method for producing evidence of the efficacy of a discrete intervention by attempting to control—through randomization—for all other factors related to an outcome of interest (Adams, 2013). Other forms of quantitative evidence that also assessed efficacy, albeit in a less controlled fashion, were included in these reviews but fell further down EBM's standard "hierarchy of evidence."

Though the language and logic of EBM and the RCT are ubiquitous in biomedicine and health policy, there is growing recognition of the limits of standard EBM approaches (Ioannidis, 2014; Hutchison & Rogers, 2012) as well as the potential contribution of qualitative evidence (Gilson et al., 2011). Those involved in health policy are increasingly linking the success of health interventions to wider questions about the complex processes of program implementation, the impact of sociopolitical contexts, resource constraints and opportunity costs, and issues of local agency, equity, and acceptability (Olivier de Sardan et al., 2017). Qualitative research is seen by many to offer a critical evidence base for addressing these questions (Lewin & Glenton, 2018).

In order to integrate qualitative research into EBM's existing evidentiary practices, some researchers have been developing methods for including qualitative evidence in policymaking in ways that are accepted as legitimate by those working within orthodox EBM frameworks. "Qualitative evidence syntheses" (or QES)—modeled on principles and methods of quantitative systematic reviews—is one such methodology. QES has been practiced on a small scale for a number of years but has only recently gained momentum as a method for integrating qualitative research into more formal processes of health policy and decision making.

The growing place of QES in health policy raises a number of important questions about new (and old) forms of evidence production, circulation, and consumption and about the ways in which these forms of knowledge practice reflect, and in turn have an impact on, forms of responsibility and accountability within health policy, and health governance more broadly. What forms of qualitative evidence will be included (or excluded) in decision making and how will this evidence be evaluated (and even ranked)? How will global policymakers understand the relationships (and differences) between quantitative and qualitative forms of evidence? How will they integrate knowledge from qualitative research about the role of local context into guidelines often understood as universal? Does the mere presence of qualitative evidence have the power to change global health decision-making processes and politics for the better, or will it simply be co-opted in service to already existing goals and perspectives?

This chapter tackles some of these questions through the lens of an ethnographic case study of the use of QES in the development of the WHO's "OptimizeMNH guidelines" (WHO, 2012) for task shifting in maternal and newborn health (MNH). The Optimize guidelines were the first WHO guidelines to officially include QES in the evidence base that informed its recommendations. It thus provides an excellent opportunity to reflect on the emergence and significance of new forms of knowledge production and decision making in global health policy. It is also an opportunity to reflect on the potential connections and tensions between the field of maternal and reproductive health and these new forms and practices of evidence-into-policy work. The ethnographic focus of the chapter is on the Optimize Technical Working Group (TWG), a collection of WHO staff and external methodologists and researchers who designed the guideline development process and carried out many of the required evidence syntheses. The TWG was a rich ethnographic site for charting the development of new methods for integrating qualitative evidence into existing health policy practices.

In the end, the OptimizeMNH guidelines were perceived by those involved to be a great success. The qualitative evidence syntheses we produced played an important role in shaping the guidelines' recommendations. The TWG enjoyed flexibility in how it approached its work as well as widespread acceptance, even enthusiasm, about its efforts among the broader group of policymakers engaged with the guidelines. The process did require negotiating an often delicate balance between existing quantitative-focused paradigms and methods for evidence synthesis and decision making, and the distinctive paradigms and methods of qualitative research. But the case study also demonstrated that EBM knowledge production practices can be more flexible and more accommodating of multiple methodological and epistemological perspectives than has been previously reported.

## A Note on Methods

I first became involved in Optimize not as an ethnographer, but as a direct participant when I was commissioned to work on several of the qualitative evidence syntheses for the guideline and join the TWG. I was initially asked to participate because of my previous research on task shifting among community health workers (CHWs). I had never conducted a QES before nor had any exposure to guideline development. Given the recency of both QES methodology and the evidence review process for Optimize, however, I was told that my lack of experience was not an issue. As soon as I got involved in the project, I became fascinated by the space for qualitative research that had apparently opened up in this particular domain of health policy. I began developing a parallel (auto-)ethnographic project to reflect on how this space opened up, how it is understood, experienced, and negotiated by those involved, and what it might (or might not) say about changing practices of knowledge production in health policy and practice. The impetus for developing this parallel project has been my ongoing experience of shifting—sometimes uncomfortably—between my anthropological lens on the world, and my public health perspective. The critical medical anthropologist in me was—and remains—suspicious of biomedicine's newfound interest in "qualitative" work; but the public health researcher in me saw—and still sees—this opening as an opportunity to be met with (cautious) good faith.

I have remained involved in a number of projects of this kind since my experience with Optimize, many of them with the same people in that initial TWG. The material presented here is based on my reflections about participating in the Optimize guideline development process as well as numerous informal conversations over the years and 12 formal in-depth interviews with several of the TWG members and others involved in QES work. My work on these guidelines began in 2011 and I have been working slowly on this parallel ethnographic project since then. My source material comes from field notes, minutes of meetings, formal review and guideline documents, and interview notes. The process of analysis has been iterative and has unfolded over time, through conference presentations and conversations with those working with me in this field. I have continued to discuss this parallel ethnographic project with the TWG group members and they have remained enthusiastic about the chance to reflect on this work. Ethics approval was provided by the University of Cape Town's Faculty of Health Sciences Human Research Ethics Committee.

## A Primer on Qualitative Evidence Synthesis

The recent growth of qualitative evidence synthesis as a method for "secondary" knowledge production emerges from the intersection of two parallel developments in global health research. The first is the aforementioned rise of evidence-based medicine and the complex set of evidentiary practices, knowledge claims, and forms of accountability and audit that have accompanied EBM (Adams, 2016). The second, less visible development has been the steady but quiet growth of "qualitative health research" in the health sciences (Pope & Mays, 2009). Though the tensions between qualitative and quantitative research in health (Inhorn, 1995; Petticrew & Roberts, 2003; Porter, 2006) persist, there has nonetheless been a slowly growing inclusion of primary qualitative research within the health sciences (Shuval et al.,

2011).[1] This inclusion of qualitative research has often been slow, grudging, and conducted on the terms of more powerful actors within health research (see, for example, the recent debate (Daniels et al., 2016; Greenhalgh et al., 2016) around the inclusion of qualitative research in the *British Medical Journal*). Nonetheless, there are significantly more qualitative health researchers, research units, academic journals, and grant-funded research projects than there were at the beginning of EBM's rise.

The focus of this chapter is not, however, on the rise of primary qualitative research in health but rather on the more recent emergence of "qualitative evidence synthesis," a term for the broad cluster of methods for systematically synthesizing the findings of primary qualitative research from multiple research studies. QES methods follow, in many ways, the basic logic of a quantitative systematic review: a thorough search of the available evidence around a specific review question, an assessment of the quality of each of these underlying studies, clear guidelines for inclusion and systematic procedures for data analysis, and the use of multiple reviewers and audit trails. However, QES approaches tailor their techniques to the important methodological and epistemological differences between quantitative and qualitative research (Hannes & Macaitis, 2012).

There has been rapid growth in QES, with nearly all of the existing reviews—now numbering in the thousands—having been conducted in the last 15 years, the majority of them in the last 5 years. Authors use a wide, sometimes dizzying range of approaches in QES (Dixon-Woods et al., 2005), reflecting the diversity of methodological and epistemological approaches that fall under the broad category of "qualitative research." Most QES authors work in applied contexts and most of the existing syntheses have been produced by researchers in the UK, parts of Europe, and Australia.

Though QES generally entail a high degree of methodological complexity and systematicity and are often published in peer-reviewed journals, they are frequently initially produced for use by health policymakers and practitioners in relation to specific policy and practice questions. Proponents of QES make several arguments for how these syntheses add an important dimension to health policymaking. They argue that qualitative evidence can answer questions that are distinct from questions asked in quantitative research, including: (1) the scope of health problems (and their causes), (2) the perspectives and experiences of different groups of people in relation to these health problems, (3) the acceptability and feasibility of interventions to address health problems, and (4) factors that affect the implementation of these interventions (Lewin & Glenton, 2018).

[1] In evidence synthesis, a distinction is typically made between "primary research" that collects and analyses new data (e.g., from interviews, observations, document reviews, and ethnography) and secondary research which synthesizes the findings from reports of previously conducted research (e.g., from journal articles, books, NGO, or government reports).

## Origin Stories: QES in OptimizeMNH

The Optimize guidelines aimed to contribute answers to all four of these types of questions in relation to "task shifting" in maternal and newborn health programs. Task shifting describes the reorganization of discrete health service tasks by moving them from one cadre of health worker to another (WHO, 2006). Though task shifting initiatives can address a variety of problems, in most cases, it is a response to the global crisis in human resources for health and an effort to realign service delivery to be more efficient and more in line with local resource limitations and capacity constraints (Lehmann et al., 2009; Mishra et al., 2015).

In this case, practitioners, program managers, and policy-makers in maternal and newborn health were confronted with a series of unanswered questions about task shifting. The WHO Departmental Director who oversaw the guideline development reported that the initial trigger for Optimize was debates around whether CHWs could safely and effectively administer misoprostol to treat postpartum hemorrhage (PPH) outside of health facilities. Misoprostol is a cheap, easy-to-use, and highly effective life-saving drug that can prevent a major cause of maternal mortality (Smith et al., 2015). Reproductive health activists were pushing for wider use of misoprostol by CHWs for those women who could not or chose not to deliver in health facilities. WHO country offices were also asking for guidance on this issue and there was a long-standing debate within the scientific literature as well. A number of contentious issues were at play, including the medical risks of improper administration of misoprostol, fears that administration by CHWs would disincentivise facility birthing, and the fact that misoprostol can also be used for medical abortion (Wainwright et al., 2016).

Though task shifting of misoprostol administration for PPH was the initial trigger for Optimize, early discussions on the scope of the guideline soon identified a wide range of other task shifting questions in maternal and newborn health around which there was uncertainty about safety, efficacy, cost-effectiveness, acceptability, and feasibility. There were questions, for example, as to whether CHWs could be trained to perform neonatal resuscitation or nurses could be trained to perform emergency caesareans. The goal of Optimize was to review the available evidence on task shifting those key tasks and cadres around which there was uncertainty. The conventional approach in this kind of scenario is for a team like the Technical Working Group to compile the existing systematic reviews of safety and effectiveness, commission systematic reviews in areas where they do not yet exist, and present all the available evidence to an independent panel, the Guideline Development Group (GDG), that would then develop the official guideline recommendations.

In the earliest discussions around Optimize, the focus was indeed on collecting quantitative evidence to address safety and effectiveness. It did not take long, however, for those involved to recognize that task shifting is as much a problem of program implementation and local context as it is one of technical training and clinical service provision. There were also larger programmatic and political issues at stake here, including: the role of community health workers in primary health care; the tensions between midwives, nurses, and doctors; the debates over facility-based versus home-based delivery; and the generally poor quality of care for women and newborns in many countries. Those involved in these early discussions recognized these were questions that could not be resolved through RCTs; they needed qualitative research to more fully understand these issues and the possible ways to address them.

This recognition of the need for qualitative research did not, however, emerge only in relation to the specific policy questions at stake in Optimize. There were a number of people, institutions, resources, and existing relationships that aligned to set the stage for recognizing the value of qualitative research in this particular set of guidelines. During informal discussions about the project, for example, TWG members often highlighted the positive influence of the Director of the Department producing the guidelines, a medical doctor with no background in qualitative research but with deep programmatic experience of the implementation of MNH services. The TWG's methodological experts had an existing relationship to this Director and were also long-standing advocates for improving how guidelines were developed and expanding the bodies of evidence guidelines made use of.

These more internal dynamics within the WHO were complemented by recent expansions in the broader conceptual vocabularies of global health policymakers and practitioners, including the rise of "health systems thinking," complexity theory, and implementation science, all important contexts for Optimize. In the years preceding the guidelines, there was growing international interest in health systems research and program implementation, and there were several initiatives just at the WHO to improve how guidelines were developed for health systems problems (Bosch-Capblanch et al., 2012). These conceptual developments in health systems research, along with the steadily growing presence of qualitative health research more generally, helped highlight the utility of including qualitative evidence in guidelines like Optimize.

Just as critical, however, was the work of individuals and research and policy institutions—like the Norwegian Knowledge Centre for the Health Services, the UK's National Institute for Health and Care Excellence (NICE), and the Joanna Briggs Institute—that had been working for years at the intersection of qualitative health research and policymaking, developing the concepts and tools, forming the personal and professional relationships, and consolidating the human and financial resources necessary for such an undertaking. Some of this foundation-laying took the form of active lobbying and awareness-raising to promote greater inclusion of qualitative evidence. For the most part, however, it was the alignment of numerous individuals, institutions, and ideas working with or, more often, adjacent to each other over time that ultimately created the window of opportunity for Optimize's engagement with qualitative evidence.

## New Hierarchies Undone by Old Methods

The core technical working group that I joined was compromised of eight members. In addition to the Department Director mentioned earlier and me, there were three other anthropologists, two with QES and guideline development experience; a nursing professor with QES methods expertise; and two medical doctors with some recent experience in conducting or reviewing qualitative research. Training in anthropology was predominant in the group and in our conversations, all of the group members (including the clinicians) frequently spoke of ethnography as both the richest and most rigorous and trustworthy form of evidence we might include in our syntheses. Though never formally codified as such, long-term, in-depth ethnographic studies stood at the top of a now-inverted hierarchy of evidence for QES.

Since there were no existing QES that addressed the guideline's focus on task shifting for maternal and newborn health, we decided to conduct three new syntheses, on lay health workers (LHWs), midwives, and mid-level providers (who occupy a space between nurses and doctors in the professional hierarchy). In each review, the primary objective was to understand the factors affecting implementation of task shifting initiatives in maternal and child health programs. These factors included both familiar concepts such as the "acceptability" of such initiatives among health-care workers, patients, family members, and others as well as concepts related to broader social and political contexts that could affect the "feasibility" of these programs.

At the start of the process, I, at least, had the sense that there was a rich ethnographic literature we would be able to draw on for the LHW and midwife reviews. I knew some of this literature already and imagined spending the next few months reading more deeply. In practice, however, rather than diving into ethnographies, I spent most of my time reading quite short, poorly conceived and poorly written qualitative health research articles based on once-off interviews and focus groups with small groups of people. In these articles, the methods section was sometimes as long as the main body of the paper and the most common analytic strategy an anodyne form of "thematic analysis." Quotes peppered the brief text but little was offered in the way of context or interpretation and discussion.

The reason we spent most of our time working through this literature was primarily methodological. The logic of systematic reviews requires a clearly defined research question and a systematic search strategy. This is consonant with the reductionist approach of the natural sciences, where the phenomenon of interest is narrowly delimited and closely examined under controlled circumstances. In our reviews, we defined our questions clearly but also, we thought, quite broadly. The LHW review, for example, was interested in any evidence on any shifting of health service tasks to or from LHWs in the context of maternal and newborn health. In theory, any ethnography that included LHWs working with women and babies would have been eligible.

In practice, however, finding such literature efficiently was next to impossible. First, few ethnographic studies define themselves narrowly around specific groups such as LHWs or specific concepts such as task shifting. Task shifting might play a key role in an ethnographic text but unless it is indexed as such in a database, it would be very difficult to find efficiently. Ethnographic research rarely sets out to answer such narrowly defined research questions using such discrete variables, and rarely frames its questions in the vocabulary of the health sciences and health policy.

Second, we had decided to not search for books, though we could include them if we knew of them already or found them during our searches and they met our inclusion criteria. This was primarily because most databases that catalogue books do not do so to the same degree of precision as journal articles. The kinds of searches that are standard practice in EBM—precise and multi-layered searches of abstracts, keywords, full-text, forward and backward citations, etc.—are generally not possible with books. The inclusion of books would have also represented a pragmatic dilemma in terms of how long it might have taken to properly read and extract the findings from multiple books.

Finally, ethnographic and other social science research articles published outside of biomedical and public health contexts could be difficult to find because of the poor quality of the database search engines that indexed these publications. The biomedical research world has, over many years, and as a result of the rise of EBM, slowly but significantly improved the platforms for indexing and searching this literature. Whereas this literature is often richly "tagged" with meta-data and is searchable with complex algorithms, the important anthropological journal database AnthroSource at the time only offered keyword searching, and frequently missed relevant articles we knew existed within its publications. Some medical anthropology journals are indexed and searchable in PubMed but this was only a limited solution to a deeper problem.

As a result, the literature that we had imagined sitting atop the QES hierarchy of evidence was precisely the literature that was least visible to the methods and tools we had at hand. Furthermore, the literature we did find from anthropology and related disciplines was most often focused on the daily lived experience and "cultural contexts" of individuals, communities, and healthcare workers. As valuable as this was, it did not meet our inclusion criteria. Ethnographic work that closely examined the process of the implementation of task shifting interventions was much harder to come by.

Throughout the search process, we thus confronted a number of obstacles in our ambition to mine the ethnographic literature. These barriers included the form and content of ethnographic knowledge itself, as well as the ways in which this knowledge is archived and made visible and accessible to other researchers. Also critical was the limiting role of time and financial constraints in determining what kinds of searches were possible and what kinds of knowledge would be feasible to include in the review.

## NerdWorld: Pragmatism, Innovation, and Ideology

I was at first frustrated by the methodological barriers to including ethnographic literature. These barriers were not merely technical but rather the result of long-standing techniques for ordering knowledge and privileging certain kinds of research questions and methods. It was also clear, however, that there was no easy way around this dilemma, not without a wholesale restructuring of the logic and methods of systematic reviews. This was something that would have not only required significant time and resources but would have also scuttled the effort to integrate QES into these guidelines.

Despite this particular methodological impasse, though, on the whole, I found the TWG's approach to methods to be pragmatic and flexible. When I started, I feared two types of methodological orthodoxy. First, I was concerned that the group members might try to mechanically and inappropriately translate techniques for quantitative systematic reviews to the qualitative literature. It was clear to me how this approach would undercut any legitimate integration of qualitative research into the guidelines.

Second, I was worried about another kind of orthodoxy, dominant in some of the qualitative health research methods literature. This part of the literature is characterized by a rigid, defensive, and even mystifying approach to qualitative research methods that tries to define itself in distinct contrast to quantitative methods. It foregrounds presumably insurmountable differences in epistemology between qualitative and quantitative paradigms and advertises the complex, thorough, and rigorous nature of qualitative data analysis (often through highly formalized procedures and complex terminology). This approach diverges dramatically from my methods training in anthropology, which like many of my generation primarily consisted of advice to just go to the field and "figure it out."

However, the TWG's methodological experts generally took a pragmatic approach. When we asked how we could adapt our search strategies, or choose a conceptual framework for analysis, or determine the difference between "empirical" research and "opinion" pieces, or draw inferences from "indirect" evidence on different but closely related topics, the methodologists generally simply asked the group what seemed most "reasonable." These kinds of questions were often debated at length in group discussions, where all sides of the issues were put on the table and a feasible but reasonable course of action eventually set out. We were always reminded at the end of these discussions to "show our work" and explain our reasoning.

Quantitative research is of course also filled with judgment and pragmatic choices like these, if mostly implicitly. It is no less shot through with the need to manage ambiguity, uncertainty, incompleteness, and the hard-to-predict impact of context. But there are well-established procedures in quantitative research—again, many of them implicit—for making this messiness much less visible. What felt different here was the absence of widely recognized, pre-existing standards against which to measure (or obscure) our pragmatic choices. In their absence, we were counseled to record and justify our approach. This imperative to "be transparent" was intended to both ensure accountability and lay the foundation for the next round of researchers to build upon and develop a community of practice for these new methodologies.

There was a great deal of positive energy and engagement in these methodological discussions, as well as an explicit contrast drawn between the routine pragmatics of methodology and broader ideological battles around knowledge production. One TWG member described the group as a bunch of "nerds" more interested in crafting a "good enough" methodology than in litigating ideological debates about qualitative versus quantitative epistemology. These methodological discussions were also characterized by an excitement around the chance to develop new methods for new problems and to be involved in the "ground-breaking" step of including QES in WHO guidelines.

The work of the TWG and the perspectives of its members were, of course, shot through with various ideologies—not least of which was the focus on innovation and the "historic" nature of the group's work—but it was not always clear which ideological frameworks were at play at a given time. Certainly, one ideological feature that often sat in tension with our pragmatic impulses was the emphasis on "evidence-based methods" and the need for vigilance in preventing unwarranted and "subjective" assumptions about methodological choices to overrule evidence-based decisions. For example, a debate emerged during the review design process about how many studies to include. Rather than aim for an exhaustive review of all the available evidence that is possibly relevant (as in a quantitative review), we did what social scientists often do—searched for and included the best evidence that would tell us the most, however, that was defined—about what we were interested in. We did this by sampling purposively from the broad set of studies identified in our original search.

This rather conventional approach generated some real hesitation among some team members about the potential for bias and the lack of an objective evidence base about how certain sampling strategies might shape the direction of our review. The anthropologists in the group countered that the possibility of alternative interpretations was a central tenet of the interpretive process—and thus not a threat, nor something that could be resolved through "evidence"—and that a random sample of eligible studies would send precisely the wrong message about how interpretation works. We also argued that reading the full set of potentially eligible studies, in some effort to avoid "bias," would likely overwhelm our capacity to effectively interpret it. Whereas "more data" is often assumed, rightly or wrongly, to be preferable in quantitative research, this is usually not the case in qualitative research.

Behind this decision to purposively sample were other factors as well, including limited funding, limited time frames, and a palpable dread within the TWG of having to deal with even more poorly done qualitative health research. These factors—time, resources, and the often-difficult lived experience of the review process—were significant forces shaping the pragmatic decisions made within our reviews.

## Show Your Work!: Transparency, Accountability, and Interpretation

While this kind of pragmatism was a welcome surprise to me, one consequence of "showing your work" was a kind of "bread crumb" approach to supporting arguments and referencing studies in our narrative. See, for example, the following excerpt from the LHW review:

> "In four USA-based studies (S16; S50; S52; S53), LHWs gave mothers, including teenage mothers and others in difficult socioeconomic circumstances, emotional and practical support and also promoted healthy behaviours during pregnancy, childbirth and in the first few weeks after birth. In one Australian study, LHWs offered emotional support and practical help to parents at risk of child abuse and neglect (S55). In approximately twelve studies, from Australia (S10), Canada (S17-18, 48), the UK (S35, S37, S44), the USA (S40, S46), Brazil (S47), Mexico (S51), India (S1), Papua New Guinea (S2) and Viet Nam (S19), LHWs carried out a package of tasks that were primarily promotional with the aim of improving maternal and child health" (Glenton et al., 2013).

This kind of analysis is at the opposite end of the spectrum from my experience in anthropology where ethnographic authority (properly established), the ethnographic vignette, and convincing theoretical argumentation are valued as the proper grounds for defending interpretations. Ethnographic claims should be defendable but not entirely or, at least, easily auditable.

The approach here, however, is organized in a way that always anticipates the audit. There was even frequent mention of the need to leave "audit trails" for future reviewers and readers. In the review narrative, however, this rhetorical strategy sits in awkward tension with conventions in qualitative interpretation. This is perhaps best seen in the strange phrase "In approximately twelve studies," a nonsensical wording (since it is *exactly* 12 studies) that attempts to combine the imperative for transparency and audit with qualitative narrative's customary resistance to quantifying individual points of information.

This approach is rooted in an idea that one can directly link interpreted findings to individual findings in the individual studies being reviewed. Instead of building holistic interpretations within studies or developing thematic, even explanatory interpretations across studies, the primary unit of analysis was the individual finding, supported by a precisely specified evidence base.

In the process, however, the cited studies appear to provide equivalent support for each claim. Each study, though, was conducted in a particular context with its own unique research question. The collected findings may have only been loosely comparable to each other. Specifying all the possible nuanced differences between studies supporting a synthesized finding is impractical (and is in fact the necessary "hidden" work of interpretation). But the demand for transparency required this kind of documenting and it often felt like the text—and our analytical ambition—was weighed down by these citations, making it difficult to draw connections across findings, evaluate patterns, and propose interpretations at a more abstract level.

Much of this effort to show our work and be transparent in our methodological judgments and interpretations was about demonstrating the legitimacy of this type of evidence production and our willingness to be held accountable for our work. This was especially important given the skepticism with which we feared some in the WHO and elsewhere would view our efforts to integrate qualitative evidence into these guidelines. Other forms of accountability and legitimacy, both new and old, were at work here as well, though. Central to the perceived legitimacy of our efforts was that we were working under the auspices of the WHO's overall Guidelines Review Committee and its *Guidelines Development Handbook*. Official institutional approval, and our accountability to the institution's procedures and standards, was vital to the legitimacy of our work, both in the eyes of the TWG members and other observers. Also important was the fact that many TWG members were affiliated with recognized research institutions and initiatives, ensuring a further layer of legitimacy and accountability.

There was one final and unexpected dynamic of accountability that may have emerged out of our careful documenting of the qualitative evidence. When this project began, I heard concerns from several people about the ways Guideline Development Groups (GDG)—the independent experts who review the TWG's work and make the formal recommendations—sometimes too easily brought their own personal experiences and perspectives to the table, using their social status within their field or the GDG to push specific policy options. This was especially true, they argued, when a GDG had only had effectiveness and safety data to work with. There have also been long-standing concerns that the experiences, needs, and preferences of patients and affected communities are not adequately represented in GDGs and that specialist panelists may too often think they can "speak for" these under-represented groups (Knaapen & Lehoux, 2016).

We certainly did not expect our qualitative syntheses to provide data-driven answers to all of the possible policy questions and options on the table. Having the evidence from our reviews readily at hand, however, may have transformed to some extent how conversations and decisions unfolded within the panel. There may have been less scope for bringing personal experiences with implementation of programs to the conversation when evidence on implementation was now available in another form. The presence of qualitative reviews may have also sat in tension with the inputs from stakeholder, advocacy, and community representatives on the GDG.

## Conclusion

So what might the aforementioned developments signify? I have described how those of us working to integrate QES in the Optimize guideline development process attempted to open up a space for a new kind of evidentiary practice—one which could in turn entail new forms of policy decision-making and practice—but were then confronted by a range of social, material, and technical limits to this project. Observers and supporters of this effort spoke often of the rhetorical importance of having QES meaningfully integrated into these guidelines, arguing that it would strike a real blow for the inclusion of new and potentially transgressive forms of knowledge within the often conservative world of health policy. I have mentioned earlier the growing strength of ideas of health systems, implementation science, and policy translation in global health as well as the slow (and still siloed) growth of qualitative research in health (Daniels et al., 2016). The decision to integrate QES into these WHO guidelines was indeed a coup for those promoting these agendas.

Of course, in practice, the project's success hinged on a careful balance between adopting conventional, quantitatively inspired methods and standards familiar to the WHO authorities overseeing the guidelines and innovating new methods that would both suit the project needs and please a different set of authorities (i.e., social scientists and other qualitative research experts). This experience raises important questions about how our understandings of EBM and EBPM may need to be revised.

For example, the integration of QES in global guideline development entails many of the same processes of *formalization* (of synthesis methods), *disentanglement* (of evidence from its underlying contexts), and *separation* (of science from politics) that have been identified by ethnographers and STS scholars of EBM (Moreira, 2007; Bohlin, 2012; Sundqvist et al., 2015). However, many of these procedures also look somewhat different from how they have been described in the literature on quantitative-focused EBM. The use of purposive sampling in QES, for example, introduces forms of judgment typically thought—albeit incorrectly—to be excluded from EBM procedures. Similarly, recognition of the critical role of local context in explaining the findings from individual studies sits in tension with the idea that EBM always works to disentangle findings from the contexts of their production. Finally, the broad scope and flexible nature of many QES review questions and the often iterative nature of QES search processes both complicate the production of "non-evidence" in EBM (Knaapen, 2013). While QES do require decisions about what should be included as "evidence" that is responsive to a particular review question, the judgments required to decide on the boundary between evidence and non-evidence look different (see Noyes (2018) for a discussion of the question of relevance when assessing evidence included in QES).

There are signs of the uptake of QES approaches in guidelines across a wide range of WHO departments (and at other institutions such as the UK's National Institute for Health and Care Excellence (NICE)). The Department Director who initiated the Optimize project identified some significant ongoing effects in his field of the integration of QES in WHO guidelines. He described a recent guideline his department produced on antenatal care (ANC) (WHO, 2016) that normally would have focused on biologically framed outcomes like ANC-related morbidity and mortality. After his department's experience with Optimize, however, the scope of the guidelines was expanded to include "positive pregnancy experiences," a phrase they even included in the guideline title and as a core guideline objective. As with Optimize, concerns with biological outcomes were integrated with social, cultural, psychological, and experiential outcomes when developing recommendations.

Such an extension of the imaginative boundaries of one or two WHO guidelines is not revolutionary. It is perhaps better understood as the result of long-term foundation-laying work in the fields of health policy and systems research—and qualitative health research more generally—as well as growing recognition of implementation processes and local contexts as critical factors in the success of any health intervention. At the very least, the growth of QES in global health policy signals that there remains room—perhaps growing room—in some spaces for a more expansive vision of what is at stake in health policy and what forms of knowledge might best contribute to decision making about health.

## References


Adams, V. (2013). Evidence-based global public health: Subjects, profits, erasures. In J. Biehl & A. Petryna (Eds.), *When people come first: Critical studies in global health* (pp. 54–90). Princeton University Press.

Adams, V. (2016). *Metrics: What counts in global health*. Duke University Press.

Bhaumik, S. (2017). Use of evidence for clinical practice guideline development. *Tropical Parasitology, 7*(2), 65–71.

Bohlin, I. (2012). Formalizing syntheses of medical knowledge: The rise of meta-analysis and systematic reviews. *Perspectives on Science, 20*(3), 273–309.

Bosch-Capblanch, X., Lavis, J. N., Lewin, S., Atun, R., Rottingen, J. A., Droschel, D., et al. (2012). Guidance for evidence-informed policies about health systems: Rationale for and challenges of guidance development. *PLoS Medicine, 9*(3), e1001185.

Daniels, K., Loewenson, R., George, A., Howard, N., Koleva, G., Lewin, S., et al. (2016). Fair publication of qualitative research in health systems: A call by health policy and systems researchers. *International Journal of Equity in Health, 15*, 98.

Dixon-Woods, M., Agarwal, S., Jones, D., Young, B., & Sutton, A. (2005). Synthesising qualitative and quantitative evidence: A review of methods. *Journal of Health Services Research and Policy, 10*(1), 45–53.

Gilson, L., Hanson, K., Sheikh, K., Agyepong, I. A., Ssengooba, F., & Bennett, S. (2011). Building the field of health policy and systems research: Social science matters. *PLoS Medicine, 8*(8), e1001079.

Glenton, C., Colvin, C. J., Carlsen, B., Swartz, A., Lewin, S., Noyes, J., et al. (2013). Barriers and facilitators to the implementation of lay health worker programmes to improve access to maternal and child health: Qualitative evidence synthesis. *Cochrane Database of Systematic Reviews, 10*, CD010414.

Greenhalgh, T., Annandale, E., Ashcroft, R., Barlow, J., Black, N., Bleakley, A., et al. (2016). An open letter to the BMJ editors on qualitative research. *BMJ, 352*, i563.

Hannes, K., & Macaitis, K. (2012). A move to more systematic and transparent approaches in qualitative evidence synthesis: Update on a review of published papers. *Qualitative Research, 12*(4), 402–442.

Hutchison, K. J., & Rogers, W. A. (2012). Challenging the epistemological foundations of EBM: What kind of knowledge does clinical practice require? *Journal of Evaluation in Clinical Practice, 18*(5), 984–991.

Inhorn, M. C. (1995). Medical anthropology and epidemiology: Divergences or convergences? *Social Science and Medicine, 40*(3), 285–290.

Ioannidis, J. P. (2014). How to make more published research true. *PLoS Medicine, 11*(10), e1001747.

Knaapen, L. (2013). Being 'evidence-based' in the absence of evidence: The management of non-evidence in guideline development. *Social Studies of Science, 43*(5), 681–706.

Knaapen, L., & Lehoux, P. (2016). Three conceptual models of patient and public involvement in standard-setting: From abstract principles to complex practice. *Science as Culture, 25*(2), 239–263.

Lehmann, U., Van Damme, W., Barten, F., & Sanders, D. (2009). Task shifting: The answer to the human resources crisis in Africa? *Human Resources for Health, 7*, 49.

Lewin, S., & Glenton, C. (2018). Are we entering a new era for qualitative research? Using qualitative evidence to support guidance and guideline development by the World Health Organization. *International Journal of Equity in Health, 17*(1), 126.

Mishra, S. R., Neupane, D., Preen, D., Kallestrup, P., & Perry, H. B. (2015). Mitigation of non-communicable diseases in developing countries with community health workers. *Globalization and Health, 11*, 43.

Moreira, T. (2007). Entangled evidence: Knowledge making in systematic reviews in healthcare. *Sociology of Health and Illness, 29*(2), 180–197.

Mykhalovskiy, E., & Weir, L. (2004). The problem of evidence-based medicine: Directions for social science. *Social Science and Medicine, 59*(5), 1059–1069.

Noyes, J., Booth, A., Lewin, S., Carlsen, B., Glenton, C., Colvin, C. J., et al. (2018). Applying GRADE-CERQual to qualitative evidence synthesis findings-paper 6: How to assess relevance of the data. *Implementation Science, 13*(Suppl 1), 51–61.

Olivier de Sardan, J. P., Diarra, A., & Moha, M. (2017). Travelling models and the challenge of pragmatic contexts and practical norms: The case of maternal health. *Health Research Policy and Systems, 15*(Suppl 1), 60.

Petticrew, M., & Roberts, H. (2003). Evidence, hierarchies, and typologies: Horses for courses. *Journal of Epidemiology and Community Health, 57*(7), 527–529.

Pope, C., & Mays, N. (2009). Critical reflections on the rise of qualitative research. *British Medical Journal, 339*, 737–739.

Porter, J. D. (2006). Epidemiological reflections of the contribution of anthropology to public health policy and practice. *Journal of Biosocial Science, 38*(1), 133–144.

Ruger, J. P., & Yach, D. (2009). The global role of the World Health Organization. *Global Health Governance, 2*(2), 1–11.

Shuval, K., Harker, K., Roudsari, B., Groce, N. E., Mills, B., Siddiqi, Z., et al. (2011). Is qualitative research second class science? A quantitative longitudinal examination of qualitative research in medical journals. *PLoS One, 6*(2), e16937.

Smith, H. J., Colvin, C. J., Richards, E., Roberson, J., Sharma, G., Thapa, K., et al. (2015). Programmes for advance distribution of misoprostol to prevent post-partum haemorrhage: A rapid literature review of factors affecting implementation. *Health Policy and Planning, 31*(1), 102–113.

Sundqvist, G., Bohlin, I., Hermansen, E. A., & Yearley, S. (2015). Formalization and separation: A systematic basis for interpreting approaches to summarizing science for climate policy. *Social Studies of Science, 45*(3), 416–440.

Wainwright, M., Colvin, C. J., Swartz, A., & Leon, N. (2016). Self-management of medical abortion: A qualitative evidence synthesis. *Reproductive Health Matters, 24*(47), 155–167.

WHO. (2003). *Guidelines for WHO guidelines*. https://apps.who.int/iris/handle/10665/68925. Accessed 1 Feb 2021.

WHO. (2006). *Task shifting to tackle health worker shortages*. https://www.who.int/healthsystems/task_shifting/TTR_tackle.pdf?ua=1. Accessed 1 Feb 2021.

WHO. (2012). *Optimizing health worker roles to improve access to key maternal and newborn health interventions through task shifting*. https://apps.who.int/iris/handle/10665/77764. Accessed 1 Feb 2021.

WHO. (2016). *WHO recommendations on antenatal care for a positive pregnancy experience*. https://www.who.int/publications/i/item/9789241549912. Accessed 1 Feb 2021.

# Part IV
# The Rise of Evidence and Its Uses

# Chapter 10
# The International Childbirth Initiative: An Applied Anthropologist's Account of Developing Global Guidelines

**Robbie Davis-Floyd**

## Introduction: A Focus on Process

As Jordan and Davis-Floyd have written, birth is everywhere socially marked and shaped, and *local realities necessitate adjusting maternity care to fit local contexts* (Jordan & Davis-Floyd, 1993). To date, much of the anthropology of policy in health has been concerned with how policies are localized and has underlined the importance of considering the economic, political, and social contexts when developing and implementing health interventions (see for instance Whiteford & Manderson, 2000). In this chapter, I draw on my personal experience as an applied anthropologist to reflect on the development of global guidelines in maternal and child health – the *International Childbirth Initiative (ICI): 12 Steps to Safe and Respectful MotherBaby-Family Maternity Care* (2018), for which I served as lead editor and wordsmith. This experience sheds light on how guidelines, at the global level, can be successfully developed and implemented with attention to local context, with the efforts of what McDougall (2016), building on the work of Sabatier and Jenkins-Smith (1993) and Keck and Sikkink (1998, 1999), terms "global advocacy coalitions."

The chapter focuses on what my colleagues and I learned from our processes: First, in addition to being guided by evidence, the guidelines grew out of earlier initiatives, described below, that cohered around shared ideas and values of the women's health and midwifery movements, including woman-centered care, a recognition of the interconnectedness of mother, baby, and family, and the understanding that women's rights are human rights. Second, the *process* of making guidelines heavily influences the final *product*, so the process must be honored, not rushed, and undertaken with commitment to see it through. Multi-level collaboration and

R. Davis-Floyd (✉)
Department of Anthropology, Rice University, Houston, TX, USA
e-mail: davis-floyd@outlook.com



L. J. Wallace et al. (eds.), *Anthropologies of Global Maternal and Reproductive Health*, Global Maternal and Child Health, https://doi.org/10.1007/978-3-030-84514-8_10

networking around a clear and shared vision, garnering input from many people with diverse voices and perspectives, and discussion and debate were essential parts of the creation of the ICI. I will elaborate further on these key lessons and others in my Conclusion. How we learned these key lessons will be clearly illustrated in what follows. In order to understand the creation of the ICI, it is first necessary to briefly acknowledge the histories of birth activism and global movements to improve the quality of maternal health within which the ICI is embedded.

## Birth Activism

The creation of the ICI and its three closely related predecessors—the *Mother-Friendly Childbirth Initiative* (MFCI) (1995), the *International MotherBaby Childbirth Initiative* (IMBCI) (2008), and the *FIGO Guidelines to Mother-Baby-Friendly Birthing Facilities* (2015) – are continuous with the deep history of activism around childbirth that has been diligently recorded and brought to light by scholars in the anthropology of reproduction, including Brigitte Jordan (1978), Emily Martin (1987), Adrienne Rich (1977), Diana Scully (1980), Nancy Stoller Shaw (1974), Sheila Kitzinger (1972, 1979, 1980), Ann Oakley (1979, 1980, 1984), Barbara Katz Rothman (1982, 1989), and others. The feminist revision of birth as presented in these early works still retains immense power and value, exposing the intense patriarchal bias in what I have long called the *technocratic* (Davis-Floyd, 1992, 2001, 2018a, b) treatment of women and their bodies throughout labor and birth. In addition to exposing the unnecessary medicalization of birth, these writers conducted research that revealed and defended the important social and cultural nature of midwifery and childbirth. Their work provided much of the inspiration for my own insights and birth activist work (see, for example, Davis-Floyd, 2018c, d), including my rather thrilling involvement with the ICI.

## The Larger Context: A Need for a Quality-of-Care-Based Initiative

The ICI guidelines are embedded within larger global movements to improve the quality of maternal care. Significant progress has been made in maternal and infant health over recent decades, yet major problems remain in both developed and developing countries. Nearly 300,000 women die each year from issues related to pregnancy and childbirth, mostly in developing regions, and many more suffer from complications of pregnancy and childbirth. The leading individual causes of maternal mortality include haemorrhage, sepsis, eclampsia, obstructed labor, unsafe abortion, and infectious diseases such as HIV/AIDS and malaria during pregnancy (Nour, 2008; Say et al., 2014). All these are socio-structurally "stratified" (Ginsburg

& Rapp, 1995) to affect the poor far more than the well-off, as their underlying causes include structural violences such as poverty, lack of access to education, malnutrition, and the lower status of women (Davis-Floyd, 2018f; Farmer, 2004). The global infant mortality rate stands at around 29/1000 (WHO, 2018a). Leading individual causes of neonatal and infant mortality include prematurity, low birth weight, birth asphyxia and injuries, infection, congenital birth defects, sudden infant death, respiratory distress, and gastro-intestinal diseases—most of which also stem from the underlying causes listed above (WHO, 2018b). Yet despite their stratified embeddedness in these larger problems, *most maternal and infant deaths are preventable* through a combination of strategies including skilled attendance during childbirth from caregivers trained in facilitating the normal physiology of birth and breastfeeding, and access to emergency obstetric care (Cheyney & Davis-Floyd, 2019).

Although a global increase has been seen in skilled birth attendance, mainly due to an increase in facility-based birth, still many women, fetuses, and babies die or develop lifelong disabilities due to poor quality of care, despite having reached a facility (see Bhutta et al., 2014; Miller et al., 2003). The use of medical interventions in pregnancy, labor, and birth can be lifesaving, but their overuse leads to avoidable complications, and causes harm and even death. Unnecessary overuse has resulted in a massive increase in health care costs, straining resources without improving birth outcomes (see Anderson et al., 2020). For example, caesarean rates in many countries far surpass the recommended upper limit of 15–20% (Miller et al., 2016; WHO Statement on Caesarean Rates, 2015). Lack of availability of caesarean section when needed costs lives, but its overuse carries serious potential short- and long-term harms, especially for mothers, including infection, blood loss, blood clots, and problems in future pregnancies. Care providers trained in intervention use are rarely also trained in the skills and knowledge required to support the normal physiology of labor and birth (Miller et al., 2016).

Ministries of Health and national governments in general see facility birth as an essential part of their overall push toward "development" and "modernization" (Cheyney & Davis-Floyd, 2019). Yet many birth facilities, particularly in low- and middle-income countries (LMICs), are overcrowded, understaffed, and have few resources. Women often choose to avoid such facilities because of abuse, coercion, and/or neglect (Sadler et al., 2016; Savage & Castro, 2017; UN, 2006). Recently there has been increasing focus among international and national organizations on examining the quality of care and highlighting the abuse/neglect of women in facilities during childbirth and the lack of professional and social accountability among facility-based care providers (Assembly UNG, 1993; UN, 1966; UN Entity for Gender Equality and the Empowerment of Women, 2009; UN High Commissioner, 2010). Evidence collected in a variety of settings has documented that the *quality of care is directly related to maternal and newborn health outcomes*, including mortality (UN, 1996, 2009; White Ribbon Alliance 2011). Therefore, many saw a need for a global initiative focused on improving quality of care, and that understanding led to the development of the IMBCI, the FIGO Guidelines, and finally the ICI—a progression that I will describe in the next section.

## Creating the International MotherBaby Childbirth Initiative (IMBCI): 10 Steps to Optimal MotherBaby Maternity Services

The Coalition for Improving Maternity Services (CIMS), founded in the United States in 1996, for a time incorporated in its membership 50 childbirth-related organizations representing over 90,000 members. Its mission was to promote a wellness model of maternity care that would improve birth outcomes and substantially reduce costs. This mission was ultimately realized as the *Mother-Friendly Childbirth Initiative (MFCI): 10 Steps to Mother-Friendly Hospitals, Birth Centers, and Home Birth Services.* I served as lead editor and wordsmith for the MFCI, with Henci Goer and Roberta Scaer as co-editors. The MFCI was modeled, in part, after the long extant (1991) WHO-UNICEF *Baby-friendly Hospital Initiative* (BFHI), and the BFHI 10 Steps to successful breastfeeding were incorporated as the final Step of the MFCI and the other three initiatives that followed it.

The MFCI was released in 1996, went global via the internet, was translated into multiple languages, and was put to work in many countries, most often by consumer organizations. In subsequent years, CIMS received many requests from organizations and advocacy groups both large and small around the world to help them create their own initiatives. To these requests, CIMS consistently responded with the message that the MFCI was freely available and could be adapted by any country to meet its own needs. We did not want to seem in any way to be "American imperialists," so we kept repeating that message. Yet over time, more and more international birth activists and practitioners, including obstetricians, kept showing up at CIMS conferences in the United States and repeating their requests for CIMS to create a global initiative that would work for all countries, insisting that they did not have the resources nor experience to create such an initiative, whereas we—supposedly—did.

Finally, in 2005, CIMS gave up protesting that each country should create its own initiative, and formally created the CIMS International Committee, which eventually morphed into the International MotherBaby Childbirth Organization (IMBCO), with Debra Pascali Bonaro (world-renowned birth activist, doula trainer, and producer of the film *Orgasmic Birth*) as its Chair, and Maureen Corry (then-Director of Childbirth Connection), Rae Davies (a doula trainer and administrator who later became IMBCO's Administrative Director), Mayri Sagady-Leslie (nurse-midwifery practitioner, researcher, and professor), and myself (an applied reproductive anthropologist) as the five original IMBCO Board members. Our initial goal would be to create a global initiative based on a worldwide survey of birth and breastfeeding organizations to assess levels of agreement with the 10 Steps of the MFCI. The survey results showed that agreement was high, so we felt we had a working mandate to create what became the IMBCI—an initiative based on a process of *extensive collaboration and networking*, which we knew were essential in order to ensure strong international support.

To jump-start our process, we obtained funding to hold a meeting in Geneva of what we called our Technical Advisory Group (TAG), which was attended by representatives from the following organizations: WHO, UNICEF, USAID, CIMS, Childbirth Connection, Lamaze International, DONA, La Leche League International, Wellstart International, the World Alliance of Breastfeeding Associations (WABA), the International Lactation Consultant Association (ILCA), the International Confederation of Midwives (ICM), the International Council of Nurses (ICN), the International Pediatric Association (IPA), and JPHIEGO. We recruited these organizations because of our profound respect for the international work they had already done, and left that 2-day meeting with an initial draft of the IMBCI. The process of finalizing the IMBCI then took a full year, during which I, as lead editor, garnered feedback from over 100 childbirth experts, practitioners, grassroots activists, and some interested lay women from many countries, and of course, from the original members of the IMBCO Board. *Gathering this broad range of feedback was essential to the IMBCI's success* and its eventual ability to serve as a template for the ICI (see below). Every individual who received a draft was able to make some kind of contribution toward its betterment, demonstrating the values of collaboration and of patience.

An important and lasting contribution of the IMBCI is the term "MotherBaby" – first used by Audrey Naylor, MD, DrPH, who was then CEO of Wellstart International. A pediatrician and longtime champion of breastfeeding in the international arena, Naylor believed that "mothers and babies are an interdependent, biologic unit…inseparable throughout the continuum of care" (Naylor, e-mail message to Mayri Sagady Leslie, August 8, 2010). Once the IMBCI was completed, we posted it on our newly created website www.imbci.org and sent it out to our IMBCO regional and country representatives. They translated the IMBCI into 27 languages and put it to work in their countries and regions. A number of smaller birthing facilities and NGOs took the IMBCI as their chartering document and implemented it in their practices and countries. (The full story of the IMBCI is told in Davis-Floyd et al., 2011.)

## IMBCO's Pilot Project: Disappointment and Setback

A common course for international initiatives is to seek to have them ratified in a formal process by all major and relevant organizations. IMBCO did not choose that course, since we recognized that international formal ratification could hold dissemination of the document up for a year or more. Instead, we chose to pilot the IMBCI at demonstration sites to test its efficacy in decreasing unnecessary interventions and improving outcomes via high quality of care. We felt that once contextually relevant evidence was available, we would have a far better chance of receiving international endorsements and funding.

We put out an international call, and received and, after careful review, accepted applications from eight hospital pilot/demonstration sites in seven countries.

However, we needed funding for practitioner training in how to implement the 10 Steps, and for statistical documentation of the results of implementation so that we could prove efficacy. Then, suddenly, the Transforming Birth Fund, our former staunch supporter, indicated that they had shifted focus to the United States and would no longer be able to fund us. Although we were devastated, three of our pilot sites in Canada, Austria, and Brazil were high-resource enough to implement on their own: the Pavillon des Naissances, Hôpital Brome Missisquoi Perkins, Cowansville, Centre de Santé et Services Sociaux La Pommeraie, in Quebec, Canada; Community Hospital Feldbach, Feldbach, Austria, Department of Obstetrics and Gynaecology; and Hospital Sofia Feldman, Belo Horizonte, Brazil. (Sofia Feldman is described in Davis-Floyd & Georges, 2018; see also Davis-Floyd et al., 2011).[1] These highly humanistic hospitals are demonstrating in practice how maternity care services can offer women optimal MotherBaby care. IMBCO also developed evaluation tools for these and future sites to utilize, including questionnaires addressed to women who had just given birth, self-assessment by caregivers, and standard statistical measurements for interventions such as cesarean or induction rates.

## MotherBaby Networks (MBnets)

As word about the IMBCI spread, many smaller independent facilities and practices began to contact us, asking how they could participate. We responded that they were perfectly free to implement the IMBCI 10 Steps on their own, yet we wanted to be connected, as by now we fully understood the importance of networking and "global advocacy coalitions." Our then-Administrative and Executive Directors Rae Davies and Rodolfo Gomez came up with the idea of linking these sites in an international network and calling them "MotherBaby networks"—"MBnets" for short. "Mbnets consist of individuals such as midwives and physicians; or a collaboration of individuals, community grassroots advocates and organisations, and careproviders; or a facility such as a birth center, clinic or hospital where women give birth... that are using the IMBCI to promote the 10 Steps in their own contextual surroundings" (IMBCO, 2020).

Two of these MBnets—the Bumi Sehat Foundation, founded by midwife Robin Lim, and Mercy in Action, founded by midwife Vicki Penwell—successfully implemented all 10 Steps of the IMBCI for years in their birth centers in Indonesia and the Philippines. They have also done so during their maternity care relief work in major disaster zones in the Philippines after Hurricane Hayan; in Aceh, Indonesia after the tsunami; and in Nepal and Haiti after major earthquakes, providing prenatal and postpartum care and assisting births in tents, with no electricity or running water! (For full descriptions, see Davis-Floyd et al., 2021; Penwell, 2018, and Lim

[1] See http://imbco.weebly.com/demonstration-sites.html

& Davis-Floyd, 2021). Their work demonstrates that *full IMBCI or ICI implementation is not dependent on the availability of high technologies.* We believe that this flexibility and non-reliance on high technology during labor and birth are two of the greatest strengths of these initiatives.

## The FIGO Initiative

From its launch in 2008 until 2015, the IMBCI was the only global initiative of its kind. Then in 2015, FIGO published its own international initiative—the *FIGO Guidelines to Mother-Baby Friendly Birthing Facilities*—in the *International Journal of Gynecology and Obstetrics.* These guidelines were developed by the members of the FIGO Safe Motherhood and Newborn Health (SMNH) Committee in collaboration with the International Confederation of Midwives (ICM), IPA, WRA (White Ribbon Alliance), and WHO. I vividly recall my reaction upon first reading them—that they contained many similarities to the IMBCI, that they were evidence-based and extremely well intentioned, and that some of their 10 Steps were a mélange of too many different things crowded together in each Step, resulting in a lack of clarity. I longed to dig my editorial fingers into these *FIGO Guidelines*—and 3 years later, to my everlasting delight, I got the chance.

## Creating the International Childbirth Initiative: 12 Steps to Safe and Respectful MotherBaby-Family Maternity Care

After launching the IMBCI in 2008, we expanded our IMBCO Board considerably to be more global and diverse. It currently consists of Debra Pascali Bonaro still as Chair; Rae Davies as Administrative Director; myself; Daphne Rattner MD, a Brazilian epidemiologist, professor, and former Director of the Women's Health Program for the Brazilian Ministry of Health; Hélène Vadeboncoeur, a longtime researcher, birth activist, and scholar who authored the first Canadian book on VBAC and helped the Quebec Ministry of Health develop the first birth centers in Quebec; Amali Lokugamage, an obstetrician and researcher from Sri Lanka who works in London; Soo Downe, a UK midwifery professor and researcher; and Kathy Herschderfer, a Dutch midwife and former CEO of the International Confederation of Midwives. It was this IMBCO Board that participated in creating the ICI.

In the fall of 2016, Board member Daphne Rattner organized a conference in Brasilia in which she took care to create a session in which both the IMBCI and the *FIGO Guidelines* would be presented. The similarities between the two were obvious to all attending, and two of our IMBCO Board members, Kathy Herschderfer and Helene Vadeboncoeur, had already begun comparing their principles and Steps. That night, FIGO SMNH representative Andre Lalonde, Debra Pascali Bonaro, and

I had dinner together in the conference hotel and followed through on the idea of formally merging them—and that job was assigned to me.

Since this was now my third initiative to serve as lead editor for (after the MFCI and the IMBCI), I had a pretty good idea of how to proceed: I immediately began to painstakingly integrate the two sets of guidelines, sentence by sentence and phrase by phrase. Early in the process, I realized that this new initiative, which we had decided to call the *International Childbirth Initiative* (ICI), was going to have to contain 12 Steps instead of 10, as the FIGO SMNH Committee members had thought of two important Steps that the IMBCI did not contain. One was staff safety and protection. It was surprising that we at IMBCO had not thought about including this issue, given that many birth ethnographers, including myself, had documented the challenges of being a compassionate caregiver when you yourself are being abused by others higher up in the system (Beck & Gable, 2012; Olza, 2013; Leinweber et al., 2017; Davis-Floyd, 2018e). The other was full financial disclosure of all hospital costs and charges in advance of a birth—we should have thought of that too, as it can be common in some LMICs to refuse to release babies until the parents have paid the hospital bill in full, even when care is supposed to be free. Lim and Legget (2021) also realized the wisdom of including Indicators for measuring the implementation of each Step – something that *FIGO Guidelines* contained but the IMBCI did not. (The lesson here: *learn from others.*)

## Resolving Disagreements in the Creation of the ICI

FIGO SMNH Coordinator Andre Lalonde informed us that one of the reasons FIGO had not just adopted the IMBCI wholesale, but created its own Guidelines instead, was the issue of pain relief. In the FIGO *Guidelines*, Step 9 said that a mother–baby-friendly birthing facility: "Educates, counsels, and encourages staff to provide both non-pharmacological and pharmacological pain relief as necessary." While creating the IMBCI, we had debated whether or not an optimal MotherBaby facility should offer both drug and drug-free pain relief options. The epidural is experienced by many women as a humanistic pain-relieving option during labor. Yet it carries risks and complications, especially if given too early in labor. In addition, the IMBCO Board felt that including pain-relieving drugs, most especially the epidural, would be to ask developing countries that cannot afford such drugs to provide them, which would be unrealistic and unfair. Thus the IMBCI suggests only non-pharmacologic pain relief options. FIGO was not comfortable with leaving out drug-induced pain relief, whereas we at IMBCO were not willing to "push epidurals." However, we could all agree that *use of pain relief measures must be the mother's choice*, and that non-drug pain relief options should be offered first. Therefore, after various drafts, that ICI Step and its associated Indicators ended up reading:

> **Step 5 PROVIDE PAIN RELIEF MEASURES. Offer drug-free comfort and pain relief measures as safe first options, explaining their benefits for facilitating normal birth.** Educate women (and their companions) about how to use these methods, including

breathing, touch, holding, massage, relaxation techniques, and laboring in water (when available). **If pharmacological pain relief options are available and requested, explain their benefits and risks.** Train staff in all comfort measures and pain relief options and to respect women's preferences and informed choices to maximize their confidence and well-being.

**Indicators**

1. Written protocols about comfort measures and pain relief, including the need for increased monitoring of MotherBaby if pharmacological pain relief is used, are in place, and made available to assessors.
2. In interviews and/or surveys, staff confirm their knowledge of these protocols and report being trained in all methods of comfort measures and pain relief.
3. Direct observations can be made as to whether comfort measures and pain relief are being offered and appropriate monitoring is being done.
4. Random record review for documenting compliance may be a possibility in some facilities/practices. New mothers can be queried about the availability of pain relief measures via questionnaires and interviews.

This wording worked for FIGO, and it worked for us, as it does not *require* facilities to have the resources to provide epidurals, etc., nor does it advocate for pharmacological pain relief, but rather leaves that entirely up to the birthing person as part of the principle of informed choice. Thus, in addition to being guided by evidence, the IMBCO and FIGO cohered around shared ideas and values of the women's health and midwifery movements, including: woman-centered high quality care; recognition of the interconnectedness of mother, baby, and family; and the understanding that women's rights are human rights. This coherence also demonstrates my point that the *process* of consensus building in the development of these guidelines heavily influenced the final *product*, so the process must be honored, not rushed, and undertaken with commitment to see it through.

Another tense issue was whether or not (and how) to refer to traditional midwives. Anthropologists tend to prefer the terms "traditional," "Indigenous," or "empirical" midwives in order to fully acknowledge their important roles in their communities as *midwives*. Yet the International Confederation of Midwives defines a "midwife" as one who has graduated from a government-approved midwifery training program, seeking to reserve that appellation for professional midwives only (ICM, 2017). Thus, ICM, WHO, UNICEF, and others refer to these practitioners as "traditional birth attendants" (TBAs), and we understood that we could not garner their support if we used the term "traditional midwife." In fact, the FIGO Guidelines made no mention at all of traditional midwives/TBAs, while the IMBCI Step 9 called for a "continuum of collaborative maternal and newborn care with all relevant health care providers, institutions and organizations" including TBAs. The carefully negotiated inclusion of the TBA in two steps of the ICI would eventually read:

**Step 4 OFFER CONTINUOUS SUPPORT. Inform the mother of the benefits of continuous support during labor and birth, and affirm her right to receive such support from companion(s) of her choice.** These include father, partner, family member, doula, TBA, or others. [Bold in original]

**Step 11 PROVIDE A CARE CONTINUUM. Provide a continuum of collaborative maternal and newborn care with all relevant health care educators, providers, institu-**

> **tions, and organizations.** Include traditional birth attendants (TBAs) and others attending at births who have been acknowledged, recognized, and/or integrated into the health services in this continuum of collaboration. [Bold in original]

I put the "and/or" in there very much on purpose, wishing to be careful not to require that TBAs had to be "integrated"—as so often they are not, hampering their ability to ensure quick access to emergency care when needed (see Roy et al., 2021). And originally, the ICI Executive Group and the various partner organizations had put "trained" in front of "TBA." We were determined to avoid wording that insisted that TBAs had to be officially trained to provide labor support, attend births, and/or accompany women to clinical facilities, and we also argued that TBA "trainings" had been shown by ethnographers to frequently be pedagogically ineffective and culturally inappropriate (Jordan & Davis-Floyd, 1993; Pigg, 1997) and that TBAs had been shown by health researchers to often be helpful adjuncts to quality maternity care (Sibley et al., 2004). I was told that in discussions among FIGO SNMH reps and representatives from WHO that WHO had not wanted TBAs to be mentioned at all. This compromise in wording is one of many examples of how anthropological knowledge and perspectives on reproduction, along with knowledge of scientific evidence, careful wording, and consensus on key principles, contributed to the successful development of global guidelines in the form of the ICI.

Another issue to negotiate was perineal shaving. In the IMBCI, it was part of **Step 6: Avoid potentially harmful procedures and practices that have no scientific support for *routine or frequent use* in normal labor and birth**. But it got left out of the ICI because, I was told, women in many countries now shave themselves—either in preparation for birth or for personal or cultural reasons. Shaving can lead to tiny abrasions where bacteria can grow, but IMBCO and FIGO collectively felt that we should pick our battles carefully and that the risks of shaving were not significant enough to include in the list of routine procedures to avoid. Much more important were the procedures that *were* included in this list in ICI Step 7 of procedures to avoid unless strongly medically indicated. They include, among others:

- Medical induction or augmentation of labor.
- Intravenous fluids.
- Withholding food and water.
- Continuous electronic fetal monitoring.
- Frequent vaginal exams.
- Supine or lithotomy position.
- Episiotomy.
- Forceps and vacuum extraction.
- Immediate cord clamping.
- Cesarean section.
- Suctioning of the newborn.
- Separation of mother and baby.

Since almost all of these procedures are absolutely routine and culturally entrenched in hospitals all over the world, it is going to take a paradigm shift of epic proportions to get practitioners to stop performing them. Yet the scientific evidence against their routine use is solid, and in some settings, the rates of these unnecessary procedures are beginning to fall. For instance, episiotomy rates in the United States fell from 25% in 2004 to 14% in 2014 (Friedman et al., 2015), as is the case in many European countries (Graham et al., 2005),

After numerous and mostly harmonious email and phone conversations between Andre and myself, I finished my tasks of wordsmithing the 12 Steps and their Indicators and merging the IMBCI and the FIGO Foundational Principles, first begun by Kathy and Helene. These principles give the ICI a solid human-rights-based, woman-and-family-centered, and midwifery model of care foundation, which we decided to rename ***The MotherBaby-Family Maternity Care Model*** (Fig. 10.1). The ICI principles include:

- Advocating rights and access to care.
- Ensuring respectful maternity care.
- Protecting the MotherBaby–Family triad.
- Promoting wellness, preventing illness and complications, and ensuring timely emergency referral and care.
- Supporting women's autonomy and choices to facilitate a positive birthing experience.
- Providing a healthy and positive birthing environment: The responsibilities of caregivers and health systems.
- Using an evidence-based approach to maternal health services based on the MotherBaby-Family Model of Care.

International
Childbirth
Initiative
**12 Steps to Safe and Respectful**
**MotherBaby-Family Maternity Care**

**Fig. 10.1** ICI logo created by graphic designer Suzie Vitez (Permission for the use of the ICI logo in this publication has been granted by the ICI Executive Committee. Logo not to be replicated without express permission from the ICI Executive Committee.)

## Endorsement and Implementation

Unlike with the IMBCI, which we wanted to put into immediate action, with the ICI we sought endorsements from professional associations, NGOs, and university-based research institutes concerned with maternal and newborn health. We quickly received endorsements from FIGO, IMBCO, the White Ribbon Alliance, the International Confederation of Midwives, the International Council of Nurses, the International Pediatric Association, Lamaze International, DONA International, the Harvard T. Chan School of Public Health, and others (for the full list, go to www.ICIchildbirth.org). These endorsements will matter as plans for implementation proceed and funding for implementation trainings and results documentation is sought—a process already underway. We are seeking active participation from endorsing partners to move the initiative forward.

Any practice or facility can implement the ICI Philosophy and 12 Steps on its own and join our MotherBaby networks; the ICI Executive Committee created an application process for sites that would like to become "early adopters" and the applications are flowing in. To quote directly from the ICI (p. 19):

> The ICI envisions that the actual implementation of the 12 Steps will vary between settings based on an assessment of current services, available resources and perceived needs. Whether or not the 12 Steps are implemented as a whole or in phases can be determined locally. The ICI Coordination Group will continually gather information on the process of implementation as it is being done in real-time, collate this information, analyze it, and feed it back to assist on-going implementation and new implementation processes. In doing so, a learning cycle will be created and maintained that will benefit implementation of the ICI Steps in all settings.
>
> Implementation can be small- or large-scale and both top-down and bottom-up. Individual facilities may be motivated and have resources to start on ICI implementation themselves, while in other situations, health managers and planners may initiate a process of implementation for a specific district or region…In general, the ICI offers the following implementation recommendations:
>
> - Work with local community groups to ensure relevance, engagement, and acceptance by the end users.
> - Ensure the involvement of local and/or national health professionals' organisations to support the valued care providers on the work floor.
> - Whenever possible, include the knowledge, skills and evidence contained in the ICI 12 Steps in continuing educational programmes and trainings to help with efficient implementation in practice.
>
> The ICI envisions that the 12 Steps will be implemented in partnerships among local and national health planners and managers, maternity care providers and communities. Ideally, the ICI 12 Steps will be embedded in local and national guidelines and recommendations and supported by governments, UN agencies,

and health funding mechanisms. The ICI endorsing partners can provide continuing support through their networks.

The key feature here is the *ICI's emphasis on the involvement of local groups and organizations*. We unanimously agreed that local grassroots community groups are the most ideally positioned to collaborate with caregivers and facilities to monitor and encourage a facility's progress toward implementation, in combination with international trainers to be sent in as needed. This approach is not only money-saving – sending international trainers is expensive – but also has the great advantage of engaging communities with the facilities that serve them, which will also enable these community representatives to ensure that implementation is contextually appropriate and culturally safe. At present, the IMBCO is developing, with the FIGO SNMH Committee, updated versions of our IMBCO Women's Questionnaires and tools for monitoring progress and self-initiated quality assurance mechanisms. The ICI Executive Committee also envisions a system of recognition for those who successfully implement the 12 Steps in any setting.

The latest update (May 2021), which I received from Debra Pascali Bonaro, IMBCO Chair and member of the ICI Executive Committee, includes the information that 61 hospitals and health centers in 19 countries are in the process of ICI implementation; three midwifery programs are engaging in curriculum development based on the ICI in the US, Kenya, and Sweden; the ICI 12 Steps were included in the *German Guidelines for Vaginal Birth at Term* in December 2020: these guidelines are for use in Germany, Austria, and Switzerland; and the ICI core documents have been translated into 23 languages, including Turkish, Croatian, Tagalog, Waray Waray, Dutch, French, Spanish, Chinese, and Mongolian. In addition, Moi University in Kenya received a UNFPA grant to develop and teach a training curriculum based on the ICI; the curriculum was prepared and taught during a 3-day training for public facility staff in October 2020. In addition, the students of the Mercy in Action College of Midwifery have developed training modules based on the ICI to teach to their partner health centers in the Philippines in 2021. The IMBCO Board has finalized ICI implementation guidance and tools for monitoring, evaluation, and learning. According to IMBCO Board and ICI Executive Committee member Kathy Herschderfer:

> We at IMBCO have created a series of webinars addressing each Step; these have been very well received. The FIGO ICI Working Group will start with a project funded by the New South Wales Government in Australia. This will involve ICI implementation in Fiji, the Solomon Islands and Papua New Guinea. A regional support team has been established in Australia and contacts have been made with key persons in the islands who will be responsible for the project. It is expected that the implementation will take place in 1-3 settings in each island and this project has been met with great enthusiasm. Because of the coronavirus pandemic, the start of the project has been postponed until (hopefully) in the fall. Preliminary preparations are being worked on with virtual communication. We are continuing to be a presence in various global communities who deal with respectful care.

## Conclusion

The ICI addresses the needs of all nations and birthing women for evidence-based and humanistic improvements in the quality of maternity care, and is both educational and instrumental in purpose. The ICI's *educational purpose* is to call global attention to the importance of the *quality of the mother's birth experience and its impact on the outcome*, the risks to mother and baby from inappropriate medical interventions, and the scientific evidence showing the benefits of MotherBaby-Family-centered care based on the normal physiology of pregnancy, birth, and breastfeeding, and on attention to women's individual needs. The *instrumental purpose* of the ICI 12 Steps is to put into worldwide awareness and practice the MotherBaby-Family Model of Care – a woman-centered, non-interventive approach that promotes the health and well-being of all women and babies during pregnancy, birth, and breastfeeding in a human rights and midwifery model of care framework, with care and compassion for MotherBaby within their family context.

To recap, my account of the development of the ICI highlights two important reflections about the development of global guidelines. First, just as the quality of care influences birth outcomes, *the process of making guidelines heavily influences the final product.* Attention to process was essential, including collaboration and networking around a clear vision and respectful and fruitful dialogue and discussion. Second, attention to key values of the women's health and midwifery movements, such as the importance of woman-centered care and women's rights as human rights, were important shared ideas and values upon which consensus could be negotiated when disagreements arose.

These findings align with McDougall's account of the work of global advocacy coalitions in maternal health. According to McDougall, advocacy coalitions are "formal or informal networks through which actors build resources and strategies to influence policy." McDougall (2016, pp. 310–311) argues that in the global case, "coalitions are understood less as geographically bounded and operating with formal political systems, but rather as loose collections of alliances made up of committed individual and institutional policy actors with dense inter-organisational and interpersonal ties working across borders to influence policy." McDougall shows that advocacy coalitions are important in facilitating cooperation among stakeholders, and can create a common platform on which many different institutions and types of stakeholders can engage. This insight applies to the creation of the ICI, as we included many different organizations and individuals in our process, and their participation did create a "common platform" for endorsement by diverse maternity-related organizations.

As McDougall (2016) emphasizes, advocacy coalitions can also compete against one another for political attention. As a result, certain "camps" and actors, values, and forms of evidence may come to dominate policy processes. Yet in FIGO's and IMBCO's process of creating the ICI, no individual nor "camp" dominated. We worked relatively harmoniously, despite the fact that FIGO is a much larger and more globally powerful organization than IMBCO, a small NGO. Our efforts resulted in the successful development of both a global advocacy coalition and a set of global guidelines in the form of the ICI.

I reiterate that this chapter describes my own experience and thus can be only partial. Others in our advocacy coalition would no doubt tell these creation stories differently. In an effort to ensure that their voices would not contrast too severely from my own, I sent this chapter to all the members of the IMBCO Board and of the ICI Executive Committee for their review; they all approved it. Of course, it remains to be seen whether or not this new global policy initiative will be successful at effecting real change on a large scale. Global guidelines, such as the Baby-friendly Hospital Initiative, have been thinly implemented in some contexts, failing to improve quality of care, owing to various challenges (see for instance UNICEF and WHO, 2017; Wieczorek et al., 2015). Researchers will be needed to study the implementation process, help to identify barriers, and document outcomes.

## *Our Ultimate Vision: Setting the Gold Standard for Optimal Maternity Care*

The full text of the ICI is available at www.ICIchildbirth.org for anyone in any country to download and work with in their area. Individuals, practices, facilities, and organizations can join our mailing list to stay informed and become involved in supporting and implementing the ICI 12 Steps as a template for their work, and use the ICI as an educational instrument and guide. Ultimately, our vision is that every birth facility and practice will operate according to the ICI 12 Steps, resulting in high quality, evidence-based, and respectful care that will dramatically reduce mortality, morbidity, and financial costs, and will physically and psychologically enhance both birth and breastfeeding outcomes for mothers, babies, and families.

## References

Anderson, D. A., Daviss, B.A, Johnson, K.C. (2020). What if 10% more women delivered at home or in a birth center? The economics and politics of out-of-hospital birth in the U.S. In B.A. Daviss & R. Davis-Floyd (Eds.), Birthing models on the human rights frontier: Speaking truth to power. Routledge. (in press).

Beck, C., & Gable, R. (2012). A mixed methods study of secondary traumatic stress in labor and delivery nurses. *Journal of Obstetric, Gynecologic, & Neonatal Nursing, 41*(6), 747–760. https://doi.org/10.1111/j.1552-6909.2012.01386

Bhutta, Z. A., Salam, R. A., Lassi, Z. S., Austin, A., & Langer, A. (2014). Approaches to improve Quality of Care (QoC) for women and newborns: Conclusions, evidence gaps and research priorities. *Reproductive Health, 11*(Suppl. 2), S5. https://doi.org/10.1186/1742-4755-11-S2-S5

Cheyney, M., & Davis-Floyd, R. (2019). Birth as culturally marked and shaped. In R. Davis-Floyd & M. Cheyney (Eds.), *Birth in eight cultures* (pp. 1–16). Waveland Press.

Davis-Floyd, R. (1992). *Birth as an American rite of passage* (1st ed.). University of California Press.

Davis-Floyd, R. (2001). The technocratic, humanistic, and holistic models of birth. *International Journal of Gynecology & Obstetrics, 75*(Suppl. 1), S5–S23.

Davis-Floyd, R. (2018a). The technocratic, humanistic, and holistic paradigms of birth and health care. In R. Davis-Floyd & Colleagues (Eds.), *Ways of knowing about birth: Mothers, midwives, medicine, and birth activism* (pp. 3–44). Waveland Press.

Davis-Floyd, R. (2018b). The rituals of hospital birth: Enacting and transmitting the technocratic model. In R. Davis-Floyd & Colleagues (Eds.), *Ways of knowing about birth: Mothers, midwives, medicine, and birth activism* (pp. 45–70). Waveland Press.

Davis-Floyd, R. (2018c). Anthropology and birth activism: What do we know? In R. Davis-Floyd & Colleagues (Eds.), *Ways of knowing about birth: Mothers, midwives, medicine, and birth activism* (pp. 361–372). Waveland Press.

Davis-Floyd, R. (2018d). Working with anthropology in policy and practice: An activist's experience. In R. Davis-Floyd & Colleagues (Eds.), *Ways of knowing about birth: Mothers, midwives, medicine, and birth activism* (pp. 373–388). Waveland Press.

Davis-Floyd, R. (2018e). Open and closed knowledge systems, the 4 stages of cognition, and the cultural management of birth. *Frontiers in Sociology, 3*(23), 1–13. https://doi.org/10.3389/fsoc.2018.00023

Davis-Floyd, R. (2018f). Mutual accommodation or biomedical hegemony? A brief anthropological overview of global issues in midwifery. In R. Davis-Floyd & Colleagues (Eds.), *Ways of knowing about birth: Mothers, midwives, medicine, and birth activism* (pp. 265–282). Waveland Press.

Davis-Floyd, R., & Georges, E. (2018). The paradigm shift of humanistic and holistic obstetricians: The "good guys and girls" of Brazil. In R. Davis-Floyd & Colleagues (Eds.), *Ways of knowing about birth: Mothers, midwives, medicine, and birth activism* (pp. 141–164). Waveland Press.

Davis-Floyd, R., Pascali, B. D., Sagady-Leslie, M., Vadeboncoeur, H., Davies, R., & Gomez Ponce de Leon, R. (2011). The *international MotherBaby childbirth initiative*: Working to achieve optimal maternity care worldwide. *International Journal of Childbirth, 1*(3), 196–212. https://doi.org/10.1891/2156-5287.1.3.196

Davis-Floyd, R., Lim, R., Penwell, V., & Ivry, T. (2021). Sustainable birth care in disaster zones: Low-tech, skilled touch. In B.-A. Daviss & R. Davis-Floyd (Eds.), *Birthing models on the human rights frontier: Speaking truth to power* (pp. 261–276). Routledge.

Farmer, P. (2004). An anthropology of structural violence. *Current Anthropology., 45*(3), 305–325.

FIGO, WRA, ICM, IPA, & WHO. (2015). FIGO guidelines to mother-baby friendly birthing facilities. *International Journal of Gynecology & Obstetrics, 128*(2), 95–99. https://doi.org/10.1016/j.ijgo.2014.10.013

Friedman, A. M., Cande, V., Ananth, E. P., Mary, E., Alton, D., Wright, J. D., et al. (2015). Variation in and factors associated with use of episiotomy. *Journal of the American Medical Association, 313*(2), 197–199. https://doi.org/10.1001/jama.2014.14774

Ginsburg, F., & Rapp, R. (1995). *Conceiving the new world order: The global politics of reproduction*. University of California Press.

Graham, I. D., Carroli, G., Davies, C., & Medves, J. M. (2005). Episiotomy rates around the world: An update. *Birth: Issues in Perinatal Care, 32*(3), 219–223. https://doi.org/10.1111/j.0730-7659.2005.00373

International Childbirth Initiative. (2018). *International childbirth initiative: 12 steps to safe and respectful motherbaby-family maternity care*. www.ICIchildbirth.org. Accessed 15 Jan 2020.

International Confederation of Midwives (ICM). (2017). *Core document: International definition of the midwife*. https://www.internationalmidwives.org/assets/files/definitions-files/2018/06/eng-definition_of_the_midwife-2017.pdf. Accessed 15 Jan 2020.

International MotherBaby Childbirth Organization (IMBCO). (2020). *What are MBnets?* http://imbco.weebly.com/mbnets.html. Accessed 15 Jan 2020.

Jordan, B. (1978). *Birth in Four Cultures: A Cross-Cultural Investigation of Childbirth in Yucatan, Holland, Sweden, and the United States*. Montreal: Eden Press.

Jordan, B., & Davis-Floyd, R. (1993). *Birth in four cultures: A cross-cultural investigation of childbirth in Yucatan, Holland, Sweden, and the United States* (4th ed.). Waveland Press.

Keck, M. E., & Sikkink, K. (1998). *Activists beyond borders: Advocacy networks in international politics*. Cornell University Press.

Keck, M. E., & Sikkink, K. (1999). Transnational advocacy networks in international and regional politics. *International Social Science Journal, 51*(159), 89–101.

Kitzinger, S. (1972). *The experience of childbirth* (3d ed.). Penguin Books.

Kitzinger, S. (1979). *Birth at home*. Penguin Books.

Kitzinger, S. (1980). *Women as mothers: How they see themselves in different cultures*. Vintage Books.

Leinweber, J., Creedy, D. K., Rowe, H., & Gamble, J. (2017). Responses to birth trauma and prevalence of posttraumatic stress among Australian midwives. *Women and Birth, 30*(1), 40–45. https://doi.org/10.1016/j.wombi.2016.06.006

Lim, R., & Davis-Floyd, R. (2021). Implementing the *International Childbirth Initiative* (ICI) in disaster zones: Bumi Sehat's experience from Aceh, Haiti, the Philippines, and Nepal. In B. A. Daviss & R. Davis-Floyd (Eds.), *Birthing models on the human rights frontier: Speaking truth to power* (pp. 253–265). Routledge.

Lim, R., & Leggett, S. (2021). Bumi Sehat Bali: Birth on the checkered cloth. In B. A. Daviss & R. Davis-Floyd (Eds.), *Birthing models on the human rights frontier: Speaking truth to power* (pp. 55–74). Routledge.

Martin, E. (1987). *The woman in the body*. Beacon Press.

McDougall, L. (2016). Discourse, ideas, and power in global health: Political attention for maternal and child health in the millennium development goal era. *Globalization and Health, 12*(21), 1–14. https://doi.org/10.1186/S12992-016-0157-9

Miller, S., Cordero, M., Coleman, A. L., Figueroa, J., Brito-Anderson, S., Dabash, R., et al. (2003). Quality of care in institutionalized deliveries: The paradox of the Dominican Republic. *International Journal of Gynecology & Obstetrics, 82*(1), 89–103.

Miller, S., Abalos, E., Chamillard, M., Ciapponi, A., Colaci, D., Comandé, D., et al. (2016). Beyond too little, too late and too much, too soon: A pathway towards evidence-based, respectful maternity care worldwide. *Lancet, 388*(10056), 2176–2192. https://doi.org/10.1016/S0140-6736(16)31472-6

Nour, N. M. (2008). An introduction to maternal mortality. *Reviews in Obstetrics and Gynecology, 1*(2), 77–81.

Oakley, A. (1979). *Becoming a mother*. Schocken Books.

Oakley, A. (1980). *Women confined: Towards a sociology of childbirth*. Schocken Books.

Oakley, A. (1984). *The captured womb: A history of the medical care of pregnant women*. Basil Blackwell.

Olza, F. I. (2013). PTSD and obstetric violence. *Midwifery Today International Midwife, 105*(68), 48–49.

Penwell, V. (2018). *Mercy in Action: A birth model for disaster care in the Philippines*. Unpublished masters thesis, National College of Midwifery.

Pigg, S. L. (1997). Authority in translation: Finding, knowing, naming, and training "traditional birth attendants" in Nepal. In R. Davis-Floyd & C. Sargent (Eds.), *Childbirth and authoritative knowledge: Cross-cultural perspectives* (pp. 233–262). University of California Press.

Rich, A. (1977). *Of woman born: Motherhood as experience and institution*. Bantam Books.

Rothman, B. K. (1982). *In labor: Women and power in the birthplace*. WW. Norton.

Rothman, B. K. (1989). *Recreating motherhood: Ideology and technology in a patriarchal society*. W.W. Norton.

Roy, B., Qadeer, I., Sadgopal, M., Chawla, J., & Gautam, S. (2021). Giving birth at home in resource-scarce regions of India: An argument for making the women-centric approach of the traditional dais sustainable. In K. Gutschow, R. Davis-Floyd, & B.-A. Davis (Eds.), *Sustainable birth in disruptive times* (pp. 217–232). Springer Nature.

Sabatier, P. A., & Jenkins-Smith, H. C. (1993). *Policy change and learning: An advocacy coalition approach*. Westview Press.
Sadler, M., Santos, M., Ruiz-Berdun, D., Rojas, G. L., Skoko, E., Gillen, P., et al. (2016). Moving beyond disrespect and abuse: Addressing the structural dimensions of obstetric violence. *Health Matters, 24*(47), 47–55. https://doi.org/10.1016/rhm.2016.04.002
Savage, V., & Castro, A. (2017). Measuring mistreatment of women during childbirth: A review of terminology and methodological approaches. *Reproductive Health, 14*(1), 138. https://doi.org/10.1186/s12978-017-0403-5
Say, L., Chou, D., Gemmill, A., Tuncalp, O., Moller, A. B., & Daniels, J. (2014). Gulmezoglu., A.M., Temmerman, and M., Alkema, L. Global causes of maternal death: a WHO systematic analysis. *Lancet, 2*(6), e323–e333.
Scully, D. (1980). *Men who control women's health: The miseducation of obstetrician-Gynecologists*. Houghton-Mifflin.
Shaw, N. S. (1974). *Forced labor: Maternity care in the United States*. Pergamon Press.
Sibley, L., Sipe, T. A., & Koblinsky, M. (2004). Does traditional birth attendant training improve referral for women with obstetric complications? A review of the evidence. *Social Science and Medicine, 59*(8), 1757–1768.
UNICEF and WHO. (2017). *Country experiences with the baby-friendly hospital initiative: Compendium of case studies from around the world*. WHO.
United Nations Educational Scientific and Cultural Organization. (2006). *Universal declaration on bioethics and human rights*. http://www.unesco.org/new/en/social-and-human-sciences/themes/bioethics/bioethics-and-human-rights/. Accessed 15 Jan 2020.
United Nations Entity for Gender Equality and the Empowerment of Women. (2009). *Convention on the elimination of all forms of discrimination against women*. http://www.un.org/womenwatch/daw/cedaw/text/econvention.htm. Accessed 15 Jan 2020.
United Nations General Assembly. (1993). *Declaration on the elimination of violence against women*. http://www.un.org/documents/ga/res/48/a48r104.htm. Accessed 15 Jan 2020.
United Nations High Commissioner. (2010). *Report of the Office of the United Nations High Commissioner for Human Rights on preventable maternal mortality and morbidity and human rights*. http://www2.ohchr.org/english/bodies/hrcouncil/docs/14session/A.HRC.14.39_AEV-2.pdf. Accessed 15 Jan 2020.
United Nations Office of the High Commissioner for Human Rights. (1966). *International covenant on economic, social and cultural rights*. http://www.ohchr.org/EN/ProfessionalInterest/Pages/CESCR.aspx. Accessed 15 Jan 2020.
United Nations Office of the High Commissioner for Human Rights. (1996). *International covenant on civil and political rights*. http://www.ohchr.org/en/professionalinterest/pages/ccpr.aspx. Accessed 15 Jan 2020.
White Ribbon Alliance for Respectful Maternity Care. (2011). *The universal rights of childbearing women*. https://www.whiteribbonalliance.org/wp-content/uploads/2017/11/Final_RMC_Charter.pdf. Accessed 15 Jan 2020.
Whiteford, L. M., & Manderson, L. (2000). *Global health policies, local realities: The fallacy of the level playing field*. Lynne Rienner Publishers.
WHO. (2015). *WHO statement on cesarean section rates*. https://www.who.int/reproductivehealth/publications/maternal_perinatal_health/cs-statement/en/. Accessed 15 Jan 2020.
WHO. (2018a). *WHO global health observatory data*. https://www.who.int/gho/child_health/mortality/neonatal_infant_text/en/. Accessed 15 Jan 2020.
WHO. (2018b). *Intrapartum care for a positive childbirth experience*. https://www.who.int/reproductivehealth/publications/intrapartum-care-guidelines/en/. Accessed 15 Jan 2020.
Wieczorek, C. C., Schmeid, H., Dorner, T. E., & Dur, W. (2015). The bumpy road to implementing the baby-friendly hospital initiative in Austria: A qualitative study. *International Breastfeeding Journal, 10*, 3.

# Chapter 11
# Selling Beautiful Births: The Use of Evidence by Brazil's Humanised Birth Movement

**Lucy C. Irvine**

## Introduction

In February 2018, the World Health Organization (WHO) published its recommendations on *Intrapartum care for a positive childbirth experience* (WHO, 2018). This technical guidance—aimed primarily at healthcare professionals responsible for developing national and local health protocols and providing care to pregnant women and their newborns—came more than two decades after its previous iteration (WHO, 1985). During this period, significant new challenges have emerged in global maternal health, many of which result from the overuse of clinical interventions in healthy pregnancies and low-risk labour. This increasing medicalisation of childbirth "tends to undermine the woman's own capacity to give birth and negatively impacts her childbirth experience" (WHO, 2018, p. 1). The WHO guidelines reflect a consensus among global maternal health experts that maternal health care should be "normalised" where possible, based on the understanding that birth is a normal physiological process that can be accomplished without intervention for most women (WHO, 2018). Whilst acknowledging the importance of life-saving obstetric interventions for women with underlying health conditions or complications, the WHO guidelines draw on a woman-centred model, which takes a holistic

This chapter is a discussion of data collected for my doctoral research (Irvine, 2021).

L. C. Irvine (✉)
Institute for Global Health, University College London, London, UK
e-mail: lucy.irvine@ucl.ac.uk



L. J. Wallace et al. (eds.), *Anthropologies of Global Maternal and Reproductive Health*, Global Maternal and Child Health, https://doi.org/10.1007/978-3-030-84514-8_11

approach to maternity care[1]. It recognises women's social, cultural, and emotional needs, and the importance of comfortable surroundings and supportive birth attendants for a positive childbirth experience (WHO, 2018). These recommendations are supported by systematic reviews of scientific evidence (Bohren et al., 2017; Downe et al., 2018) and are echoed in recommendations from leading health institutions, such as England's National Institute for Health and Care Excellence (NICE), and comprehensive research, such as the *Birthplace in England* study (Birthplace Collaborative Group, 2011).

While the women-centred model of respectful maternity care informs the development of institutional practice and public policies around the world, service provision is far from adequate in many health systems, with huge variation between and within countries. In many high-income contexts, obstetric-led hospital-based care has become the standard model for healthy women with healthy babies, despite the evidence-base favouring care in a midwifery-led unit. In over-medicalised settings, such as private hospitals in the United States, the Dominican Republic, and Egypt (Boerma et al., 2018), women are at risk of a "cascade of interventions," in which one minor medical intervention, such as an induction of labour using synthetic oxytocin, can require further monitoring with a cardiotocograph (CTG), a move from midwifery-led to obstetrician-led care, and ultimately delivery by forceps or c-section (Jansen et al., 2013). In other health systems, such as rural regions of West and Central African countries, technological interventions are not accessible for women who need them, resulting in preventable deaths and illness (Cavallaro et al., 2013). Women may also be poorly treated by health professionals, particularly in societies where doctors are revered and their decisions rarely questioned (WHO, 2015; Manning & Schaaf, 2019)—this disrespect and abuse is often termed *obstetric violence* (Jardim & Modena, 2018). Although the term remains contested, activists use obstetric violence to refer to both the excessive or inappropriate use of clinical interventions, and the disrespectful treatment of women during pregnancy and childbirth.

The most alarming example of the overuse of interventions is caesarean sections. The global rate of c-section has almost doubled in the years between 2000 and 2018 and is now estimated to be the mode of delivery for 21.1% of births, despite the WHO's recommendation that rates above 10–15% are excessive (Boerma et al., 2018). C-sections are "associated with an increased risk of uterine rupture, abnormal placentation, ectopic pregnancy, stillbirth, and preterm birth" (Sandall et al., 2018). Short-term risks for newborns include altered immune development, an increased likelihood of allergies, and reduced intestinal gut microbiome diversity (Sandall et al., 2018).

[1]This model emerged from social movements for midwifery and homebirth in the 1970s and 1980s in the United States and Canada. There is not one single definition of 'woman-centred care', but generally it requires health professionals to respond respectfully to a woman's unique needs, women to be well-informed and play a central role in planning and making decisions about their care, and creating a calm birth environment (Morgan 2015).

It is now a global health policy priority to *optimise* the use of c-sections and other interventions that may cause harm to women and their newborns. In this chapter, I focus on these efforts in Brazil, where maternal health care in both public and private hospitals is highly medicalised, and "aggressive management" with excessive intervention is the norm (Diniz et al., 2018). My research involved following the *movement for humanised care in childbirth*—a national social movement that formed in the early 1990s, whose members seek to reduce unnecessary clinical interventions and promote a "humanised" model of childbirth where women are respected and birth is normalised as far as possible (Davis-Floyd, 2018). I focussed on the movement's activities between 2015 and 2018 when it was starting to see measurable progress, with rates of c-section and episiotomy falling in São Paulo's public municipal and private hospitals. The movement's profile grew as national celebrities opted for normal births, and women from different areas of the country and different social classes sought alternatives to the highly medicalised norm.

Key actors in the movement—including academics, humanised health professionals, and women seeking obstetric services—have been involved in the development and implementation of policies to promote humanised birth, including the *Rede Corgonha* national policy plan in the public health system (*Sistema Único de Saúde* or SUS), and a large number of local-level programmes and interventions in specific municipalities and hospitals (Diniz et al., 2018). I followed three policy case studies: (1) *Parto Adequado,* a partnership between *Hospital Einstein* (the largest private hospital in Brazil), the Brazilian health regulatory authority, and the US-based *Institute for Health Care Improvement*, which sought to reduce the rate of c-sections in participating private hospitals by training health professionals in normal deliveries; (2) *Parto Seguro*, a policy implemented by the research institute CEJAM (*Centro de Estudos e Pesquisas "Dr. João Amorim"*) and the São Paulo Municipality health department, which implemented humanised protocols based on international best practice guidelines, including freedom of movement, non-medical analgesia, delayed cord clamping, and breast-feeding support; and (3) the *Volunteer Doula programme*, a pilot intervention to train and integrate volunteer doulas into municipal hospitals, providing women with continuous support during labour.

My findings provide a local-level analysis of what Storeng and Béhague (2014) identify as "evidence-based advocacy" (EBA) in their ethnography of the *Safe Motherhood Initiative* (SMI). EBA represents a shift in the tactics used by the SMI over the past 20 years, where actors now use quantitative scientific evidence instead of moral arguments to call for policy change in global maternal health (Storeng & Béhague, 2014). I found that members of the humanised birth movement strategically used the power and perceived objectivity of science and evidence-based medicine (EBM) to further their goals in a similar way to the SMI actors. Storeng and Béhague also identify ways in which some safe motherhood experts are resisting and modifying these authoritative paradigms, and "couching [their] ideological and moral convictions in the language of scientific evidence for the sake of political expediency" (2014, p. 274). My findings suggest that the humanised birth movement has employed this strategy from its beginnings in the 1990s (Irvine, 2021). Throughout this time, key members have explicitly framed their campaigns as *combining* evidence-based and women's reproductive rights perspectives (Diniz & Chacham, 2004; Rattner et al., 2010). For instance, movement members would use the term "obstetric violence" to indicate that they saw the poor treatment of Brazilians as a violation of rights, in addition to describing the issue as a public health problem (the c-section "epidemic"), and references to systematic reviews that supported a humanised model (such as Sandall et al.'s 2016 systematic review of midwifery-led care). The decision of which strategy to use (or whether to use them all in the same speech, legal document, or social media post) depended on its perceived effectiveness and on who the audience was. This research is, therefore, also a contribution to what Ecks has called "evidence-based medical anthropology", where evidence use is performative, strategic, and "always used in relation to a particular audience" (2008, p. S85).

In the same way that some SMI actors expressed frustration with the "technocratic narrowing" of the policy agenda through prioritising particular forms of evidence (Storeng & Béhague, 2014), some members of the humanised birth movement were exasperated that pro-c-section doctors and the powerful medical lobby resisted the movement's activities and policy reforms, and firmly rejected the scientific support for humanised birth and moral claims that their actions constituted obstetric violence. In response, some members of the movement also used other tactics to raise public awareness about these issues and to stimulate private sector demand for humanised services. I discuss this alternative strategy and briefly reflect on its implications for the accessibility of natural/normal birth care.

## Methods

My methodological approach is informed by Wright and Reinhold's approach of *studying through* policy (2011). This method enables researchers to "follow a process of contestation as it tracks back and forth across different sites in a policy field and over time" (Wright & Reinhold, 2011, p. 88). It captures how policies develop and the real-life impact they have as they are implemented, how they are perceived, potentially manipulated, and shape people's everyday lives—aspects that are often missing in more traditional methods of studying policy (as covered in Walt et al., 2008).

From October 2015 to February 2018, I made several trips to São Paulo, for a total of 12 months of fieldwork. Upon arrival, I constructed a map of the policy community at the local level in central São Paulo, as well as key figures in the national movement I met at conferences in São Paulo and the capital Brasília, and who were vocal on social media. The movement can be conceptualised as an "issue network" (Walt et al., 2008) with a dominant core of stakeholders who were instrumental in the development of multiple, clearly defined policy programmes. The movement is composed of peripheral groups and individuals working towards a common cause (humanising childbirth in Brazil), who have differing values (such as choosing to work in the private sector or public sector) and levels of participation (from weekly participation in policy development meetings to occasional comments on Facebook groups).

I chose research sites to conduct observation based on their association with the movement. These included: five municipal public hospitals implementing humanised policy programmes; three humanised birth clinics that ran regular antenatal classes; a private hospital; state health council meetings; health conferences and campaigning events. I observed clinical training sessions for *Parto Adequado* and the integration of volunteer doulas into the hospital wards. The ethical approval I obtained from the public hospital administrations permitted me to conduct participant observation on the obstetric wards, but not to conduct formal interviews, which seemed appropriate given that women there were either in labour or had recently given birth. I was, however, able to informally discuss their experiences of care to document how they perceived existing services and new policy interventions.

I conducted in-depth semi-structured interviews (n45) and shorter informal interviews during participant observation (n4) with: women who were pregnant or had recently given birth in the public or private sector (n8), doulas and trainee doulas (n15), midwives (n10), obstetricians (n5), senators and politicians (n4), academic researchers (n4), and the policy programme leads (n3) at CEJAM, Hospital Einstein and the São Paulo municipal health department. I conducted two focus groups—one with a group of trainee doulas from the private sector, another with trainee doulas from the volunteer doula programme. The majority of my interviewees explicitly identified as being part of the humanised birth movement and would refer to themselves or their style of healthcare provision as *humanizada,* as opposed to the *cesarista* (pro-caesarean) doctors.

I recruited participants by identifying key members of the movement at academic conferences, at the municipal government health department, and at Hospital Einstein. I used snowball sampling to meet other stakeholders, most of whom were humanised health professionals. I asked key contacts to post on relevant social media groups about my research, asking if any mothers or women who were currently pregnant if they would be interested in participating. This meant that I was mainly speaking to mothers who were self-selecting for participation, potentially bringing about some bias in their positive attitudes toward the movement. I controlled for this by asking interviewees to reflect on the negative aspects of the movement and its relevance for different population groups. My attempts to interview *cesarista* doctors were unsuccessful, as despite the objective position set out in my research questions it was likely they assumed I was involved with the movement and that they would face criticism (studies of the c-section epidemic and/or the movement have, for the most part, painted obstetricians in a negative light—see McCallum & dos Reis, 2008; Diniz et al., 2018; Lansky et al., 2019).

I developed a standard set of interview questions that generally covered: how the interviewee perceived the humanised birth movement, why they thought there was more demand for humanised birth, how they sought to influence policy or improve services, the importance of scientific evidence, political and social rights, and supporting laws in achieving this, and what they thought of specific programmes (Irvine, 2021). I used *NVivo* qualitative data analysis software to organise and code interview transcripts to compare interviews through connected themes. I coded my paper fieldnotes thematically and referred back to these to triangulate my data.

Being non-Brazilian meant I was able to navigate a politically delicate field and ask sensitive questions that I may not have been able to if I was positioned inside the policy community (Walt et al., 2008). I found that having some clinical experience as a trainee midwife in the UK made people feel comfortable discussing their experiences of delivering and receiving obstetric care. I personally support the normalisation of birth, whilst also recognising the need for life-saving interventions where necessary. To account for my positionality, I would remain impartial in interviews until explicitly asked about my own opinion. Many people were curious about the NHS in England because it is internationally recognised for its model of midwifery-led care. In response to questions, I would direct people to key research studies on this topic, framing my own experiences as my subjective viewpoint.

## The Intervention Epidemic in Brazil

There is strong evidence to support the humanised birth movement's claims that the excessive use of procedures in Brazil is driven by political, economic, and convenience factors rather than genuine clinical need. C-sections and other clinical procedures are overused due to a combination of factors that include: financial gain for clinicians or hospitals, patient demand, cultural, and professional norms, and a lack of practice by clinicians of difficult vaginal deliveries (Irvine, 2021).

Throughout the 1970s and 1980s, Brazilian maternal health care became increasingly medicalised, at the same time as services were privatised and deregulated, particularly in the rapidly industrialising cities. Private obstetricians promoted c-sections as a "safe, painless, modern, and ideal form of birth" (de Mello e Souza 1994, p. 358). Over this period, Brazil's c-section rate soared, with many private hospitals in the wealthy south-eastern states delivering 80–95% of babies operatively (Leal et al., 2012). Rates of c-section in the private sector remain between 80–90%, and around 30–40% in public sector hospitals (Secretaria Municipal da Saúde, 2015). Research into c-section rates (Alonso et al., 2017) and private insurance coverage (in Paim et al., 2011) suggests that around 75% of the population deliver in SUS facilities. These excessive rates are referred to as the "caesarean epidemic" in national (Ferey & Pelegri, 2018) and international media (Associated Press, 2015), as well as by Brazilian politicians and in leading academic journals (Barros et al., 2018).

Monetary reward for physicians is a key driver of high c-section rates. In an attempt to lower the rate of c-section, government policy dictates that doctors are paid less per procedure for a c-section than a normal birth. They can, however, still earn more overall by carrying out c-sections by performing multiple operations per day. Elective c-sections can also more easily be performed during normal working hours, meaning doctors do not have to work nightshifts, on weekends or holidays. Private obstetricians will have multiple clients, all of whom expect them to be present to deliver their babies, which can lead to scheduling difficulties. Elective c-sections are thus preferable and more convenient for many doctors, being easier to plan than normal birth (de Bessa, 2006).

Because of the high rates of c-section in teaching hospitals and the use of out-of-date training manuals (Hotimsky, 2008), few doctors have the opportunity to practice complex vaginal deliveries such as breech position, making them less inclined to perform one. Obstetricians are also expected to be proactive and "hands-on" in a delivery, and to treat any problem that does emerge aggressively—which normally means exhausting all options for intervention. Doctors who do not intervene in a normal birth with a poor outcome risk being sued, meaning that very few will attempt vaginal delivery with intermittent monitoring (the suggested approach in a woman-centred model for low-risk pregnancies). C-section is, therefore, the preferred mode of delivery for many doctors, despite the risk of serious adverse effects for the woman and newborn (Souza et al., 2010).

A key factor driving patient demand for c-section is the poor quality of care offered during normal birth, especially in the public sector. While c-section rates are far lower in the SUS, care is still highly interventionist, and clinical procedures such as the shaving of pubic hair, induction of labour using synthetic oxytocin, continuous monitoring with a CTG, and episiotomy (a surgical cut at the opening of the vagina) are routinely practiced (Leal et al., 2014). For instance, 56.1% of low-risk women undergo episiotomy in Brazil across the public and private sectors (Leal et al., 2014), despite the lack of clinical evidence to support its routine use (Jiang et al., 2017). Some SUS hospitals are infamous for institutionalised maltreatment of women, particularly women of colour and low economic status (Diniz et al., 2018). There are reports of inappropriate or disrespectful behaviour towards women by medical staff, most often in the form of verbal bullying and coercion into unnecessary treatment. Anaesthesia is rarely used in public sector births, despite the frequent use of oxytocin to induce and augment labour, which increases the intensity of contractions. Because of this, many women closely associate vaginal deliveries with pain and suffering. Those that can will avoid this risk by paying for an elective c-section in the private sector (McCallum & dos Reis, 2008; Béhague, 2002). Women in the public sector have also negotiated with clinicians to access the kind of care they prefer and avoid pain. In Bahia, women persuaded doctors to use medicalised interventions, such as foetal monitoring, because they knew this was more likely to clinically justify a c-section delivery (Béhague et al., 2002). Women seeking care are therefore not merely passive patients or consumers of care, but themselves deploy strategies in order to access particular services and interventions.

On top of this, Brazilian women face substantial legal, financial, and practical challenges to accessing alternative types of care, such as midwifery-led care or homebirth services. Only 16.2% of vaginal births are carried out by a nurse or nurse-midwife, with the rest performed by doctors (Gama et al., 2016). The University of São Paulo began the first direct-entry midwifery (*obstetriz*) degree in 2005, but graduates have faced obstacles to entering the workforce. The conservative medical lobby has blocked midwives' appointments to public hospitals. The Brazilian Nursing Council has resisted licensing and regulating midwives (Gualda et al., 2013). Private hospitals have refused doulas entry for questioning the overuse of clinical interventions. These competing professional interests create barriers to the employment of health professionals adequately trained in women-centred and evidence-based care (Gualda et al., 2013).

Further, contracting a team of humanised health professionals is costly. From my interviews, I gathered that in São Paulo hiring a humanised doctor and obstetric nurse for their services in a hospital costs between US$1600 and US$2400, a team of midwives for a homebirth around US$2000, and a doula US$350–US$500 for either home or hospital birth. These are considerable expenses given that the average monthly salary is around US$1000 (IBGE, 2019). Some women seek humanised care at normal birth centres, most of which are free at the point of use, but this can mean travelling a considerable distance, as there are few in existence. At the time of my fieldwork, there was only one freestanding normal birth centre in operation in São Paulo city. Across the country, some public hospitals have been refurbished with normal birth centres under the *Rede Cergonha* policy, but not all hospitals are participating in these programmes. So far, seven out of eighteen municipal hospitals in São Paulo have brought in humanised protocols and retrained obstetricians and obstetric nurses under the *Parto Seguro* programme. Four municipal hospitals are trialling the volunteer doula programme.

These financial barriers to accessing humanised birth services reinforce the existing unequal distribution of obstetric care. Poorer women using SUS hospitals are more likely to experience poor quality care or obstetric violence unless they live close to one of the hospitals participating in *Parto Seguro* or another humanised policy programme. In contrast, upper-class women can opt for an elective c-section with a private obstetrician and also have the option of contracting their own humanised birth team at home, or delivering at a private hospital that permits humanised births.

## The Movement for Humanised Care in Childbirth

The movements' diverse members are united by their goal to normalise vaginal delivery for low-risk births and to humanise care more broadly. "Non-expert" members include pregnant woman and mothers who have sought out a humanised birth. "Expert" members include academics, politicians in regional government health departments, and humanised health professionals—doctors, midwives, nurses, anddoulas who practice according to this model (Diniz, 2005; Diniz et al., 2018). The movement is active across the country, with many different permutations (see Béhague, 2002; McCallum & Dos Reis, 2008). Members are predominantly upper- and middle-class women, educated, *branca* (of European descent), and carry "cultural capital", understood as the capacity to critically challenge certain social regulations (Carneiro, 2015).

Diniz (2005), who has studied the movement extensively, describes how it grew slowly over the 1970s and 1980s, when dissident health professionals were inspired by indigenous childbirth practices and the global feminist movement. From the late 1990s the humanised birth community met several times a year at conferences and communicated via email, and more recently, social media platforms (Irvine, 2021). Important milestones included the first humanised public maternity hospital in Rio de Janeiro in 1994; the creation of prizes for humanised maternity wards, based on adherence to WHO recommendations for promoting normal birth; and the introduction of freestanding normal birth centres. The movement has played a central role in influencing public policy and some members have worked closely with the government to develop humanised policy interventions and guidelines (see Diniz et al., 2018 for a comprehensive list of these).

## Strategies for Humanising Policy and Practice

Movement members transitioned between personal and professional spheres, employing different strategies as they moved between sites and spoke with a range of audiences. Different factions within the movement prioritised particular activities for influencing policy over others. Some members—mostly academics working at universities and in national and local government departments—directed their attention towards using research to inform public policies, campaigning and lobbying for the rights of women to have access to humanised services in SUS hospitals, and sharing information about humanised birth with women in poorer areas of the city through outreach programmes. Within this group, actors tended to support their arguments either with scientific evidence and/or rights-based arguments grounded in national and international law.

### *Obstetric Violence*

Obstetric violence was commonly discussed among movement members—and it was one of the primary reasons that women sought humanised care or became involved with the movement. One woman, a nurse, described its long-term impact: "I suffered obstetric violence from an obstetric nurse…in 35 years I haven't been able to forget…It's the same for all of us [women]. During labour, we are abused". Women described specific clinical interventions that are contraindicated in best practice guidelines (such as routine use of episiotomy) as obstetric violence: "women, principally black women from the periphery, suffer [obstetric violence] the most…we have cases where women have had the cut on the perineum without anaesthesia, and this is recurrent". Until recently, the term "obstetric violence" was present in formal policy documents, including in a memo written in 2014 by the São Paulo State Ministry of Health which defined it as: "the appropriation of women's bodies and reproductive processes by health professionals through dehumanised treatment, drug abuse and pathologisation of natural processes" (Ministério Público do Estado de São Paulo, 2014, p. 1).

Obstetric violence was a central theme of public academic events with high-profile speakers from academia and government. For example, a conference held at The University of São Paulo's Faculty of Public Health was entitled "Best practices to counter obstetric violence". At this event, Professor Simone Diniz (who is frequently cited in this chapter) spoke about the evidence of the effect of obstetric violence on physical and mental health indicators, and the State Secretary for Health gave a plenary session which detailed the "gold standards and best practices" to reduce obstetric violence. The title and content of these talks very literally brought together the discourses of obstetric violence and scientific evidence.

The idea of the right to quality humanised care and freedom from violence also came up frequently in interviews. In her discussion of the Volunteer Doula Programme, a leading academic who ran advocacy groups argued: "if health is a right, and not a product—doulas improve outcomes for babies and women, so a doula should be a right in the SUS". Similarly, one of the few working midwives described the movement as a "battle for rights", another explained that women had "the right to a homebirth" and another still stated that a woman has "the right to a professional companion of her choice". These activists' claims were supported with references to clinical evidence that supported the interventions referred to—for instance, the doula who insisted women have a right to homebirth went on to talk about how "studies confirm it".

However, the changing political environment influenced which strategies activists were using. Two senior politicians explained that they had worked with the movement to create a progressive course for the volunteer doula training programme, "about elements of humanised birth, feminism, and principally to combat obstetric violence". But when the conservative mayor of São Paulo, João Doria, came into office in January 2017, "the feeling of the course changed completely…the content of the course has been tamed…they said you cannot teach obstetric violence in a doula course". Obstetric violence was clearly politically controversial and had to be removed from the volunteer doula training programme in order for it to run during the Doria administration. The term recently has been revoked and disallowed in policy by the Ministry of Health under President Jair Bolsonaro, to the ire of the humanised birth movement (Cancian, 2019). The Brazilian Medical Association argued that the term is too judgemental and attributes the poor quality of care solely to doctors. In the eyes of most humanised birth activists, this was an accurate attribution. When movement members met this kind of resistance from the medical establishment and politicians, they would turn to the authority of scientific evidence to bolster their claims.

## *Using Evidence in Humanised Policy Design*

The movement worked to bring in evidence-based policy-making (EBPM) to national decision-making. In 2011, CONITEC (the National Committee for Health Technology Incorporation) was established to make recommendations for the use of medicines and procedures in the SUS based on the best available scientific evidence. According to a midwifery professor involved in the movement, CONITEC is directly modelled on similar health technology assessment (HTA) initiatives from other countries, such as NICE and the Belgian Health Care Knowledge Centre. A public consultation process brought in several thousand professionals and members of the public (many of whom were members of the movement) to advise CONITEC on the creation of best practice guidelines for c-section and normal birth.

Clinical evidence-based guidelines were a tool the movement used to negotiate. They informed the overarching goals and the design of specific policy programmes, including the installation of normal birth centres under *Rede Cergonha* and local level initiatives, such as *Parto Seguro*. These were the result of key figures championing humanisation within the Municipal Health Secretariat or the support of research institutes and private hospitals (Diniz et al., 2018). For instance, both the *Parto Seguro* and *Parto Adequado* programmes created normal birth facilities in hospital wards and implemented humanised birth protocols in São Paulo that were based on WHO recommendations and NICE guidelines such as freedom of movement and positioning during labour, water birth facilities, non-medical analgesia, delayed umbilical cord-cutting and breastfeeding support. *Parto Seguro*'s stated aim was to "ensure high quality humanised obstetric and neonatal care based on scientific evidence" (CEJAM, 2019, no page). Its director repeatedly stressed the importance of clinical evidence and internationally recognised models of care that had been incorporated into its programme design: "We're leaving the biomedical model behind and advancing towards the humanised model. And what helps us in this process are our indicators and goals". She makes a clear distinction between the "biomedical model", which is not supported by internationally recognised assessment metrics, and the "humanised model", which is.

The volunteer doula policy authors frequently referred to scientific research on the benefits of non-clinical emotional support during labour (such as Bohren et al., 2017) that was disseminated in online humanised birth groups by a group of doulas in Rio (Núcleo Carioca de Doulas, 2012). Volunteer doulas received training on how to apply this evidence in their practice—for example, their manual sets out the equipment and techniques doulas can use for non-clinical analgesia (Kozhimanni et al., 2013). One of the authors explained: "Trials, scientific evidence—I think this is aligned [with the policy's aims]. The scientific point of view is something that helps our actions". Another doula who was involved in lobbying for the professionalisation of doulas explained: "Science says that a trained companion...is the sole intervention with the most significant impact on outcomes...Fewer c-sections, less use of anaesthesia, pain killers, medications". She describes doula care as an "intervention" with clear outcomes for maternal health, taking up the scientific language typically used to convey the results of clinical trials.

Several interviewees explicitly linked research done by health professionals linked to humanised/natural birth movements around the world with the growth of EBM, with one humanised doctor explaining that "Cochrane, and the evidence movement, arose with the humanised birth movement…The first research was done by midwives, because of the demand for midwife-led birth". In Brazil, the stubbornly high maternal mortality ratio (MMR) has been an important tool for the movement, precisely because epidemiologists have found an association between Brazil's poor performance and the excessive use of clinical interventions (Barros et al., 2018). One humanised doctor explained that "the government evaluated [the MMR]…in neighbourhoods with lots of c-sections…c-section can lead to preventable deaths, due to haemorrhage, infection. So this led to their focus on reducing the c-section rate and unnecessary interventions".

Some of the evidence being used in advocacy was generated by Brazilian public health and midwifery researchers who were involved with the movement (Diniz & Chacham, 2004; Rattner et al., 2010; Niy & Delage, 2015; Diniz et al., 2018). One doula explained that many women who had opted for humanised birth were part of a particular educated, middle-class social group who also "produced scientific evidence", through their professional roles as academics, adding to the pool of knowledge about humanised birth. Senior politicians (such as the now-former Brazilian Minister of Health, Gilberto Magalhães Occhi) published comment pieces in the *Lancet* about "Brazil's strategic measures to reduce the c-section rate", referencing *CONITEC*, *Rede Cergonha,* and *Parto Adequado* by name (Occhi et al., 2018).

## Contesting Evidence, Overcoming *Cesaristas*

Non-expert members of the movement accessed and shared clinical evidence through social media and personal networks to disseminate information and attract new members. The movement's frequent citation of scientific papers and best practice guidelines meant that women who sought out humanised care, but were not clinically trained, were nonetheless familiar with and confident using scientific terminology. A midwife explained:

> …women already know how to translate this information. What is a meta-analysis, what a study with *x* amount of participants means…this entered into the imagination of women, and they began to use these terms, and these became part of the political strategy of these [humanised] groups.

Her observation that the scientific method "entered into women's imagination" hints at how women have taken up the powerful discourse of clinical research to legitimise their support for normal birth. One mother also explained:

> Evidence has power, because it's not me just thinking it's the best. Studies have shown that those are the best policies. Those have the better outcome for health, for results, so we need to use that. Because that information is being shared…that is what's driving the change.

Mothers and pregnant women involved in the movement had taken to using evidence to promote its messages among friends. One middle-class mother who had opted for humanised birth with a doula explained that she would share WHO recommendations with people: "I bought a book just about c-sections. I would bring the book with me and would tell my friends who are pregnant". Others explained key "inspirations" they had from friends who had homebirths or "very natural birth stories", who had introduced them to the movement, and shown them key materials, such as the *Rebirth of Birth* documentary.

Links to research article summaries, open access articles, and Cochrane reviews were regularly posted on Facebook and in humanised birth WhatsApp groups, framed by comments encouraging people to read them and a liberal scattering of emojis. One woman who had a humanised birth in a public hospital explained that Facebook was a tool for the movement: "you have information exchange, you report on your [birth] experience, and let people know if you had a doctor who claimed to be humanised but turned out not to be". The membership of these online groups ranged from around 10,000 to 200,000. Even though they had initially only been accessible to wealthier women, this was changing with the proliferation of cheap smartphones. According to one influential member of the movement, social media was important in building bridges to reach poorer women in the *periferia*. These women, most of whom used SUS services, were not as familiar with EBM terminology as middle-class members of the movement—but were certainly aware of the positive stories passed on from friends and relatives about certain humanised protocols that had been introduced, such as the use of birthing pools and being able to move around freely.

Doulas in particular prided themselves on being up-to-date with the latest international evidence. In a doula training course at one of the private humanised birth centres, every technique was taught alongside the evidence that supported it, including the "emotional work", such as reassuring touch and creating a relaxed birth environment. A Cochrane review on the benefits of continuous support during childbirth was regularly referred to (Bohren et al., 2017). One doula also described the success of an informative booklet she had helped produce and distribute in the public sector—"It has all the information…[about] women's rights, birth positions, nutrition".

Access to scientific knowledge about pregnancy and birth gave non-clinical professionals and their clients greater power in encounters with resistant doctors, however, the movement's members experienced varying degrees of success in confronting *cesarista* doctors. One doula described her use of a birth plan "as the WHO recommends" with a woman she was supporting: "The woman did not want an episiotomy—I told the doctor this and showed him the birth plan and he said "Oh but it's just a little cut" and does it anyway".

Humanised obstetricians, midwives, and doulas claimed *cesarista* doctors were aware of evidence-based guidelines, but that they often refuted them on personal or political grounds:

> There are lots of doctors who unfortunately think that this evidence is not reliable, that its manipulated…The oldest ones, the professors, defend caesarean…It's difficult for someone to change, who has practiced in a certain way for their whole life…

> The doctors have access to the same scientific evidence that we doulas and humanised doctors have. But they keep telling the pregnant women that episiotomy is better, that it's necessary…They lie.

One doula told me she had shown multiple doctors best practice guidelines only for them to shrug her off and say "Brazilian women are different—this doesn't apply here". Another told me of the countless instances a doctor had performed a c-section because of "foetal distress" when none had been recorded, or because the baby's umbilical cord was wrapped around its neck (not an indication for c-section). Scientific evidence was effective up until a point: when *cesarista* doctors were powerful enough to refute it.

Interviewees in the movement blamed the self-interest of doctors and considerable political influence of the Brazilian Medical Council (CFM) for the resistance to evidence-based policy change. Doctors were known to have considerable political influence over policy-making and implementation and to fight aggressively for their professional interests over those of patients and other health professionals. One midwife explained: "In Brazil, doctors are very mixed up in politics. So when you offend the doctors, you lose votes…and the doctors are strong, they have money, they have power".

CONITEC should arguably have become a centrally important institution in determining evidence-based policy guidelines for Brazil—as NICE has in the UK. But, according to movement activists, from the outset it was given limited political power, and health professionals and hospital management teams resistant to change often ignore its recommendations.

Some of my interviewees seemed unsure about the future direction for humanised birth policy in an increasingly conservative national policy environment. When I asked government officials in the São Paulo health secretariat what actions they would take to continue the movement's progress, they often replied that all they could do was to continue producing evidence and developing "technocratic" answers to policy problems.

## Marketing Beautiful Births

One subgroup of the movement was deeply disillusioned with trying to change public policy with appeals to evidence and women's rights. These members tended to work as doulas or doctors in private humanised birth centres and sought to influence hospital practice and public opinion by inducing a rise in demand for humanised birth, believing that private services would necessarily adapt. São Paulo was a consumer society, they argued, and, therefore, the way to change hospital policy and practice was to stimulate demand for humanised services among paying clients. These activists essentially marketed humanised birth as a "lifestyle product" to paying clients, primarily on social media, through humanised birth websites, and at private humanised birth centres as well as on posters and flyers displayed at organic supermarkets and yoga centres in São Paulo's bohemian neighbourhoods. Clients—normally wealthy and influential women—would then request humanised services from private obstetricians and hospitals, and as a result, hospital administration would modify hospital regulations. The humanised health professionals who engaged in this strategy claimed it was highly effective:

> It's a question of the market exactly...Past experiences have shown me that if you approach doctors trying to change their behaviour it won't work at all. You have to create a demand; the doctors then understand that if they don't change they are going to lose their clients.

> the hospitals are going to start changing, once the pregnant women, the clients, start complaining, more than if we go and try to change policy.

Private sector doulas and midwives spoke about their own role in increasing the demand for humanised birth:

> I believe in creating an attractive product...One day our society will evolve so that it doesn't function anymore in this product mentality. But at the moment it works like this. Creating desires. Working with image.

These activists clearly describe birth as a commodity that could be marketed in an attractive way to women. The implication of this is that women can pay to achieve their desired outcome in childbirth. In some instances, this has the negative effect of women feeling disappointed or even as though they have failed if they do end up genuinely requiring clinical intervention—something I observed in postnatal groups in São Paulo, and which Rossiter (2017) discusses in her work on the ecstatic birth movement in the United States.

These movement members were still aware of the evidence-base and would inform women about best practice guidelines, as well as their rights during childbirth—but they suggested that for the particular audience they were targeting (women who were attracted to alternative health and lifestyle practices and wanted or could afford private care) the positive experience of humanised birth was as, if not more important than the scientific evidence supporting it. Further, some attested that behaviour change among *cesaristas* would only occur through financial incentivisation.

Women who had opted for private humanised services spread awareness about and generated further demand through sharing their own experiences online, particularly "birth reports" posted online on Facebook or Vimeo, and widely distributed. The majority of the women I met at private humanised birth clinics captured their births in this way and said it helped to change opinions about what birth could (and in their opinion should) be like.

Interviewees described specific ways in which marketing humanised birth had proven to be effective. Humanised doulas and midwives working in the private sector confirmed there had been a steady rise in demand for their services, with a sharper increase from 2010 onwards. According to the managers of two of the private humanised birth centres, they had gone from running one or two doula training courses each year to one every month, each with a cohort of 20 doulas, the majority of whom were able to find steady employment. Some humanised obstetricians attributed specific policy changes in certain private hospitals (such as whether or not they allowed humanised doctors to practice there, or if they allowed doulas into the delivery room) to the rise in demand from women. One humanised doctor told me about the changes in private hospitals: "Ten years ago, rupturing membranes to induce labour was considered absurd in these hospitals. This has changed a lot…In 2006 [Hospital], São Luis opened the first *sala de parto* [normal birth room]". She explained that two of São Paulo's largest private hospitals implemented these humanised protocols because women "who inform themselves don't want another kind of assistance".

I observed some minor tensions between the different factions of the movement, for instance, some members focussing on public policy expressed frustration that more activists did not attend public hearings and campaign for the rights of all women to access humanised services (rather than just those who could pay). But for the most part, relations were amicable and many members worked collaboratively on research projects and campaigning efforts.

## Discussion

Brazilian authors have studied the humanised birth movement over the course of its history (Tornquist, 2004; Diniz, 2005; Rattner, 2009; Carneiro, 2015; Diniz et al., 2018 among others) and provide a comprehensive review of the public policies and private sector initiatives the movement has helped shape and deliver. To contribute to this literature, I have focussed on *how* the movement has changed policy and practice, critically analysing what I see as specific strategies its members employ. I have discussed several of these in this chapter: the use of the term obstetric violence and rights-based arguments; the strategic use of scientific evidence in developing specific policy programmes and lending authority in clinical encounters; and the marketing of humanised birth as a desirable product to increase demand among wealthier women.

In their study of EBA, Storeng and Béhague (2014) explain how at the global level, maternal health agencies and researchers responded to the global growth of EBM and EBPM by removing moral arguments from the policy-making process—though more recently, some actors have resisted this trend and strategically obfuscate ideological debates and subjective values as scientific and objective. In Brazil, rights-based arguments have been employed *alongside* evidence-based justifications for improving maternal health services since the beginning of the humanised birth movement's activism (Irvine, 2021).

Using the term "obstetric violence" in official policy documentation has been central to this activism, and indicates its legitimacy at high levels of government. Movement members also positioned themselves in alignment with global best practice guidelines, bolstering their cause. At public talks, on social media, and in conversation, the movement clearly distinguished the humanised model of care (scientifically proven, safe, best for women) against pro c-section doctors and hospitals. The terminology of EBM and EBPM was used by many non-clinical professionals, including doulas and women, giving them greater power to negotiate in clinical settings. This finding has been reported by others studying the humanised birth movement, for instance, Tornquist (2004) showed that movement members had publicly accused doctors of being ignorant about international evidence when they tried to block the opening of normal birth centres. This behaviour was also observed by McCullum and dos Reis when a senior medic in their study insisted that the WHO recommendations on oxytocin did not apply to public maternity hospitals in Brazil (2008). Scientific evidence was, therefore, not advancing over-medicalisation of childbirth but instead supporting the optimal use of medical technology in childbirth. This is in direct contrast to authors who have written of their concerns that EBM supported and even extended an excessively empirical and clinical approach to complex global health problems (Adams, 2013) and obstetric care (Wendland, 2007).

Resistant health professionals and the institutions that represented their interests were in some circumstances able to reject global best practice guidelines, refuting their suitability for Brazilian women in their care. Brazilian evidence-based institutions such as CONITEC have thus far failed to build a national culture of support for EBM, as seen in other countries such as the UK and Belgium. This led to some members of the movement arguing that behaviour change would only occur among *cesaristas* through a rise in demand for private humanised birth services as an alternative "product" to elective c-section. Anecdotal evidence suggests that these strategies have been reasonably effective in increasing demand for humanised birth (measured, for instance, by the growing number of job opportunities for doulas and midwives in the private sector, the greater number of private hospitals allowing humanised obstetricians to deliver on their wards and growing membership of humanised birth groups online). This strategy seemed to have increased the number of wealthy women accessing humanised birth. It could be seen as what others have described as the "commodification of" or "consumerism in" childbirth, motherhood, and midwifery-led care (Taylor et al., 2004; Davis-Floyd, 2004; Macdonald, 2006). At the same time, there is a risk that investing time in selling the notion of beautiful births diverts attention away from the core principles of equity and justice espoused in the humanised birth movement, and in broader efforts towards universal health coverage. Some in the movement have voiced concerns that poorer and disadvantaged women will continue to face financial barriers to accessing high-quality care during childbirth and the risk of obstetric violence. This concern was somewhat alleviated by a trend I observed among the recently trained doulas I interviewed, almost all of whom expressed their desire to address inequalities of access and to provide their services at an affordable cost, or for free, for women from the poorer *periferia* of the city. This does not, however, address the more fundamental issue of tackling embedded and systematic differences between the SUS and private hospitals.

With the election of the right-wing President Jair Bolsonaro in October 2018, much of the progress made by the humanised birth movement is now under threat. As part of a broader movement to restrict women's rights and cut funding for social services, members of Bolsonaro's government are passing increasingly conservative legislation. In 2019, a São Paulo state deputy allied with Bolsonaro was accused by movement members of colluding with the CFM after a video circulated in which she promised to represent their interests in government—supporting the widely held beliefs that *cesarista* doctors are politically powerful. The Ministry of Health has recently attempted to remove the term "obstetric violence" from legislation and prevent policymakers from referring to it. This is in contrast to the global health arena where there is widespread expert consensus that best practice is normalised, woman-centred, respectful care where possible, and policymakers are beginning to return to moral and rights-based approaches *with support from* the evidence base. My fieldwork ended in the run up to the 2018 election in Brazil, but the shift towards populist conservatism and the widespread public frustration with "politics as usual" was already visible. These events confirm the necessity for those working in global maternal health to consider contextually specific factors that facilitate or hinder the implementation of evidence-based guidelines. This chapter adds to the ethnographic literature that shows that evidence itself is not necessarily enough to support change.

If the global c-section epidemic and the widespread disrespectful treatment of women around childbirth are to be adequately addressed, the barriers to implementing policies focussed on improving the quality of care must be understood. In São Paulo, we have seen how the political power and social authority of doctors allow for the complete rejection of scientific evidence and the gravity of widespread obstetric violence. Looking at the strategies of local movements like the humanised birth movement might aid future efforts to normalise birth.

## References


Adams, V. (2013). Evidence-based global public health: Subjects, profits, erasures. In J. Biehl & A. Petryna (Eds.), *When people come first: Critical studies in global health*. (pp. 54–90). Princeton University Press.

Alonso, B. D., Silva, F. M. B. D., Lattore, M. D. R. D. O, Diniz, C. S. G., Bick, D., et al. (2017). Caesarean birth rates in public and privately funded hospitals: A cross-sectional study. *Rev. Saúde Pública, 51*, 101. https://doi.org/10.11606/S1518-8787.2017051007054

Associated Press. (2015, January 7). Brazil unveils new rules to curb country's caesarean 'epidemic'.

Barros, F. C., Neto, R., & D.dL., Villar, J., et al. (2018). Caesarean sections and the prevalence of preterm and early-term births in Brazil. *BMJ Open, 8*, e021538. https://doi.org/10.1136/bmjopen-2018-021538

Béhague, D. (2002). Beyond the simple economics of cesarean section birthing: Women's resistance to social inequality. *Culture, Medicine and Psychiatry, 26*, 473–507.

Béhague, D. P., Victora, C. G., & Barros, F. C. (2002). Consumer demand for caesarean sections in Brazil: Informed decision making, patient choice, or social inequality? A population-based birth cohort study linking ethnographic and epidemiological methods. *BMJ, 324*(7343), 942–945. https://doi.org/10.1136/bmj.324.7343.942

Birthplace Collaborative Group. (2011). Perinatal and maternal outcomes by planned place of birth for healthy women with low risk pregnancies: The Birthplace in England national prospective cohort study. *BMJ, 343*, d7400. https://doi.org/10.1136/bmj.d7400

Boerma, T., Ronsmans, C., Melesse, D. Y., Barros, A. J., Juan, L., Moller, A., et al. (2018). Global epidemiology of use of and disparities in caesarean sections. *Lancet, 392*, 1341–1348. https://doi.org/10.1016/S0140-6736(19)30717-2

Bohren, M. A., Hofmeyr, G. J., Sakala, C., Fukuzawa, R. K. & Cuthbert, A. (2017). Continuous support for women during childbirth. *Cochrane Database of Systematic Reviews, 7*, CD003766.

Cancian, N. (2019, May 7). Ministério da Saúde veta uso do termo 'violência obstétrica'. *Folha de São Paulo.*

Carneiro, R. G. (2015). *Cenas de Parto e Políticas do Corpo.* Fundaçao Oswaldo Cruz.

Cavallaro, F. L., Cresswell, J. A., França, G. V., Victora, C. G., Barros, A. J., Ronsmans, C., et al. (2013). Trends in caesarean delivery by country and wealth quintile: Cross-sectional surveys in southern Asia and sub-Saharan Africa. *Bulletin of the World Health Organization, 91*(12), 914–922D. https://doi.org/10.2471/BLT.13.117598

CEJAM. (2019). *Parto Seguro Homepage.* https://cejam.org.br/o-cejam/parto-seguro/. Accessed 10 Oct 2019.

Davis-Floyd, R. E. (2004). Consuming childbirth: The qualified commodification of midwifery care. In J. Taylor, L. Layne, & D. Wozniak (Eds.), *Consuming motherhood* (pp. 211–248). Rutgers University Press.

Davis-Floyd, R. E. (2018). *Ways of knowing about birth: Mothers, midwives, medicine, and birth activism.* Waveland Press.

de Bessa, G. H. (2006). Medicalization, reproductive agency, and the desire for surgical sterilization among low-income women in urban Brazil. *Medical Anthropology, 25*(3), 221–263. https://doi.org/10.1080/01459740600840263

de Mello e Souza, C. (1994). C-sections as ideal births: The cultural construction of beneficence and patients' rights in Brazil. *Cambridge Quarterly of Healthcare Ethics, 3*, 358–366. https://doi.org/10.1017/s096318010000517x

Diniz, S. G. (2005). Humanization of childbirth care in Brazil: The numerous meanings of a movement. *Ciencia e Saúde Collectiva, 10*(3), 627–637. https://doi.org/10.1590/S1413-81232005000300019

Diniz, S. G., & Chacham, A. S. (2004). "The cut above" and "the cut below"- the abuse of caesareans and episiotomy in São Paulo, Brazil. *Reproductive Health Matters, 12*(23), 100–110. https://doi.org/10.1016/s0968-8080(04)23112-3

Diniz, S. G., Rattner, D., d'Oliveira, A. F. P. L., Aguilar, J. M. & Niy, D. Y. (2018). Disrespect and abuse in childbirth in Brazil: Social activism, public policies and providers' training. *Reproductive Health Matters, 26*(53), 19–35. https://doi.org/10.1080/09688080.2018.1502019

Downe, S., Finlayson, K., Oladapo, O., Bonet, M., & Gülmezoglu, A. M. (2018). What matters to women during childbirth: A systematic qualitative review. *PLOS ONE, 13*(4), e0194906. https://doi.org/10.1371/journal.pone.0194906

Ecks, S. (2008). Three propositions for an evidence-based medical anthropology. *Journal of Royal Anthropological Institute, 14*, S77–S92.

Ferey, M. –P., & Pelegri, A. (2018, October 12). Brasil é o segundo país com maior taxa de cesáreas do mundo. *Folha de São Paulo.*

Gama, S. G. N., Viellas, E. F., Torres, J. A., Bastos, M. H., Brüggemann, O. M., Filha, M. M. T., et al. (2016). Labor and birth care by nurse with midwifery skills in Brazil. *Reproductive Health, 13*, 123.

Gualda, D. M. R., Narchi, N. Z., & de Campos, E. A. (2013). Strengthening midwifery education in Brazil: Education, regulation and professional association of midwives. *Midwifery, 29*, 1077–1081. https://doi.org/10.1016/j.midw.2013.08.002

Hotimsky, S. N. (2008). A formação em obstetrícia: Competência e cuidado na atenção ao parto. *Interface – Comunicação Saúde Educação, 12*(24), 215.

IBGE – Instituto Brasiliero de Geografia e Estatistica. (2019). *São Paulo – Trabalho*. https://cidades.ibge.gov.br/brasil/sp/sao-paulo/. Accessed 22 May 2019.

Irvine, L. C. (2021). *Citizenship, sisterhood and scientific evidence: Strategies for 'humanising' childbirth policy and practice in São Paulo*. Doctoral thesis, University College London.

Jansen, L., Gibson, M., Bowles, B. C. & Leach, J. (2013). First do no harm: Interventions during childbirth. *Perinatal Education, 22*(2), 83–92. http://dx.doi.org/10.1891/1058-1243.22.2.83

Jardim, D. M. B., & Modena, C. M. (2018). Obstetric violence in the daily routine of care and its characteristics. *Revista Latino-Americana de Enfermagem, 26*, e3069.

Jiang, H., Qian, X., Carroli, G., & Garner, P. (2017). Selective versus routine use of episiotomy for vaginal birth. *Cochrane Database of Systematic Reviews, 2*, CD000081.

Kozhimannil, K. B., Johnson, P. J., Attanasio, L. B, Gjerdingen, D. K. & McGovern, P. M. (2013). Use of nonmedical methods of labor induction and pain management among U.S. women. *Birth, 40*(4), 227–236. https://doi.org/10.1111/birt.12064

Lansky, S., Souza, K. V., Peixoto, E. R. M., Oliveira, B. J., Diniz, C. S. G., Vieira, N. F., et al. (2019). Obstetric violence: influences of the Senses of Birth exhibition in pregnant women childbirth experience. *Ciência & Saúde Coletiva, 24*(8): 2811–2823.

Leal, M. C., Silva, A. A. M., Dias, M. A. B., Gama, S. G. N., Rattner, D., Moreira, M. E., et al. (2012). Birth in Brazil: National survey into labour and birth. *Reproductive Health, 9*(15).

Leal, M. C., Pereira, A. P. E., Domingues, R. M. S. M., Filha, M. M. T., Dias, M. A. B., Nakamura-Pereira, M. et al. (2014). Intervenções obstétricas durante o trabalho de parto e parto em mulheres brasileiras de risco habitual. *Cad Saúde Pública*, S17–S32. http://dx.doi.org/10.1590/0102-311X00151513

Macdonald, M. (2006). Gender expectations: Natural bodies and natural births in the new midwifery in Canada. *Medical Anthropology Quarterly, 20*(2), 235–256. https://doi.org/10.1525/maq.2006.20.2.235

Manning, A., & Schaaf, M. (2019). *Disrespect and abuse in childbirth and respectful maternity care*. White Ribbon Alliance. https://www.healthynewbornnetwork.org/resource/disrespect-and-abuse-in-childbirth-and-respectful-maternity-care/. Accessed 5 Oct 2021.

McCallum, C., & dos Reis, A. P. (2008). Users' and providers' perspectives on technological procedures for 'normal' childbirth in a public maternity hospital in Salvador, Brazil. *Salud Publica Mex, 50*, 40–48. https://doi.org/10.1590/s0036-36342008000100010

Ministério Público do Estado de São Paulo. (2014). "Carta de São Paulo sobre a Violência Obstétrica". São Paulo, 17 de Novembro de 2014.

Morgan, L. (2015). Conceptualizing women-centred care in midwifery. *Revue Canadienne de la recherche et de la pratique, 15*(1), 8.

Niy, D. Y., & Delage, D. R. A. (2015). Hospitais de ensino em obstetrícia: campo de violação dos direitos das mulheres. In D. Stefano & M. L. Mendonça (Eds.), *Direitos Humanos no Brasil 2015 – relatório da Rede Social de Justiça e Direitos Humanos*. Outras expressões.

Núcleo Carioca de Doulas. (2012). *Por que Doula? Suporte contínuo baseado em evidências científicas*. https://doulasrio.wordpress.com/2012/12/18/evidenciadoula/. Accessed 6th October 2021.

Occhi, G. M., Netto, T. L. F., Neri, M. A., Rodrigues, E. A. B. & Fernades, A. L. V. (2018). Strategic measures to reduce the caesarean section rate in Brazil. *Lancet, 392*, 1290–1291. https://doi.org/10.1016/S0140-6736(18)32407-3

Paim, J., Travassos, C., Almeida, C., Bahia, L. & Macinko, J. (2011). The Brazilian health system: History, advances, and challenges. *Lancet, 377*, 1778–1797. https://doi.org/10.1016/S0140-6736(18)32407-3

Rattner, D. (2009). Humanização na atenção a nascimentos e partos: Ponderações sobre políticas públicas. *Interface, 13*(S1). https://doi.org/10.1590/S1414-32832009000500027
Rattner, D., Santos, M. L., Lessa, H. & Diniz, S. G. (2010). ReHuNa – The Brazilian network for the humanization of childbirth. *Rev Tempus Actas Saúde Col.*
Rossiter, K. (2017). Pushing ecstasy: Neoliberalism, childbirth, and the making of mama economicus. *Women's Studies, 46*(1), 41–59.
Sandall, J., Soltani, H., Gates, S., Shennan, A. & Devane, D. (2016). Midwife-led continuity models versus other models of care for childbearing women. *Cochrane Database of Systematic Reviews, 4*, CD004667.
Sandall, J., Tribe, R. M., Avery, L., Mola, G., Visser, G. H. A., Homer, C. S. E., et al. (2018). Short-term and long-term effects of caesarean section on the health of women and children. *Lancet, 392*, 1349–1357. https://doi.org/10.1016/S0140-6736(18)31930-5
Secretaria Municipal da Saúde de São Paulo. (2015). *Saúde em Dados: Bulletim CEInfo*. Ano XIV, no 14, Junho/2015.
Souza, J. P., Gülmezoglu, A., Lumbiganon, P., Carroli, G., Fawole, B., Ruyan, P., et al. (2010). Caesarean section without medical indications is associated with an increased risk of adverse short-term maternal outcomes: The 2004–2008 WHO Global Survey on Maternal and Perinatal Health. *BMC Medicine, 10*(8), 71. https://doi.org/10.1186/1741-7015-8-71
Storeng, K., & Béhague, D. (2014). "Playing the numbers game": Evidence-based advocacy and the technocratic narrowing of the safe motherhood initiative. *Medical Anthropology Quarterly, 28*(2), 260–279. https://doi.org/10.1111/maq.12072
Taylor, J., Layne, L. & Wozniak, D. (Eds.) (2004). *Consuming Motherhood*. New Brunswick, NJ: Rutgers University Press.
Tornquist, C. S. (2004). *Parto e poder: análise do movimento pela humanização do parto no Brasil*. Tese de doutorado em Antropologia, UFSC.
Walt, G., Shiffman, J., Schneider, H., Murray, S. F., Brugha, R. & Gilson, L. (2008). 'Doing' health policy analysis: Methodological and conceptual reflections and challenges. *Health Policy Plan, 23*(5), 308–317. https://doi.org/10.1093/heapol/czn024
Wendland, C. L. (2007). The vanishing mother: Cesarean section and "evidence-based obstetrics". *Medical Anthropology Quarterly, 21*(2), 218–233. https://doi.org/10.1525/maq.2007.21.2.218
WHO (1985). Appropriate technology for birth. *Lancet, 2*, 436–437. https://doi.org/10.1016/S0140-6736(85)92750-3
WHO (2015). *The prevention and elimination of disrespect and abuse during facility-based childbirth*. WHO.
WHO (2018). *WHO recommendations: Intrapartum care for a positive childbirth experience*. WHO.
Wright, S., & Reinhold, S. (2011). 'Studying through': A strategy for studying political transformation. In C. Shore, S. Wright, & D. Però (Eds.), *Policy worlds: Anthropology and the analysis of contemporary power* (pp. 86–104). Berghahn Books.

# Index





L. J. Wallace et al. (eds.), *Anthropologies of Global Maternal and Reproductive Health*, Global Maternal and Child Health, https://doi.org/10.1007/978-3-030-84514-8

The manufacturer's authorised representative in the EU is Springer Nature Customer Service Centre GmbH, Europaplatz 3, 69115 Heidelberg, Germany. If you have any concerns regarding our products, please contact ProductSafety@springernature.com

Printed and bound by CPI Group (UK) Ltd, Croydon, CR0 4YY
30/09/2026
02225324-0005